FORGOTTEN BODIES

MEDICAL ANTHROPOLOGY:
HEALTH, INEQUALITY, AND SOCIAL JUSTICE

Series editor: Lenore Manderson

Books in the Medical Anthropology series are concerned with social patterns of and social responses to ill health, disease, and suffering, and how social exclusion and social justice shape health and healing outcomes. The series is designed to reflect the diversity of contemporary medical anthropological research and writing, and will offer scholars a forum to publish work that showcases the theoretical sophistication, methodological soundness, and ethnographic richness of the field.

Books in the series may include studies on the organization and movement of peoples, technologies, and treatments; how inequalities pattern access to these; and how individuals, communities, and states respond to various assaults on well-being, including from illness, disaster, and violence.

For a list of all the titles in the series, please see the last page of the book.

FORGOTTEN BODIES

Imperialism, Chuukese Migration, and Stratified Reproduction in Guam

SARAH A. SMITH

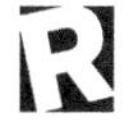

RUTGERS UNIVERSITY PRESS
New Brunswick, Camden, and Newark, New Jersey
London and Oxford

Rutgers University Press is a department of Rutgers, The State University of New Jersey, one of the leading public research universities in the nation. By publishing worldwide, it furthers the University's mission of dedication to excellence in teaching, scholarship, research, and clinical care.

Library of Congress Cataloging-in-Publication Data

Names: Smith, Sarah A. (Medical anthropologist), author.
Title: Forgotten bodies : imperialism, Chuukese migration, and stratified reproduction in Guam / Sarah A. Smith.
Description: First edition. | New Brunswick, New Jersey : Rutgers University Press, [2023] | Series: Medical anthropology | Includes bibliographical references and index.
Identifiers: LCCN 2023007329 | ISBN 9781978832602 (paperback : acid-free paper) | ISBN 9781978832619 (hardcover : acid-free paper) | ISBN 9781978832626 (epub) | ISBN 9781978832640 (pdf)
Subjects: LCSH: Medical anthropology. | Imperialism—Health aspects. | Women, Chuukese—Guam—Social conditions. | Birth control—Government policy—Guam. | Chuukese (Micronesian people)—Social life and customs. | Ethnology—Micronesia (Federated States)
Classification: LCC GN296 .S588 2023 | DDC 306.4/61—dc23/eng/20230602
LC record available at https://lccn.loc.gov/2023007329

A British Cataloging-in-Publication record for this book is available from the British Library.

∞ The paper used in this publication meets the requirements of the American National Standard for Information Sciences—Permanence of Paper for Printed Library Materials, ANSI Z39.48-1992.

rutgersuniversitypress.org

For Kiki. May you rest in power.

CONTENTS

FOREWORD

LENORE MANDERSON

The Medical Anthropology: Health, Inequality, and Social Justice series is concerned with the diversity of contemporary medical anthropological research and writing. The beauty of ethnography is its capacity, through storytelling, to make sense of suffering as a social experience and to set it in context. Central to our focus in this series, therefore, is the way in which social structures, political and economic systems, and ideologies shape the likelihood and impact of infections, injuries, bodily ruptures and disease, chronic conditions and disability, treatment and care, and social repair and death.

Health and illness are social facts: the circumstances of the maintenance and loss of health are always and everywhere shaped by structural, local, and global relations. Social formations and relations, culture, economy, and political organization as much as ecology shape experiences of illness, disability, and disadvantage. The authors of the monographs in this series are concerned centrally with health and illness, healing practices, and access to care, but in the different volumes, the authors highlight the importance of such differences in context as expressed and experienced at individual, household, and wider levels. Health risks and outcomes of social structure and household economy (for example, health systems factors), as well as national and global politics and economics, all shape people's lives. In their accounts of health, inequality, and social justice, the authors move across social circumstances, health conditions, geography, and their intersections and interactions to demonstrate how individuals, communities, and states manage assaults on people's health and well-being.

As medical anthropologists have long illustrated, the relationships between social context and health status are complex. In addressing these questions, the authors in this series showcase the theoretical sophistication, methodological rigor, and empirical richness of the field, while expanding a map of illness, social interaction, and institutional life to illustrate the effects of material conditions and social meanings in troubling and surprising ways. The books reflect medical anthropology as a constantly changing field of scholarship, drawing on research in such diverse contexts as residential and virtual communities, clinics, laboratories, and emergency care and public health settings; with service providers, individual healers, and households; and with social bodies, human bodies, biologies, and biographies. While medical anthropology once concentrated on systems of healing, particular diseases, and embodied experiences, today the field has expanded to include environmental disasters, war, science, technology, faith, gender-based violence, and forced migration. Curiosity about the body and its vicissitudes remains a pivot of our work, but our concerns are with the location of bodies in social life and with how social structures, temporal imperatives, and shifting exigencies shape life courses. This dynamic field reflects the ethics of the discipline to address these pressing issues of our time.

As the subtitle of the series indicates, the books center on social exclusion and inclusion, social justice and repair. The volumes in this series illustrate multiple ways in which globalization and national and local inequalities shape health experiences and outcomes across space; and how economic, political, and social inequalities influence the likelihood of poor health and its outcomes in different settings. At the same time, social and economic relations enable the institutionalization of poverty; they produce the unequal conditions of everyday life and work, and, hence, powerfully influencing who gets sick and who is most likely to survive. The books challenge readers to reflect on suffering, deficit, and despair within families and communities, while they also encourage readers to remain alert to resistance and restitution—to consider how people respond to injustices and evade the fissures that might seem to predetermine their lives.

The nineteenth and twentieth centuries might be characterized for much of the world by the institutionalization and then the formal undoing of European colonialism, the twenty-first century by the challenges of redressing and repairing its enduring inequalities. But while most countries worldwide struggle to undo colonialism's aftereffects, in some settings existing governance, laws, institutions, and rights continue as colonial structures through the networks of colonial relationships. Here—including in a limited number of U.S. outposts—the health and well-being of local populations, and the everyday relations between peoples and places, are shaped by the continued explicit artifacts of colonialism. This is marked in Micronesia, a vast and largely neglected network of islands, lagoons, atolls, and open seas, populated by linguistically and culturally distinct populations whose lives are determined by the differential political arrangements that determine their relationships with the United States and one another. Micronesia, and one troubled fragment of it, is the focus of Sarah Smith's book *Forgotten Bodies: Imperialism, Chuukese Migration, and Stratified Reproduction in Guam.*

European visits to the largest of Micronesia's islands date from Spanish sojourns in the 1500s; colonization and Christian conversion and institutionalization was then sustained by Germany, Britain, America, and Japan. But in the twentieth century, especially from the late 1940s, the political geography of the region took shape under U.S. dominance, when the network of islands in the northwest Pacific proved strategically important as a base for U.S. air and naval forces. Today, many of the islands are independent nations, but in some cases, islands are bundled together in a Compact of Free Association with the United States. Chuuk is one such state in the Federated States of Micronesia (FSM); its neighbor island, Guam, along with the Commonwealth of the Northern Mariana Islands and Wake Island, is constitutionally part of the United States. Being in a Compact of Free Association—able to visit and work in the United States but without citizen rights or services—or being part of the United States makes all the difference to the people who live across this necklace of islands, atolls, and reefs.

Guam's population of indigenous Chamorro and immigrant Filipinos, Japanese, Koreans, and Americans all identify, are treated, and enjoy rights as U.S. citizens, with resources and services that render them distinctly advantaged from others in the region. As Sarah Smith illustrates in *Forgotten Bodies*, for those who live on or are from Chuuk, Guam offers the first steps toward an American dream of vocational and higher education; contemporary employment opportunities; and modern medical, health, and welfare services, and people from Chuuk travel there to take advantage of its services and resources. They are not, however, welcomed; Guam residents treat Chuukese people who migrate to Guam with hostility, suspicion, and resentment. This anti-immigrant sentiment shapes the everyday lives and health outcomes of people from Chuuk—poor-quality and overcrowded housing, low-paying jobs, persistent poor health, and shocking child and maternal health outcomes. Women's life circumstances, the events that mark their passage from childhood to maturity, and the options and choices they make regarding education, employment, and marriage are all set by the inequities of national political status that distinguish Chuuk, other islands in Micronesia, and Hawai'i and the U.S. mainland from one another. These inequities are reinforced through everyday acts of aggression on Guam.

In this compelling and troubling account of embedded and embodied colonialism, Sarah Smith illustrates how women's lives and health are shaped by structural inequality, political ambiguity, economic precarity, gender inequality, and racism. Chuukese women fly on the Island Hopper from their home in the FSM to Guam, United States, for a variety of reasons, including for what they expect to be superior health care during pregnancy and childbirth. Guam's reproductive health statistics prove otherwise. Chuukese women on Guam experience more pregnancies with untreated gestational diabetes than other women on Guam, nearly double the rate of cesarian sections, over half of Guam's fetal deaths, and 20 percent of Guam's infant mortality. And as Sarah Smith describes, Chuukese women are treated with disrespect and rudeness in day clinics and hospital settings; they are routinely humiliated and derided, denied services, and subject to diffident care. Health workers and others on Guam describe Chuukese women in derogatory terms of sexual license, subject to sexually transmitted infections, hyperfertility, and gender-based violence, and use this as an explanation for women's poor health outcomes. The neglect that Chuukese women experience, in consequence, is less benign than explicit, targeted, and cruel.

As anthropologists, we have increasingly been called to task for and have engaged in conversations regarding the role of the discipline in facilitating and ignoring colonialism's reach and savage vestiges, and for our inadequate efforts to decolonize intellectually if not in practice. But as *Forgotten Bodies* demonstrates so powerfully, colonialism continues to affect women's social lives, political rights, and physical bodies in direct ways. The final chapter captures the considerable energy, determination, jubilance, and political savvy of many Chuukese women and other Micronesians. But still, U.S. imperialism determines how and where Chuukese women and their children live, what kinds of care they provide and receive, and their autonomy and agency, all of which shape their reproductive and everyday experiences and outcomes. *Forgotten Bodies* provides a deeply unsettling account of the toxic ways in which structural vulnerability, stratified reproduction, racism, and sexism intersect with political ambiguity, contested rights, and neglect in Chuukese society as well as on Guam and beyond. The uneasy lesson for readers is that Chuuk is only the most obvious and forgotten example of systemic structural violence.

ABBREVIATIONS

CDC	Centers for Disease Control and Prevention (U.S. Department of Health and Human Services)
CIMA	Coordinated Investigation of Micronesian Anthropology
CNMI	Commonwealth of the Northern Mariana Islands
COFA	Compact of Free Association
CWC	Chuuk Women's Council
DPHSS	Department of Public Health and Social Services
FAS	Freely Associated States (including FSM, RMI, and ROP)
FSM	Federated States of Micronesia
GHURA	Guam Housing and Urban Renewal Authority
GMH	Guam Memorial Hospital
HIV/AIDS	Human Immunodeficiency Syndrome/Acquired Immune Deficiency Syndrome
HPV	Human papillomavirus
IMR	Infant mortality rate (per 1,000 live births)
IPV	Intimate Partner Violence
MIP	Medically indigent program
MMR	Maternal mortality ratio (per 100,000 live births)
RMI	Republic of the Marshall Islands
ROP	Republic of Palau
SIM	Scientific Investigation of Micronesia
SNAP	Supplemental Nutrition Assistance Program (U.S. Department of Agriculture)
STI	Sexually transmitted infection
TANF	Temporary Aid to Needy Families (U.S. Department of Health and Human Services)
USAPI	United States-Associated Pacific Islands
USTTPI	U.S. Trust Territory of the Pacific Islands
WHO	World Health Organization
WIC	Special Supplemental Nutrition Program for Women, Infants and Children (U.S. Department of Agriculture)

FORGOTTEN BODIES

INTRODUCTION

Imperial Chuukese Bodies, Transnational Migration, and Stratified Reproduction in Guam

"Can I get a copy for the doctors in Guam?" Serena asked her health-care provider after a lightning-fast prenatal checkup. Her provider, in Chuuk's public health clinic on the central island of Wééné, saw over one hundred patients a day sometimes: a quick measurement of fundal height, a vaginal exam, and a verbal report to the nurse to enter the information on the patient's chart was standard operating procedure. Often, the patient and provider did not speak at all, so Serena's question slowed things down a bit. "Yes, of course. When are you going?" asked the provider. Serena told her in two weeks. She was already thirty weeks pregnant, but the provider did not question her ability to fly. Plenty of women simply hide their belly on the plane with larger skirts and dresses to ensure they could do so, and the flight from Chuuk to Guam is under two hours. It was also a much more comfortable journey than the boat rides from other islands in Chuuk lagoon (or on the bigger boats coming from outside the lagoon) to Wééné, the central port island of Chuuk.

The provider told the nurse to make a copy of the records and asked Serena to go back to the waiting room so that the next patient could be seen. As Serena tried to pull down her long skirt and roll to her side to help herself back up, she started to tell me about her plans to get to Guam. Her belly made the task of getting up an arduous one, and I offered a hand. Serena got down from the table, and I followed her out to the sea of pregnant women waiting their turn to be seen in Chuuk's public health clinic that day. We found a seat and continued chatting; she told me she came from the island of Tol, about an hour or so by boat—depending on the weather and point of departure—to get to this appointment. She rode on a small outboard motorboat that belonged to a neighbor, giving him gas money for payment; these small fishing and traveling boats were basically the taxis of Chuuk.

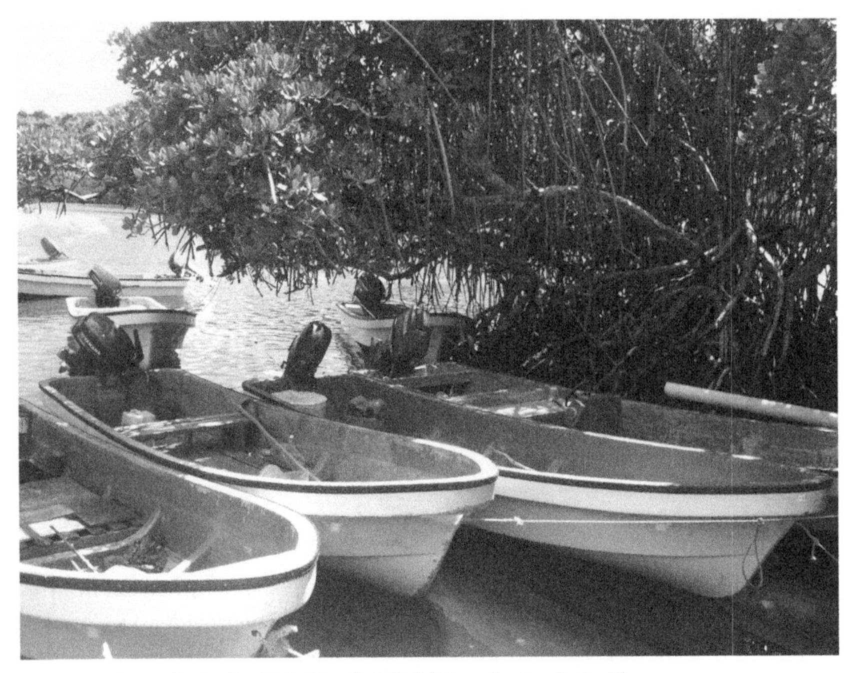

FIGURE 1. Boats docked in Tol, Chuuk, FSM. Photo by Sarah Smith.

Typical commuting boats in Chuuk lagoon are pangas,[1] which are medium-sized outboard motorboats in which the driver sits at the back with a tiller on the motor for steering (see figure 1). They are usually about eighteen to twenty-two feet with around 40-horsepower motors. They are small and agile little boats for island commuting or chasing schools of tuna. In Guam, these boats are nicknamed mosquitoes, a derogatory term referring to the way they can buzz around the larger charter boats and their association with Micronesian migrants who move there and buy fishing boats familiar to them. While easy to maneuver, they are not the most comfortable mode of transportation and bounce quite a bit.

Serena said she would stay with relatives in Wééné until her flight; she was done with the very bumpy lagoon boat rides in her condition. For her, it was now just a few car rides on the unfinished roads of Wééné, and then she would get on the quick United Airlines flight to Guam's paved roads and higher-technology hospital. However, like most women I spoke with, Serena was waiting on money pooled and sent by relatives abroad to buy her ticket. While some extended family members in the continental United States had already transferred funds via Western Union, those in Guam and Saipan were expected to just deposit money into her Bank of Guam account. Bank of Guam has branches all over Micronesia, allowing easy remittances to family members. Serena was headed to the Chuuk branch of Bank of Guam after her appointment to see how much they had deposited. Once she collected the approximately $350 for a one-way ticket to Guam, she would walk down to the United Airlines counter and buy the ticket. She did not have regular access to the Internet—and even if she did, Chuuk's Internet is notoriously slow, so buying tickets online is uncommon.

Serena told me she loved Chuuk and had no intention of moving to Guam despite purchasing a one-way ticket. Her husband insisted she go there to give birth, and she agreed that it was the safest choice. For Serena, it was very familiar; she had spent a few years of junior high school in Guam when her parents were working there, and she spoke English fluently. To her, it was a metropolis version of Chuuk, as it had the same flora and fauna but with more concrete, bureaucracy, and technology. It was not difficult to get there, in great contrast to Hawai'i or the U.S. mainland, where many of her relatives resided. Some two months after the birth—or however long it took for the infant to get a social security number and thus a passport and the ability to travel—Serena would save and collect funds for her return ticket to Chuuk, where she wanted to raise the baby.

Serena was one of many women I met both in Chuuk and Guam who traveled while pregnant to access the better hospital care of Guam. This usually happened in the second or third trimester of their pregnancy. For women, the short flight between Chuuk and Guam was well worth the enhanced feelings of safety, and everyone had some relative in Guam to stay with while waiting out the last weeks of pregnancy. While Serena and several other women planned to return home soon after delivery, others planned to stay in Guam, or would simply end up staying longer than expected. They often imagined spending a few months there to work and save up money but then extended the trip by a few months, over and over, until suddenly they had been in Guam for years. For some, it was then time for their children to enter elementary school, which was also considered superior in Guam. Other Chuukese women simply lived in Guam when they got pregnant and chose to stay there to get good health care. Safe reproductive health care was one of many reasons for Chuukese people to migrate to Guam, which is what I wanted to investigate when I traveled there in January 2011.

For me, the trip to Guam was a bit longer than Serena's, but I was not pregnant and could more comfortably endure the twenty-seven hours and four airports I traversed from Tampa, Florida, where I began my journey. I arrived exhausted at A.B. Won Pat International Airport in Guam. It was a Sunday, so it was quiet. As I rode through Guam that first time, I was struck not only by the concrete strip malls, parking lots, and car-centric environment but also by the beauty of big island skies and the lush green tropical spaces, full of mango and coconut trees.

Travel writer Chloe Fox wrote an article about Guam in which she began with a question: "What happens when you mix Texas with Hawaii?" Her answer was that you get Guam. She continued: "In many ways, Guam seems like a wonderfully unique contradiction. It's a remote island and an international melting pot;

it's an American territory, and the gateway to Asia; it's home to an intensely local culture, but it's filled with outsiders. And to top it all off, it's just beautiful" (Fox 2014). In many ways, Fox is correct. Guam is a web of contradictions, and while it is far away from the Americas, it is also an American territory. And there *are* stunning vistas of cliff lines, beaches, and mountains on this old volcanic island of the Pacific. Further, references to Texas and Hawai'i make sense sometimes. It felt like Texas every New Year's Eve, when I would hear gunshot celebrations on people's ranches. Trucks and jeeps are the most popular vehicles to get around this largely suburban island of mid-twentieth-century concrete houses and strip malls, many of which don stickers with slogans conveying both American and Guamanian pride.[2] But it is also a Pacific Island with a long seafaring tradition. Many people still love to fish the reefs and at sea. A form of tortillas called titiyas—from the Spanish occupation—are served at every gathering, but so are Spam musubi and Filipino pansit and lumpia. Beautiful old Catholic churches are in major village centers, serving the 95 percent Catholic community. People have strong family and community ties as well as vibrant annual fiestas honoring village patron saints. These are just surface images of this complex island, however. While this imagery is consistent in many ways, Fox and others who have written about Guam have also exoticized its remoteness, perpetuating forms of otherness and difference that set it apart from the United States and downplay the imperial circumstances that shape life in Guam and the "melting pot" they describe.

Once I arrived where I was staying, I quickly dozed off. The next morning, the weather was hot and humid—a comfort for someone who was born and raised in Florida. I found my way onto the Internet and opened my browser to check the day's news. The headline story was that Guam Memorial Hospital (GMH)—the only civilian hospital on Guam at the time—was out of epidural medication and was not getting more anytime soon because, it was reported, the hospital had not paid its bills. As a reproductive health scholar, I had arrived to investigate how and why women from Micronesia were flying to Guam for what they perceive to be a better, high-tech birth. I was surprised to learn that this standard biomedical intervention for birthing women was unavailable. Why would women from all over Micronesia come to a hospital that cannot even get basic medication due to its debts?

I arrived interested in U.S. imperialism, migration, gender, and reproductive health. I wanted to understand how migrants are treated differently on this colonized island and how these differences are embodied in women's reproductive health outcomes. I was especially interested in people from Chuuk, one of the four groups of islands that constitute the Federated States of Micronesia (FSM). Chuukese people were always in Guam newspapers for costing money through their use of Guam's education and health systems and, it was alleged, for committing crimes. Little research was available on the health disparities of Micronesian migrants in Guam,[3] even less so specifically on Chuukese migrants. What was available told me that while Micronesian women represented only 9 percent of women of childbearing age on Guam, they accounted for over half of all deliveries with no prenatal care (Haddock et al. 2008). Micronesian women suffered gestational diabetes at greater rates than others in Guam, and had more cesarean deliveries (Alur et al. 2002). These few sources and anecdotal information indicated that Chuukese and other Micronesian women faced reproductive health inequities in the very place they traveled to seek improved care.

What I could not discern from the U.S. mainland, given the lack of published material, was why there were such widespread disparities in access and health outcomes, and, in light of this, why women like Serena believed they would receive better health care in Guam. During my initial trip in 2011, I met with employees of Guam's Department of Public Health and Social Services (DPHSS), which provides women's health care and sexually transmitted infection (STI) prevention, testing, and treatment. Members from these departments showed me the work they were doing and shared their concerns about Micronesian migrants. They believed that people from the FSM—mostly from Chuuk—had more STIs, experienced more complications in pregnancy, and were generally sicker and poorer than their clients who were indigenous Chamoru or Filipino/a,[4] the ethnic groups that make up the majority of residents on Guam. They also believed that the Chuukese women who came to Guam to have babies had diverse motives, from wanting safer health care to gaining American citizenship and welfare benefits for their children. These anti-immigrant discourses over Chuukese motivations for migration were not limited to Guam's newspapers and these workers; they also percolated in the community. These conversations confirmed the paradoxical circumstances in which women travel to seek better care and yet suffer the worst outcomes on the island. I decided to investigate this paradox; I moved to Guam later that year to start data collection. In this book, I illustrate how U.S. imperialism shapes cultural narratives about the movement of Micronesian peoples, discourses about gender and reproduction, and healthcare experiences in Guam, and ultimately how these layers of social life stratify Chuukese women's health. I also consider how and why Chuukese bodies are largely forgotten in the U.S. federal landscape through an intentional strategy I call the politics of benign neglect.

HOPPING FROM CHUUK, FEDERATED STATES OF MICRONESIA, TO GUAM, UNITED STATES

Chuuk is one of four states in the FSM, a small island nation that was believed to be inhabited around 2000 B.P. (Carucci and Poyer 2002). Chuuk has been tied to the United States since the end of World War II, when the United Nations designated its islands one of six strategic trust territory districts to be administered and supported by the United States on the path to independence. The FSM gained independence and entered a Compact of Free Association (COFA) with the United States in 1986. The COFA is an agreement that provides U.S. financial and logistical assistance for the FSM to build an independent nation, thus supporting the government, education and health systems, and the economy. In return, the United States retains military control over its vast Pacific waters. While this relationship, supposedly intended as supportive for development, began in the mid-1940s and continued through the COFA agreement, the FSM and especially Chuuk continue to suffer endemic poverty, a deteriorating healthcare infrastructure, a failing education system, and virtually no economic opportunities for its residents. This is largely a result of the imperial circumstances facilitating the agreement of their supposed postcolonial sovereignty and the politics of benign neglect, which I elaborate on in chapter 1. For these reasons, many Chuukese citizens leave the state for other settings, in search of improved access to education, higher-tech biomedical health care, and jobs.

Chuukese citizens can leave Chuuk because of a stipulation in the COFA agreement that enables the mobility of FSM citizens (and those from other Micronesian nations with COFAs) throughout U.S. jurisdictions. COFA-country citizens can enter the United States anytime as "nonimmigrants," a designation that means they are citizens of their own nations, and while not on a path to permanent U.S. residency or citizenship, they have an ease of entry unlike any other noncitizens. They can simply arrive in U.S. jurisdictions with their FSM passport; fill out an I-94 (Arrival/Departure Record) form; and live, work, and go to school with no permit or visa required. This flexible mobility enabled by the COFA resulted in a mass exodus to places like Guam and Hawai'i soon after it was ratified (in 1986), and it is estimated that at least one-third of the approximately 102,000 FSM citizens live in U.S. jurisdictions (Hezel and Levin 2012).[5] Movement is most intense in Guam, Saipan, and Hawai'i; these U.S. locations are known in the COFA Amendments Act of 2003 as "affected jurisdictions" (COFA 2003).

COFA citizens do not, however, simply move away and forget where they came from. They maintain connections at home and abroad, emulating what anthropologists and other scholars have deemed transnational migration (see, for example, Glick-Schiller, Basch, and Blanc-Szanton 1992; Glick-Schiller 2003). Inspired by increased globalization in the 1990s, anthropologists began to focus more on population mobility and on how identities are shaped and reshaped by people moving across increasingly globalized flows of capital, culture, and politics (Inda and Rosaldo 2008; Glick-Schiller 1995).[6] The term "transnational" elucidated how migrants continue to participate in their community of origin in meaningful ways while also forming new experiences and meanings abroad, creating multi-stranded social relations. In doing so, migrants link spaces together and have a dual identity or connection with cultural, political, and economic ties in two nations.[7] The concept of transnationalism contributed to understanding how relations of power and domination and hegemonic constructions are maintained and contested across nations (Basch, Glick-Schiller, and Blanc 1994; Kearney 1995). Chuukese women are one example; they create multi-stranded social relations in transnational spaces, negotiating relations of power and domination—in this case, between Chuuk and Guam. This contributes to their vulnerabilities in Guam, but it also demonstrates their agency in a place often hostile to their arrival.

ARRIVING IN GUAM

Guam and Chuuk are just one stop away from each other on United Micronesia's Island Hopper flight.[8] Chuukese migrants dominated migration to Guam from the outset of the COFA; others, such as those from the Marshall Islands, moved to Hawai'i in greater numbers, taking advantage of the frequency of flights to and from their islands (Hezel and McGrath 1989; Rubinstein and Levin 1992). After nearly forty years of open migration, the Chuukese now constitute nearly 72 percent of all FSM migrants in Guam and nearly 7 percent of Guam's overall population (U.S. Census Bureau 2022).

Guam is the largest island in Micronesia, with approximately 153,836 residents (U.S. Census Bureau 2022). It is home to the indigenous Chamoru, who are hypothesized to have arrived from Southeast Asia around 3500 B.P. (Carucci and Poyer 2002). It has endured four centuries of colonization, the most recent being the United States, which took control from Spain in 1898 following the Spanish-American War (Rogers 1995). Since 1950, after years of the Chamoru fighting for greater autonomy, Guam was designated an unincorporated territory instead of a possession (Perez 2002; Camacho 2011; Diaz 2010). Even so, Guam lacks autonomy over many legal processes, and its residents, who are U.S. citizens, lack some of the social and economic benefits and rights given to citizens in U.S. states. In chapter 1, I outline Guam's and Chuuk's imperial histories and present circumstances, providing context to the role of the United States and other former imperializing powers in Micronesia (Spain, Germany, and Japan) in shaping Chuukese women's lives.

One of Guam's most popular island slogans is "Where America's day begins!" evoking pride in a connection to the United States (see figure 2). Vince Diaz pointed out that the Japanese invasion—and after WWII—color television, "glued" Chamorus to America (2010, 182). While the TV programs at the time were a week late, he reported, the Guam community took pride in always being a day ahead of the mainland. The mainland rarely returned the attention, however. While Guam is part of the United States, whenever I discuss my work with mainland U.S. residents outside my discipline, they ask, "Where exactly is Guam?" To them, Guam is far away, with unclear, possibly military connections to the

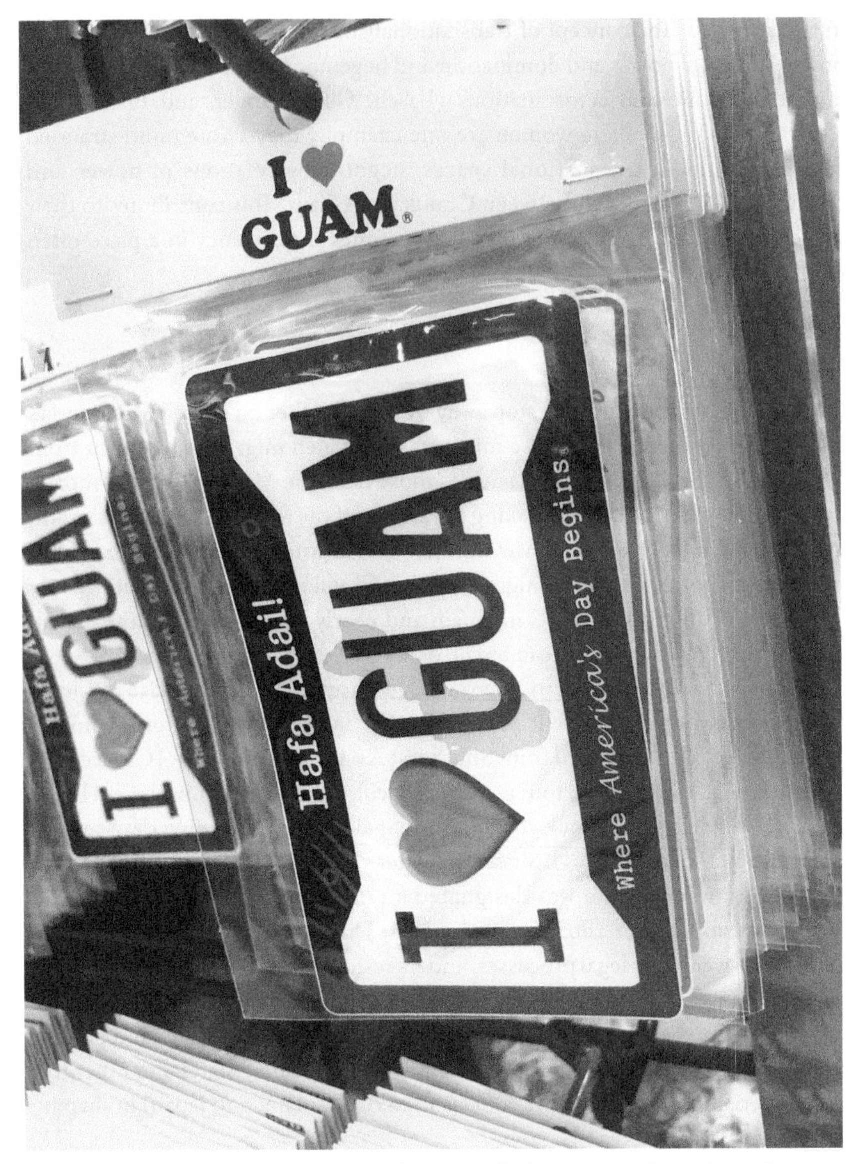

FIGURE 2. Guam memorabilia with popular slogan: "Where *America's* Day Begins." Photo by Chloe Weilbacher.

United States; in addition, many have never heard of Chuuk. Guam's invisibility is a common strategy of empire maintenance; it leaves people uncertain of the status of the island and therefore unconcerned about conditions on the island. Invisibility, or strategically forgetting these bodies, allows empires to use colonial outposts such as Guam to manage movement while securing the mainland.[9]

Like the slogan "Where America's day begins!" Guam is also where American territories in the Pacific begin for many migrants. One way in which the United States has used the unincorporated territory of Guam both directly and indirectly throughout the last century is as a migrant processing station (see chapter 1). With so much authorized migration in and out of Guam, the indigenous Chamoru population now represents just 33 percent of the total island population (U.S. Census Bureau 2022). Tensions between Chamoru and non-Chamoru populations are likely due to this lack of control (Diaz 1995, 2010). While each affected jurisdiction has had some negative reaction to all COFA migrants, the Chuukese are the focal point of this rhetoric in Guam. As I describe in chapter 3, resentment and discrimination toward COFA migrants has taken several forms. Anti-immigrant sentiment consistently focuses on blaming indigent COFA migrants for budget shortfalls in hospital, health, education, and housing services. Because of the lack of infrastructure in the FSM and particularly in Chuuk, Hawai'i, Guam, and other jurisdictions to which Micronesian citizens migrate are noted "catchment" areas for the health problems of Micronesians (Pobutsky et al. 2005, 64). With very poor health outcomes, the Chuukese represent a political and social body of invaders who bring sickness, babies, and increased costs to the Guam government without adequate compensation by their colonizer, which sanctions the migration.

Guam has the best biomedical health care in Micronesia, spending thirteen times what Chuuk does on health care per capita (Haddock 2010). But despite Guam's superior care when compared with that of Chuuk, it is also in need of much improvement. The healthcare system is substandard compared with the rest of the United States (Haddock 2010). With only 161 acute care beds and with 87 full and part time hospital physicians at the only public hospital, Guam is considered a Health Professional Shortage Area (HPSA) and a Medically Underserved Area (MUA) (Health Resources and Services Administration 2021). Both of the hospitals open to civilians (one public and one private) regularly report nursing vacancies from 20 to 40 percent, with over a hundred registered nurse positions available between the two facilities (Hattori-Uchima and Wood 2019).[10] Many specialized healthcare needs are unavailable, requiring medical referral to Japan, the Philippines, Hawai'i or the US mainland (Health Resources and Services Administration 2021). Privately insured residents of Guam also seek regular annual check-ups in the nearby Philippines; medical tourism such as these annual visits are often reimbursable by private insurance.

The only public hospital—GMH—experiences profound problems, including inadequate staffing and space, a crumbling physical infrastructure, and massive debt (Akimoto 2019; Limtiaco 2019a; Eugenio 2019). It sits on a cliff overlooking the Philippine Sea, a gorgeous view on a windy bluff that makes the site ripe for the most expensive real estate, in a central location of Tamuning near the tourist destination of Tumon (referred to by some as "little Waikiki," a

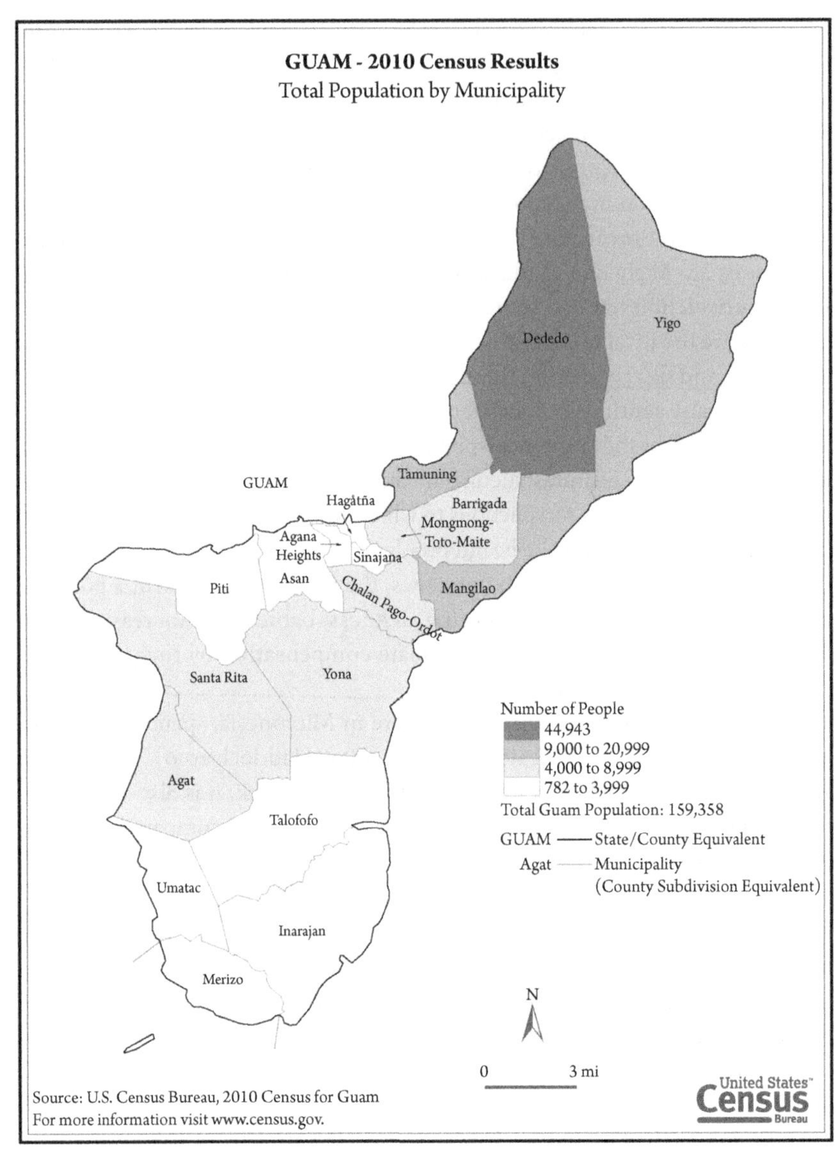

FIGURE 3. Guam map by village and population. Source: https://www.census.gov/newsroom/releases/img/cb11cn179_ia_guam_totalpop_2010map.jpg

very developed strip of high-rise beachfront hotels, restaurants, tourist shops, bars, and massage parlors; see figure 3 for a map of Guam by village). While nearby properties with this cliff view are million-dollar homes of the wealthiest residents, the hospital is a set of old, dingy concrete buildings (see figure 4). When you walk from the large parking lot in front of the building into the lobby, you predictably encounter a construction site. At all times, some part of this

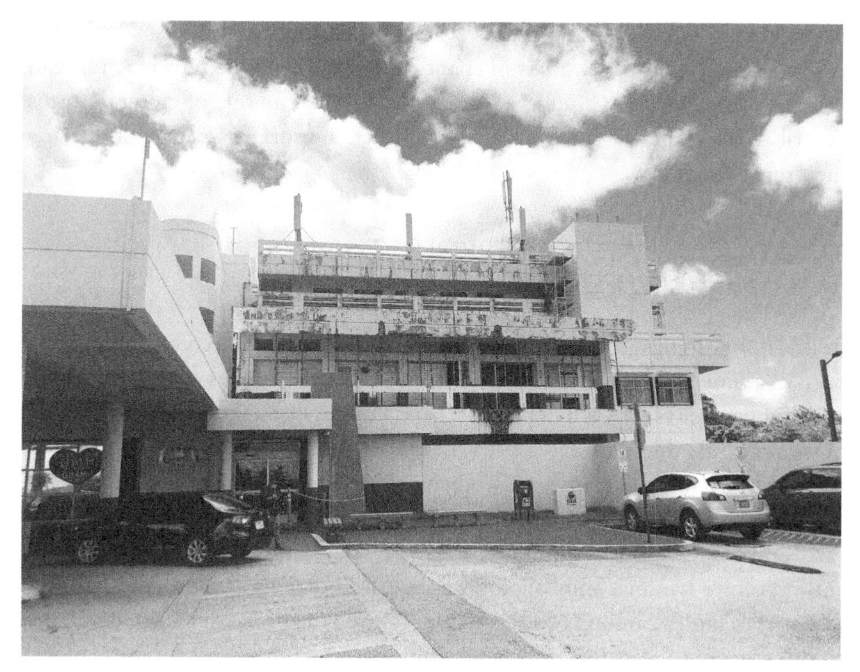

FIGURE 4. Guam Memorial Hospital under construction. Photo by Chloe Weilbacher.

decaying building is getting a facelift, but it never makes much of a difference. The duality of being one of the best health systems in Micronesia and one of the worst in the United States is a product of Guam's unique position in the U.S. and Micronesian political landscape.

While the public health system's struggles inevitably have an impact on Chuukese women, these women first struggle with other structural barriers, such as getting an appointment at the local public clinic and arriving on time in a place with limited public transportation. Once they arrive, the clinic seems rushed, overburdened, and underfunded, causing tension for employees and patients alike. Chuukese women struggle to communicate their needs and questions to healthcare workers because of the unequal power dynamic, language differences, and the rushed environment. Moreover, anti-immigrant discourses operate in these spaces. Symbolic manifestations of Chuukese women's bodies (their clothing, language, betel nut chewing, and hyperfertility) are the focus of conversations among healthcare workers, who frequently express frustration at having to serve this group. In chapter 6, I illuminate these barriers and show how even healthcare workers with the best intentions often discussed Chuukese culture as different and as negatively influencing care. They often referenced women's shyness with providers and the male partners' excessive number of sexual partners when explaining women's outcomes. I sought to learn to what degree Chuukese cultural norms shape their reproductive health and how much of healthcare workers' descriptions were simply "culturalist racism" (Bridges 2011, 132). In doing so, my focus in chapters 4 and 5 is on the reproduction and sexual relationships of Chuukese women. I consider the role of cultural norms described by women—some indigenous, others imported—play in stratifying their reproduction.

STUDYING STRATIFIED REPRODUCTION IN A TRANSNATIONAL SPACE

In this book, I engage with the politics of reproduction, a theoretical tradition born of a time in which second-wave feminist anthropologists sought to correct an ethnographic record full of male bias and limited one-dimensional portrayals of women.[11] As they replaced these missing or problematic data and rewrote the ethnographic record to include women, many found themselves focused on reproduction (Ginsburg and Rapp 1991, 1995; Rapp 2001). Drawing from these early and growing works on reproductive practices and the growth of medical anthropology, feminist anthropologists theorized that studying reproduction is essential to understanding gender inequality and is a key factor of analysis in the study of kinship.[12] A study of the politics of reproduction allows for the exploration of gendered processes, kinship and the family, medicalization, social hierarchies, and concerns regarding control of the social and individual body and the body politic all at once (Ginsburg and Rapp 1991, 1995; Rapp 2001). Reproduction is essentially represented and experienced in all aspects of human social life.[13] In following this tradition, this study of Chuukese transnational reproduction examines each layer of social life.

Chuukese communities have a clan-based matrilineal structure, and reproduction signifies perpetuating the clan and heirs for the land.[14] This means reproduction can give women power, as they enhance their status by having children and ensuring the survival of the clan and its land. Pregnancy is a time when women are indulged and pampered.[15] Husbands and other family members are expected to take over some of the domestic work of pregnant women[16] and meet any special requests. As I describe in chapter 4, the importance of reproduction can be both empowering (through reproducing) and disempowering (without reproduction) in a community in which this is perceived as women's primary goal. In Chuuk, women say they are powerless unless they are grandmothers, seemingly in charge of the family. Gender inequities and this focus on pregnancy helps us to understand poor sexual and reproductive health outcomes.

The importance of reproduction and women's social responsibility to the family means that they are less able to leave Chuuk, for they must stay near and protect the land that they and their female children inherit; men can go farther because they have no ties to the land.[17] As a result, Guam is a place of compromise for women, for it is much closer to home than Hawai'i or the U.S. mainland (Bautista 2010). It is also where women go to seek better healthcare.

Major causes of death in the FSM include infant prematurity and complications during pregnancy and labor (Government of the FSM 2012a).[18] For this reason, women may migrate from Chuuk to Guam hoping for better pregnancy and birth outcomes. A woman named Mary told me, unprompted: "If ever that I will have another baby I would prefer to give birth off island. . . . Because I'm scared . . . I would prefer to go to Guam. . . . It's closer [than Hawai'i or the mainland] and . . . the airfare is cheaper" (Smith 2019a, 349). In Chuuk, I regularly witnessed women like Serena asking for lab results and proof-of-prenatal-care documents from their provider before boarding the plane to Guam. But while some women travel to Guam for this health care, others are already there: they moved to Guam for a job, for school and work, for adventure, or to help a relative, and they became pregnant while living there. Regardless of the circumstances in which they conceive, their fertility is often a matter of concern among Guam's other residents.

Social narratives about who is reproducing reinforce ideas about who deserves to reproduce (Briggs 2017). The concept of stratified reproduction illuminates how inequity and the unequal distribution of power shape the reproductive lives differently among desirable or undesirable groups (Colen 1986). It demonstrates how reproduction differs according to inequalities of race, class, ethnicity, gender, place in the global economy, and migration status (Colen 1995, 78). Inequities in society stratify reproduction, but the resulting inequalities are also duplicated through reproduction, reinforcing the inequities in which they are grounded. Further, public discourses over the economy, race, foreign policy, and family values often center around reproduction and sexuality, including those related to immigration (Briggs 2017). Studying reproduction in the context of migration elucidates relationships between migrants and the state through analyses of reproductive health services; it also allows scholars to assess the extent to which migration reshapes or reinforces existing community discourses of gender, power, and social life.[19] The concept of stratified reproduction reflects the circumstances shaping Chuukese women's experiences as they migrate to and reside in Guam. I use this theoretical lens, in conjunction with the politics of benign neglect—a framework informed by the concepts of structural vulnerability and critical interpretive anthropology, both of which are multilayered approaches to analyzing social life.

VULNERABILITIES RESULTING FROM THE POLITICS OF BENIGN NEGLECT

Structural vulnerability is a theoretical framework that includes political and economic vulnerability as created by conditions of structural violence. It integrates social and cultural norms that reinforce inequities and reflect symbolic violence as well as individual experiences and the constraints within which agency operates. In their seminal article proposing this model, James Quesada, Laurie Kain Hart, and Philippe Bourgois (2011) first outline the history of structural violence—originally labeled by Johan Galtung, later adopted by critical medical anthropologists, and popularized by Paul Farmer—as a key framework for understanding how political exclusion, economic exploitation, and larger structural forces shape people's lives (and health). They then expand the concept of structural violence to include how those who are economically exploited or politically subordinated internalize their status and embody their place in society; this embodiment is considered a form of symbolic violence (Bourdieu 2001). People's vulnerability results not only from class oppression and economic exploitation (structural violence) but also from their position in the social hierarchy of various power relationships of race, gender, sexuality, and migrant status (symbolic violence); people embody these social locations as a form of habitus (Bourdieu 2001). Vulnerabilities at structural, social/symbolic, and individual levels are approached as operating together to shape a person's health. Since this model gained traction, a structural vulnerability tool was created for clinicians (Bourgois et al. 2017), meant to replace efforts to use problematic cultural competency measures in clinical settings (see chapter 6). This tool has been illustrated to be particularly valuable for clinicians working with migrants, signaling its importance and pragmatic accessibility outside anthropology (Caruth et al. 2021).

In conjunction with structural vulnerability, my work is informed by Margaret Lock and Nancy Scheper-Hughes's (1987, 1996) critical interpretive medical anthropology, a particularly valuable framework to analyze the discourses that exist between transnational migration and stratified reproduction (see also Unnithan-Kumar and Khanna 2014). Both structural vulnerability and critical interpretive medical anthropology use three levels of analysis; in the case of critical interpretive medical anthropology, they do so with a body-focused framework (Lock and Scheper-Hughes 1996; Scheper-Hughes and Lock 1987). At the first level of analysis is the individual body. Attempting to break free from conventional Euro-American understandings of the physical body and mind as separate, Scheper-Hughes and Lock (1987) argue that the individual body can represent a consciousness, or sense of being in the world. The second level of analysis is the social body, an instrument of both symbolism and habitus (see also Scheper-Hughes 1993, 231). This body concept is drawn from Mary Douglas (1966, 1970) and her argument that the body serves as a metaphor, or symbol, for social life. The healthy body is often symbolic of a healthy society, and the diseased body, of a malfunctioning society. Embodiment or habitus is also part of the social body, drawing on Bourdieu's (1977) understanding of habitus as the habits and actions unconsciously enacted and reproduced by humans as social beings. Bridging these individual and social bodies, Scheper-Hughes and Lock (1987) demonstrate how relationships between the two are mediated by power and control, or the body politic (23). Their third level focuses on Foucault's (1978) concept of biopower, or the control and regulation of bodies.

These approaches informed my early thinking of this region of *forgotten bodies*, as did the concept of "benign neglect" (Kiste 1994b, 230), a well-known strategy of American imperial management of Micronesia. While Micronesia is routinely embroiled in U.S. political interests, the body politic of these nations and territories is expendable or forgotten; the people are neglected. Benign neglect is thus the slow and limited attention to political, economic, education, and health infrastructures in the region, and the resulting (intentional) creation of dependency on the occupying power that results (see chapter 1). By using the concept *politics of benign neglect*, I refer to the intentional forgetting of the body politic, the political maneuvering in which social bodies are both forgotten and hypervisible depending on the need, and the resulting imprint on the physical bodies and everyday lives of people that result. It is the reflection of this slow, limited attention and its structural and social impacts on bodies that render such bodies vulnerable.

Using these theoretical approaches, in this book I examine the intersection of Chuukese transnational women's reproductive experiences and individual vulnerabilities in imperial spaces that neglect them (individual body); symbolic representations of their reproductive bodies in society, including the symbolic violence of xenophobia and gender inequality (social body); and the control and movement of their reproductive bodies through forms of structural violence, namely imperial citizenship, capitalist exploitation, slow and limited support, and the biomedical management of health (body politic). Each of these layers represents the effects of the imperial strategy of the politics of benign neglect. It renders these bodies vulnerable to poor reproductive and sexual health outcomes, stratifying their reproduction.

FINDINGS ANSWERS THROUGH ETHNOGRAPHY

In this book I draw on nine years of research in Guam and Chuuk. I began this multisited work with my dissertation research (2011–2014), and then conducted follow-up studies from 2015 to 2019. I lived in Guam from December 2011 to August 2015 (except for the five months I spent in Chuuk), conducting ethnography of both the community and the clinic; I returned for three monthlong trips annually from 2016 to 2019.[20] To engage with communities, I volunteered for organizations serving Chuukese migrants, attended women's groups meetings, and connected to families I met through an adjunct teaching position at the

University of Guam. Networking with these communities in more than one way was necessary due to their insulated social location. Most Chuukese women interact with their extended families and church groups; otherwise, they do not have extensive social contacts in Guam. I also needed to be flexible in order to spend time with women, as their work, funeral obligations, and family schedules ebbed and flowed. Over time, I made lasting connections with the women I met; many I regard as dear friends.

My methodology is both critical and feminist in approach. These approaches are theoretical (as previously noted) and methodological and require creating collaborative relationships that put the researcher in the study, avoiding objectification and exploitation. My methods are multisited to reflect the transnational nature of Chuukese women's lives and understand what is remade as people move (Marcus 1995; Tsing 2008). I conceptualize these places as not just across nations (Guam and Chuuk) but also across cultural sites (the clinics and the communities). Methods include one year accompanying Chuukese women seeking health care in women's clinics in Guam, and five non-consecutive months in the Chuuk State Department of Public Health Services. The initial study also included in-depth reproductive life history interviews with fifteen Chuukese women and semi-structured interviews with twenty-four healthcare workers. In later studies, I interviewed women about family planning decision-making ($n = 33$), action and power gained through women's groups ($n = 24$), and experiences living in mixed-citizenship-status households (that is, when some members of the household are FSM citizens and others are U.S. citizens) ($n = 7$ families). In total, the qualitative data that inform this book include over one hundred interviews with Chuukese women, their families, and their healthcare workers.

Chuukese migrants are some of the most impoverished and marginalized people in Guam (Rubinstein and Levin 1992; Bautista 2010), as already suggested. Further, Guam is a marginalized territory of the United States, and the healthcare workers who are indigenous or migrants are often further marginalized by their ethnic and class statuses. I was in an environment where I yielded power as an educated, white U.S. citizen—that is, as an American researcher. I was reminded of this constantly, as I was regularly mistaken for a military and federal government employee who might be overseeing a clinic (for example, someone from the Centers for Disease Control and Prevention). I wrestled with these unequal power dynamics. I also wrestled with anthropology's colonizing history and my role in a colonized space. Guam and Chuuk are communities written about by many colonial outsiders. With this project, I wanted to work with—not on—Chuukese women. Hence, as much as this is an ethnography of reproduction, it is primarily an ethnography of imperialism and colonialism. I attend to issues around my positionality as I consider anthropology's colonial past in chapter 2.

OUTLINE OF CHAPTERS

The role of the U.S. imperial project in shaping Micronesian colonial history is long and insidious, reflecting how empires maintain sovereignty through controlling colonial outposts. Micronesia's colonial history also shaped social and economic conditions and relationships between islanders from different islands. In chapter 1, I explore the historical and contemporary colonial settings of Guam, United States, and Chuuk, FSM, and the role of several empires—most recently the United States—in shaping the lives of Micronesians from these two places.

In chapter 2, I follow the lead of Ann Laura Stoler (1995) and Laura Briggs (2003), who have been among many urging scholars to study the role of sexuality as a discourse for empire, particularly in U.S. imperial zones. I examine the role of U.S. imperialism in creating and exoticizing discourses on Chuukese sexuality and reproduction, as well as contemporary efforts to control it through the discourses of development. I consider the role of Christian missions and U.S. patriarchal institutions in reshaping and reinforcing gender and, specifically, reproduction and sexuality. I also examine the role of anthropology in contributing to the imperial project as well as the colonizing history of this discipline. Anthropologists' depictions of Chuukese sexuality—particularly during the trust territory days—are reviewed and critiqued for their exoticizing ramifications and their role in colonizing Chuuk. Communities negotiated and adopted or rejected these new ideas about gender in ways that shifted power, and these discourses had an impact on Chuukese women in Chuuk and on their migration to Guam.

Gender inequities and relationships shape women's decisions to move from Chuuk and shape their everyday lives in Guam in ways that contribute to their vulnerability to poor reproductive health outcomes. In chapter 3, I explore women's motivations for moving. Drawing on Rosie's and Kaylyn's accounts, I also describe Chuukese women's experiences once they arrive in Guam. Chuukese women encounter anti-immigrant sentiment and social exclusion that mirror those that prevail in the United States. Findings focus on being Chuukese in Guam: I analyze how resentment, discrimination, and notions of belonging shape Chuukese women's identities and their relationships with the greater Guam community. Women's experiences in Guam help us understand the larger experience of Chuukese migrants, and the social vulnerabilities that structure women's poor health outcomes and constrain their reproductive and sexual choices.

Chuukese women's reproductive bodies are not only shaped by the conditions that foster migration and hostility in host communities and clinics; they are also shaped by social ideas about gender, health, and reproduction. In chapter 4, I consider the reproductive life histories of Praise, Mary, Siera, and others to elucidate the role of stigma and shame as strategies to control women's sexuality and reproduction. I explore the lessons on sexual purity that women receive around the time of puberty and consider how those lessons shape their entire sexual lives. I consider how the symbolic value of children and socially sanctioned pregnancies matter to women like Mary, who was taught to get pregnant the "right" way and then show strength and power in her birthing process. I illuminate the connections between land and mothering as a powerful source of women's strength in Chuuk, which may be lost when they migrate away from their land. Their stories, retold in this chapter, demonstrate the ways in which colonial histories, migration, and gender inequities stratify reproduction.

Pregnancy and birth are just one part of a study of reproduction. In chapter 5, I expand on the ways in which women can control their own reproduction and negotiate intimate relationships. First, I describe women's knowledge, access, and experiences of trying to plan their families. These plans are often made in conjunction with or completely by their intimate heterosexual partners. Such relationships are also an important part of chapter 5, as they reflect cultural constructions of the social hierarchy of gender (Bourdieu 2001), elucidating inequities in power and control over women's bodies. I illustrate this by discussing Maureen's attempted abortion, Nelly's contraction of an STI from her husband through an extramarital partner, and Jasmine's trauma from marital sexual violence. Their stories attend to some of the risks that women face, which inevitably structure their poor reproductive and sexual health outcomes.

Gender and transnational mobility also shape women's experiences of health care in Chuuk and Guam. In chapter 6, I enter the public clinics with Chuukese women and explore how biomedicine, publicly funded services, and wider Chuuk and Guam contexts play out in their care. The benign neglect and resulting deteriorating healthcare system of Chuuk motivate women to come to Guam, but once they arrive, women face new structural, social, and individual constraints that inhibit their care. I begin with an account of Marilynn's pregnancy loss to elaborate on what is at stake and what women can lose when they receive inadequate care. I then turn to Pamela to explore how much work it takes to even get in the doors of the clinic to start receiving care. Women face challenges getting insurance, making an appointment, blocking out time, finding transportation, and having adequate time and interpreter services to ask questions of their providers. Yet many women persevere in these neglected spaces, seeking to establish agency in this complex, often hostile setting. Through the lens of the clinic, I demonstrate how colonial histories of benign neglect, migration experiences, reproductive norms, sexual inequities, and clinical encounters intersect to structure Chuukese migrant women's lives and stratify their sexual and reproductive health outcomes.

In chapter 7, I pivot to explore women's agency to function within the confines of their structural, social-symbolic, and individual constraints, and consider the actions that women have taken to change their own lives. Grassroots organizations in Chuuk and Guam counteract anti-immigrant sentiment and gender inequities and, through social support, work to redefine narratives about Chuukese communities. They also contribute to changing laws reflecting gender and sexual inequities, circumvent failing health systems, and foster new creative means to get women access to care. Women's and community groups have been at the forefront of activist work in both island jurisdictions.[21] In this final chapter, I discuss the actions taken by Chuukese women's groups to improve their circumstances.

1 • IMPERIAL OCCUPATIONS

In his annual State of the Island address in 2014, then governor of Guam Eddie Calvo discussed the relationship of Guam and greater Micronesia to the United States. He chastised Guamanians who said any U.S. states were better than Guam, and reminded everyone that "the best of America is right here on Guam. And they're Americans who also call ourselves Guamanian" (Calvo 2014). In this speech, Calvo implored people to collectively fight the poverty caused by U.S. policy, some of which was a result of the migration of citizens from the Freely Associated States (FAS) of Micronesia to Guam:

> It's one thing for a society to face poverty caused by its own conditions. Things get more complicated when poverty migrates in. It is estimated that over a third of the new families on food stamps in the last three years are FAS immigrants. I don't believe that the solution is to refuse services and hospitality to our neighbors. We are connected, my dear people.... The problem is poverty.... Whether his intentions were good or bad, Uncle Sam has a habit of forgetting his stated obligations to the Micronesian islands he saw fit to administer and use for geopolitical reasons. In other words, rather than waiting around ... for the U.S. government to finally build those schools in our neighboring islands, let's just band together as Micronesians and take care of these problems on our own two feet.... We're not victims of circumstance. We ARE Micronesians. We have it within us to build a strong region, where all of us contribute to each other's success.

Calvo's speech elucidated the complex identities of Guam residents and how they conceptualize their position in the U.S. empire ("the best of America is right here on Guam"), their autonomy to control their own destiny as part of greater Micronesia ("let's just band together ... and take care of these problems on our own two feet"), and the developmental neglect Micronesia faces from "Uncle Sam," who "has a habit of forgetting his stated obligations." In doing so, the then governor both articulated anti-immigrant sentiment in the community—by referring to poverty that "migrates in"—and combated this sentiment by arguing the shared sense of subjugation of Guam and greater Micronesia by the paternalistic U.S. government ("Uncle Sam") (see also Smith and Castañeda 2021). He also acknowledged the interconnectedness of Guam and greater Micronesia ("we are connected, my dear people") and perhaps a kindred identity with other Micronesians. These contradictory messages—at times blaming Micronesian migrants and at other times blaming the U.S. government for the collective, shared oppression of the residents of Guam and greater Micronesia—were typical of perceptions, interactions, and discussions throughout Guam regarding Compact of Free Association (COFA) migration. Relationships, policies, practices, and everyday interactions between COFA migrants and Guam's other residents reflect the complex interplay of identities, which partly results from their disparate colonial history and neocolonial relationships with the United States. Interactions between COFA migrants and Guamanian residents are part of a long history of interisland and colonial relationships, which separated and connected greater Micronesia and Guam at different points in time. This history is critical to understand the social, political, and economic context of Chuuk and Guam, as well as the modern-day relationships between those who associate their heritage with these two regional entities.

COLONIZING AND NAMING MICRONESIA

The region called "Micronesia" is composed of exceptionally diverse political, social, and economic histories, although the islands of the region share common experiences of colonization (Petersen 1998; Rainbird 2003). The name Micronesia was devised by European colonizers in the nineteenth century to reflect the many tiny (micro) islands characteristic of the region. This region encompasses over one million square miles of Pacific Ocean, most located just north of the equator. The idea of tiny islands, however, reflects the imposition of outsider perspectives on this region. Indigenous scholar Gonzaga Puas (2021) demonstrates the ways in which the term "Micronesia" reinforces the perception of islands as miniscule, disconnected places while ignoring the deep connections between them and the big oceans for Micronesians.[1] The name has remained, however, partly as a useful contrast to the other (problematically) named regions of the Pacific: Melanesia and Polynesia. American Micronesia comprises the archipelagos of the Mariana Islands, including Guam and the Commonwealth of the Northern Mariana Islands; the Marshall Islands (now a republic); and the Caroline Islands, including the Federated States of Micronesia and the Republic of Palau (Rainbird 2003; Kiste 1999, 433) (see figure 5).[2]

Occupying Guam

In 1521, the Portuguese explorer Ferdinand Magellan led a Spanish expedition to Guam in what would be the first official Pacific encounter between Micronesians and Europeans (Rogers 1995). During this encounter, indigenous Chamoru

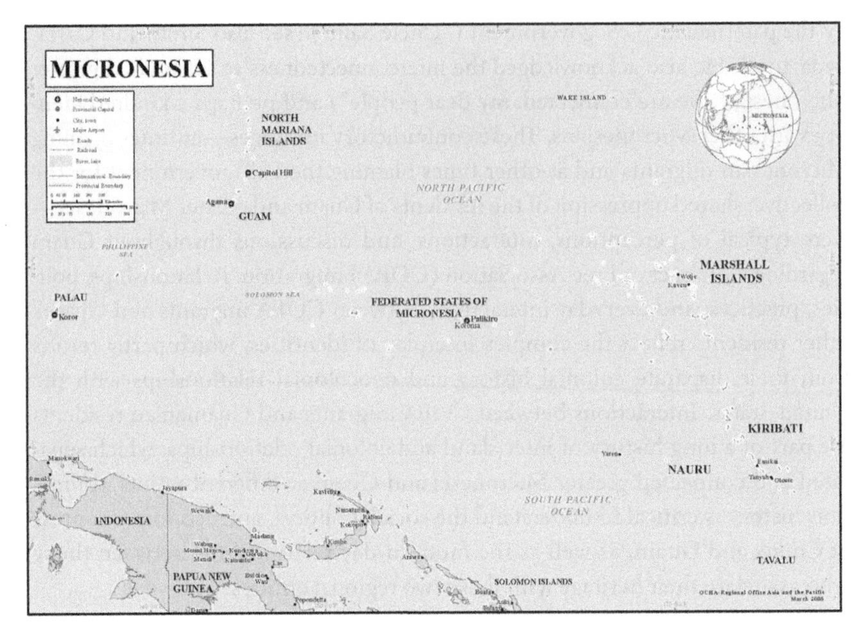

FIGURE 5. Map of the Micronesia region. Source: https://reliefweb.int/map/guam/national-reference-map-micronesia-federated-states

approached the ship that was anchored offshore, boarded it, and took goods, including a small boat. Magellan retaliated by leading a raid onshore, burning several homes and killing seven Chamoru men (Rogers 1995). He and his men then left, but soon after, the Spanish returned to the archipelago. Magellan named this great ocean the "Pacific Ocean" due to his relatively easy travel on this particular trip (he somehow encountered no major storms, typhoons, earthquakes, or volcanic eruptions, all of which are common) (Kiste 1994b). But that is not the only thing he named as a result of this trip; the Marianas archipelago, including Guam, was dubbed by Magellan "Las Islas de los Ladrones" (The Islands of Thieves). Spain officially claimed the island in 1565. It took another century to establish the colony, when missionary interest spiked (Diaz 2010).

In 1662, the Spanish Jesuit missionary Diego Luis San Vitores was on a Manila-bound ship that stopped at Guam for rest and to exchange metal articles (knives, iron) for food. Apparently "with tears streaming down his face" he noted how overwhelmed he was by the "poor naked natives" not yet blessed by Christianity (Diaz 2010, 1). He returned in 1668 to establish a Jesuit mission, thereby creating a more permanent presence. The Spanish installed governors to take control of the island and its people. They brought to Guam crops from other colonies and oversaw agricultural projects, but they largely focused on what was to be a long campaign of missionization. It was then that San Vitores was killed by chief Matå'pang of the Chamorro village of Tomhom (now Tumon) because he baptized Matå'pang's daughter against her father's wishes (Diaz 2010). This precipitated the thirty-year Spanish-Chamoru Wars (1668–1698). The fighting and the introduction of new diseases from Spanish troops and missionaries led to an estimated reduction in the Chamoru population by 90–95 percent (Hattori 2004). Today, Guam is 95 percent Catholic, and San Vitores is a martyr who is perceived to have died while saving the souls of Guam. Catholicism is more than just a religion; for Chamorus, it is a "political and cultural force" of life (Diaz 2010, 20).

Beyond the missionizing goals, Spain's choice to claim Micronesia was driven by what scholars have deemed the strategic denial of access or occupation of these islands by its French and Dutch rivals.[3] At this time, Spain controlled more of the Pacific than any other imperial nation. Located between the Spanish colonies of Mexico and the Philippines, Guam was a key waypoint, offering respite to ships sailing to and from these destinations in Spain's far-flung empire. As the largest island in the region, Guam was critical to Spanish sovereignty in the Pacific.

Despite claiming the majority of Micronesia, Spain's imperial attention remained focused on the Marianas (named after the Spanish Queen Mariana of Austria), particularly Guam, for most of more than two centuries of rule (1667–1898) (Rogers 1995) (see top of figure 5). This was one of the earliest instances in which colonial occupation disrupted connections between Chamorus and greater Micronesia. Archaeological evidence and early Spanish accounts demonstrate trade networks between the Caroline and Mariana Islands, which supported interisland connections (Berg 1992; Quimby 2011). However, the early Spanish occupation of Guam contributed to eliminating these traditional trade networks. This initiated a centuries-long separation of relationships between these island groups, leading to distinct identities, expressed through interethnic conflict between Guam and COFA citizens today. As Puas (2021) notes, colonization created boundaries in Oceania that divided islanders; they could no longer travel the seas and sustain old ties without outside interference.

Occupying Chuuk

The Federated States of Micronesia (FSM), including Chuuk, make up the Caroline Islands archipelago (Carucci and Poyer 2002) (see figure 6).[4] The indigenous peoples of the Caroline Islands encountered Europeans as early as the 1520s, when both Portuguese and Spanish expeditions reached the area. European accounts describe these initial encounters with the inhabitants as hostile, and thereafter little contact occurred until Spain laid claim to the islands in 1686, naming them after King Carlos II (Hezel 1995). Attempts to convert the inhabitants of the Caroline Islands to Christianity led to the killing of a priest, after which Spain was largely absent until 1787.[5] The entire region was known for resisting colonial outsiders from the beginning (Falgout, Poyer, and Carucci 2016). However,

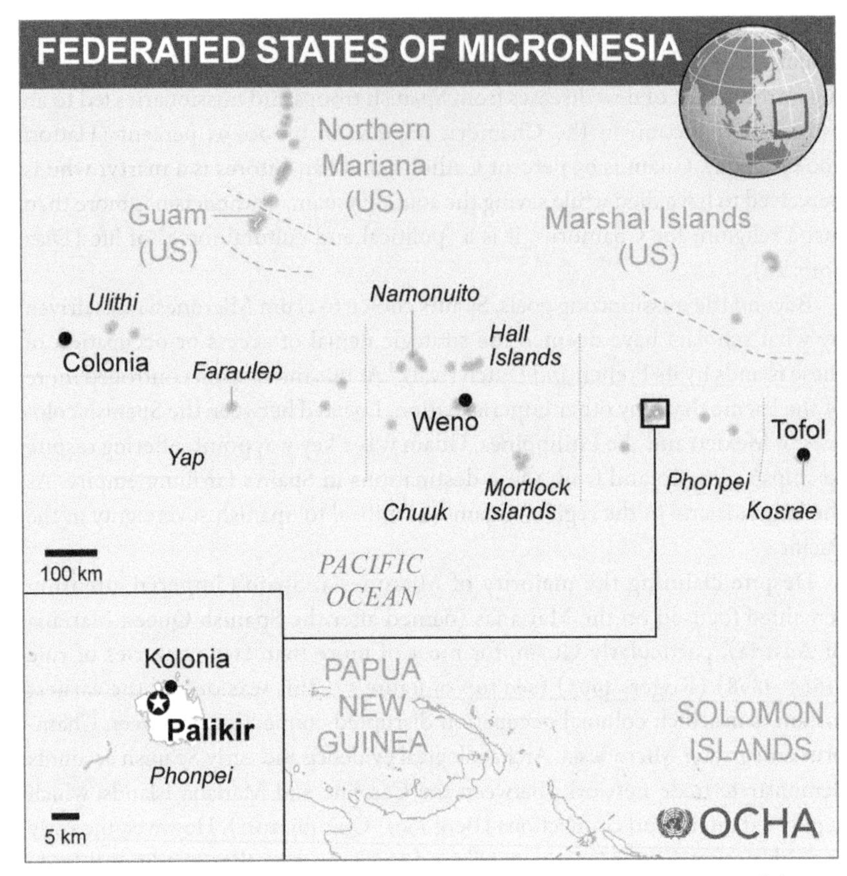

FIGURE 6. Map of the Federated States of Micronesia, including region Guam and the Marshall Islands. Source: Based on OCHA/ReliefWeb: https://reliefweb.int/map/micronesia-federated-states/federated-states-micronesia-location-map-2013

American whalers and various merchants sailed through the region and established trade networks, and missionaries founded churches throughout the nineteenth century (Hezel 1995).

The Chuuk Islands (colloquially referred to as Chuuk, previously Truk) is a unique area in this region, in that the Chuukese gained a particular reputation for hostility toward early European contacts (Hezel 1995; Kim 2007; Puas 2021).[6] The geography of Chuuk also differs from other parts of the Caroline Islands. Chuuk state is comprised of a lagoon (see figure 7) with twenty-three inhabited islands, plus several outer island chains (see figure 6). Unlike neighboring Pohnpei or Yap, it lacks a particularly large island that historically holds centralized authority over smaller satellite islands.[7] Oral histories depicted pre-contact Chuuk as egalitarian, with both descent line and order in which clans settled in a district determining ranks (Kiste 1994b). This may better explain why Chuuk, in

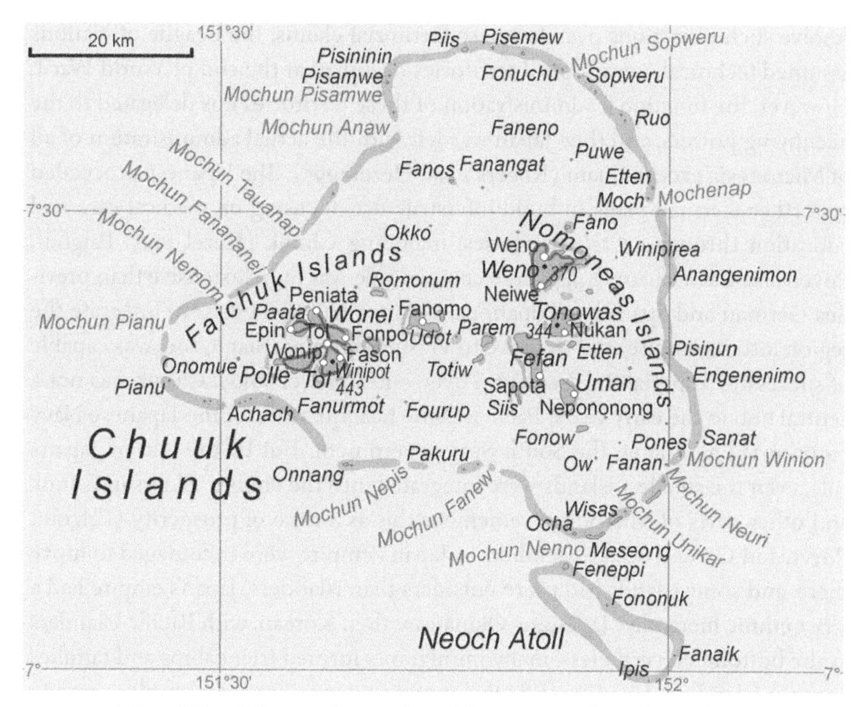

FIGURE 7. Map of Chuuk lagoon. Source: http://commons.wikimedia.org/wiki/File:Map_Chuuk_Islands1.png

great contrast to Guam, was largely left alone by outside forces until the late eighteenth and nineteenth centuries. Spain never established a permanent settlement on any island in Chuuk, even when settlements were founded on other Caroline Islands.

IMPERIAL WARS IN MICRONESIA

U.S. victory over Spain in the Spanish-American War of 1898 resulted in the dissolution of the remnants of Spain's empire, with major ramifications in Micronesia. The Treaty of Paris in 1898 transferred "ownership" of Guam from Spain to the United States. The treaty also provided for the burgeoning German empire to "purchase" the Caroline Islands and most of Micronesia from Spain in 1899, making it the region's dominant colonizer in the early twentieth century (Hanlon 1994). Under German rule, Chuuk experienced its first present and active occupation; colonizers built some infrastructure and supported increased missionary work. However, German control of Chuuk and its other Micronesian holdings was short-lived. At the outbreak of World War I in 1914, Japan declared war on Germany and seized control of its Micronesian territories; at the end of the war, Japan made claim to the entire area. The United States objected, and to resolve such objections over Japanese territorial claims, the League of Nations assumed technical control of all territories occupied at the end of World War I. However, the functional administration of these territories was delegated to the occupying powers, and thus Japan was left with the actual administration of all of Micronesia except Guam (Rogers 1995; Hezel 1995). The Japanese proceeded to further German plans to build infrastructure, focusing on medical care and education throughout the territories, including Chuuk (Hezel 1995; Falgout, Poyer, and Carucci 2016). Japanese colonial rule was more extensive than previous German and Spanish occupations, as Japan had two goals: to integrate the region into its empire, and to prove to Western empires that it, too, was capable of successful imperialism (Falgout, Poyer, and Carucci 2016). Chuuk was not a central hub in the early years; Palau was the headquarters for the Japanese Navy (1914–1922) and, later, the South Seas government. But by the end of Japan's rule, even the smallest islands were integrated into the empire. Elders in Chuuk and other parts of Micronesia remember this as a time of prosperity (Falgout, Poyer, and Carucci 2016). Members of Japan's empire were encouraged to move there, and some islands had more outsiders than islanders. Japan's empire had a strict ethnic hierarchy: Japanese, Okinawan, then Korean, with Pacific Islanders at the bottom. Nevertheless, many immigrants formed friendships and families with the islanders; Japanese and Okinawan last names are commonplace among Chuukese families today (Falgout, Poyer, and Carucci 2016). Fortification of the islands did not appear to take place until the late 1930s, as World War II approached. At that point, Chuuk became Japan's central naval office in the region. In 1940–1941, Japanese forces built two airfields and a communications center, and harbored a large portion of its naval fleet in the lagoon (Falgout, Poyer, and Carucci 2016).

As the Chuukese experienced massive changes at the hands of German and Japanese rule, citizens of Guam adjusted to their new status as colonial subjects of the United States and quickly began asserting their rights for self-government. The first formal request for Guamanian self-government under U.S. imperial control was brought to the U.S. Congress in 1901, when thirty-two prominent Chamoru men signed a petition requesting the United States to send a commission to study the possibility of a civilian government (Rogers 1995).[8] It was denied. Subsequent requests by local leaders made over the next four decades were also denied, largely because the U.S. Navy considered such proposals a threat to national security interests given Guam's strategic location. The efforts of Guam residents were particularly energetic after other U.S. possessions were given citizenship rights and some levels of self-government (Puerto Rico in 1917, the U.S. Virgin Islands in 1927, the Philippines in 1934). Nonetheless, the U.S. Navy continued to argue the importance of Guam as a unique strategic possession, justifying its desire to maintain control and limit local autonomy, and perpetuating the legacy of strategic denial first started by the Spanish (Rogers 1995).

The relationship between Spanish rulers and the Chamoru population was one that did not decimate the Chamoru language or family values, partly because some of these values mirrored Spanish traditions (such as matrilineal naming). Further, many Chamoru last names are of Spanish origin, reflecting the intermixing of Chamoru residents and Spanish occupiers. The U.S. occupation was different at first. The U.S. rulers recognized a racial hierarchy, discouraged marriages between Chamoru women and American Navy personnel, and punished Chamoru language use. This led to more tensions between this occupier and the Chamoru people, although the United States attempted to portray itself as a benevolent savior (Hattori 2004). That changed, however, after World War II.

The Japanese occupation of Guam (1941–1944) had a lasting impact on its residents. Collective memories of the war convey the violence Guamanians experienced at the hands of Japanese soldiers, including mass killings and rape of Chamoru women (Rogers 1995; Poyer, Falgout, and Carucci 2001). Rape occurred in villages at random but also through systematic means. While most Japanese "comfort women" (trafficked women from their occupied territories) were brought to Guam, some were taken from the Chamoru community. They were known as the Monday ladies, because that was the day of the week that they reported for a medical checkup (Rogers 1995).

Chuuk lagoon, in contrast, was already controlled by Japan and was central to the Japanese war effort, making it a target for U.S. forces. While the war between the United States and Japan raged throughout Micronesia, the Chuukese and other Micronesians experienced significant hardship and persevered through subsistence in an increasingly chaotic and resource-scarce environment (Hezel 1995; Poyer, Falgout, and Carucci 2001). At first, the Chuukese were expected to support the war by providing food and labor, and though they were treated as fourth-class citizens in Japan's racial hierarchies, they were not treated as prisoners of war, as were Guam's Chamoru people. But tensions escalated as the war continued and U.S. troops approached the region. Every island in Chuuk suddenly had Japanese troops on it, and the land's food was all appropriated for them (Falgout, Poyer, and Carucci 2016). As the war progressed, food ran out, and the Japanese were increasingly violent toward their colonial subjects. People were beaten for taking food from their own land or challenging Japanese military rules (Falgout, Poyer, and Carucci 2016). As food became increasingly scarce, rumors of Japanese cannibalism spread throughout Chuuk.

On February 17–18, 1944, the United States invaded Chuuk with a major airstrike called Operation Hailstone, which resulted in significant destruction of the Japanese fleet, which consisted of more than two hundred planes and forty ships—many of which still lie at the bottom of Chuuk lagoon. By the time of Japan's surrender and American occupation of the islands, the Chuukese people were starving. Some told stories of the remaining Japanese troops planning to kill the Chuukese people and themselves before the arrival of the Americans.

Chuukese people hid in caves up in the mountains and slowly came out to meet their new occupiers. With this new occupation, they expected more violence—as warned by the departing Japanese—but American troops quickly brought food and medical care, attempting to gain favor over their new imperial subjects (Poyer, Falgout, and Carucci 2001; Falgout, Poyer, and Carucci 2016). As these actions mirrored the ways in which chiefs (historically) took over newly acquired territory in Micronesia—bringing provisions to the occupied community—the Chuukese people could relate to this new group of outsiders (Falgout, Poyer, and Carucci 2016). The remaining Japanese, Okinawans, and Koreans were forced to leave, separating families. Chuukese elders report complaining to first Japanese and then American occupiers to stop waging wars that had nothing to do with them (Falgout, Poyer, and Carucci 2016).

After the military success of Operation Hailstone, the United States extended control in the Pacific. On July 21, 1944, U.S. forces recaptured Guam as part of Operation Forager in the second Battle of Guam (Poyer, Falgout, and Carucci 2001). Given residents' experiences of mass physical and sexual violence during Japanese occupation, the return of the United States near the end of the war was perceived as liberation rather than occupation.

Evidence of these wars linger throughout Micronesia, with unexploded ordinances, rusting tanks, and wartime bunkers remaining part of the landscape (see figure 8). I saw old tanks and equipment all over Chuuk and Guam when hiking or exploring. One time, when my family friends and I were on a beach in Guam, we found an old World War II hand grenade. One of the Micronesian family members with us—a weapons expert in the U.S. Army—examined it and determined that it was no longer dangerous. It became yet another World War II find displayed in someone's house.

As Vince Diaz argues, Japan's violent occupation of Guam did in three years what U.S. Navy officials had tried to do in the preceding fifty years and Spanish priests had tried to do for three hundred years before that it: "fused the Chamorros to their colonial overseer, with religious zeal and cultural prescriptions of gratitude and loyalty" (Diaz 2010, 13). This is most evident each year on July 21, when Guam residents across the island celebrate this liberation as an official holiday. Families stake out space for the annual parade in the early hours of the morning and follow this with family fiestas. American and Guam flags fly side by side, and the military typically participates in the parade, celebrating its (re)invasion of Guam. My own experience with Liberation Day festivities is reminiscent of Independence Day in mainland United States: a parade of floats full of waving leaders of local businesses, schoolchildren dancing or playing in their bands, and onlookers in lawn chairs on the side of the road, trying to keep cool on what is always a hot, steamy, and sometimes rainy holiday.

Around this time each year, local newspapers, the University of Guam, and community organizations repost oral histories and host events centered on

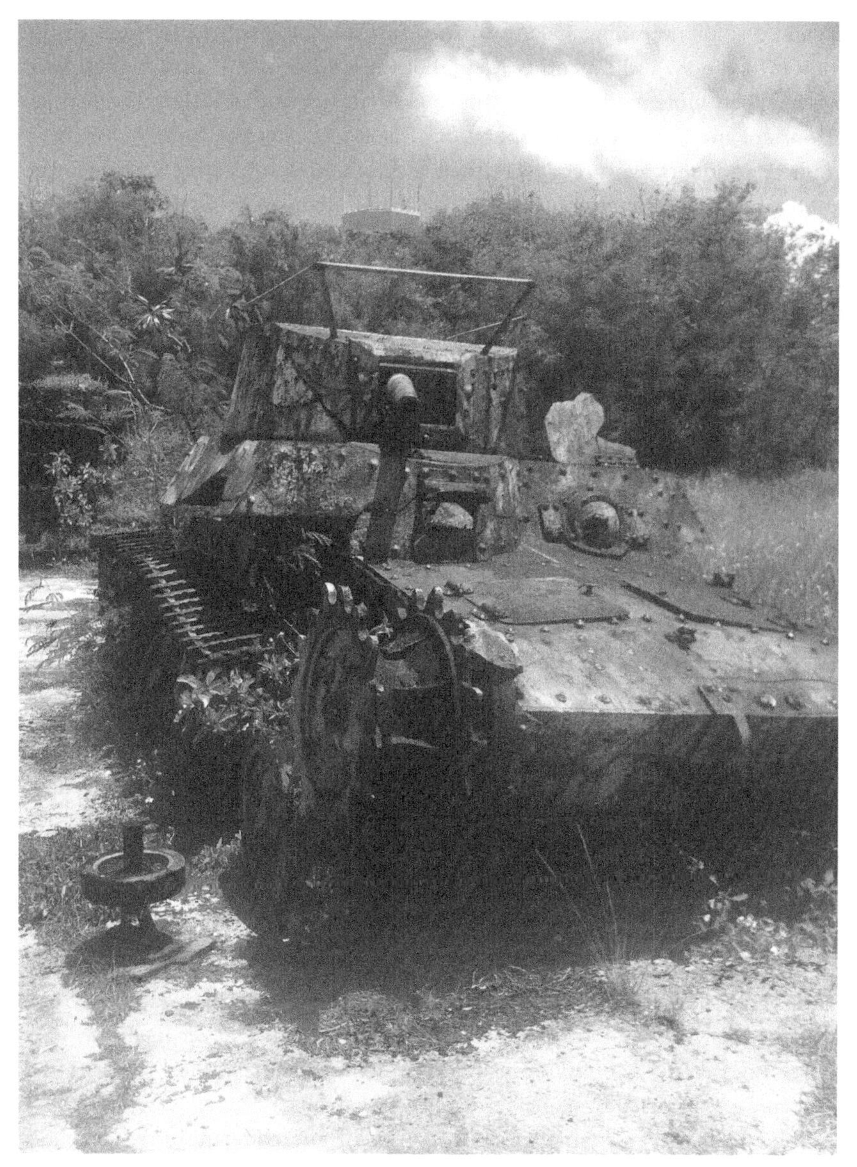

FIGURE 8. Evidence of the wars in Micronesia are everywhere. Photo by Sarah Smith.

and celebrating the remaining survivors of World War II. In these forums and oral histories, elders and their descendants discuss the violence experienced at the hands of the Japanese in Guam, such as the sexual assault of Chamoru women and forced (physical and sexual) labor camps. They also tell listeners how, as the Japanese ran out of food and supplies on the island and the threat of U.S. invasion loomed, violence toward the Chamoru people escalated. They tell of

Japanese soldiers leading Chamoru men into the jungle, forcing them to dig their own graves, and executing them. For these reasons, Chamoru elders who experienced violence by the Japanese firsthand consider Liberation Day an important marker of Guam's liberation. But it is a complex holiday for many younger residents, who recognize their lack of autonomy (DeLisle 2016). The holiday highlights conversations on what liberation means to Guam, and activist organizations take advantage of the occasion to discuss Guam's lack of self-determination with the United States, pointing out that Guam is not yet actually liberated (see, for example, Bevacqua 2019).

AMERICAN MICRONESIA

The U.S. Navy was quick to capitalize on the prevailing sentiment among Guam residents after World War II that U.S. military power had liberated the island. This was used to justify military land appropriations under the pretext that such actions would further protect the island (Rogers 1995). Despite initial positive feelings toward the U.S. government, as the military presence grew on the island, the people of Guam began to assert their rights for greater autonomy. In 1949, the Congress of Guam organized a walk-out protest, in which congressional members refused to return to work until the United States clarified the island's status. This action led to the passage of the Organic Act of 1950, which transferred rule of Guam from the U.S. Navy to the U.S. Department of the Interior, made Guam's governorship civilian instead of naval (but still appointed), and gave congressional (instead of constitutional) citizenship to people born in Guam (Perez 2002; Camacho 2011; Diaz 2010). Because their citizenship is given only by legislation requiring a simple majority in Congress, it can also be revoked this easily, making it much more precarious than that formalized by the U.S. Constitution.[9] Yarimar Bonilla (2015), describing the similar citizenship status for Puerto Ricans, illustrates well the complexity of having a U.S. passport in a territory. She describes how one holds a passport "with a shaky hand, never feeling wholly represented or fully confident in political membership that feels tenuous and unguaranteed" (xii). The same is true for Guamanians.

The Organic Act also made Guam an unincorporated territory rather than a possession, which means that the island is not considered integral to the United States and has no path to statehood or a status that approaches statehood in its future. Congressional citizenship and unincorporated status allow Guamanians to become American citizens, but it does not give them the right to all social and economic benefits available to residents of U.S. states, nor does it allow them to vote in U.S. presidential elections. The concept of graduated citizenship, in which there is not a simple citizen–noncitizen dichotomy but rather multiple forms of ambiguous belonging (Ong 2006), manifests in neoliberal empire-building. As my colleague and mentor Heide Castañeda and I argue, the ambiguities inherent in this form of citizenship better enable imperial control over borderlands and subnational jurisdictions like Guam through processes like migration (Smith and Castañeda 2021; see also Mountz 2011).

Further, creation and manipulation of subnational jurisdictions invite opportunities for increased militarization and enhancement of geopolitical power, without the responsibility of providing full rights or citizenship to local citizens (Baldacchino 2010). The military continues to build up Guam's bases with more troops and appropriate more land for military use (Gelardi 2021). Recognized as a key military position for U.S. presence in the Pacific, it is also the site of threats from other nations hostile toward the United States. A recent example of this occurred in 2017, when North Korea threatened to fire nuclear ballistic missiles at Guam. During this incident, Guam's residents and public servants were in full response mode. Healthcare workers I knew from the clinics told me they had to be "activated" for duty and take their emergency kits home; all were already trained in knowing where to take people in the event of a bombing. Yet during this 2017 incident, U.S. news agencies regularly misreported Guam as a U.S. military base in a foreign land, listing only military personnel as U.S. citizens at risk. Guam residents expressed frustration with their forgotten citizenship status, particularly as they lived under the threat of attack specifically because of their U.S. connection. The incident serves to illustrate how the application of graduated citizenship allows empires to strategically remember or forget who its citizens are and who belongs (Smith and Castañeda 2021). This was not isolated, however. A similar threat occurred in 2012 when I lived there, and there were others before and after. In another, more recent example, China launched four ballistic missiles into the South China Sea in August 2020, nicknaming one of them (DF-26) "Guam Killer" (J. Aguon 2022). During my most recent trip to Guam (March 2023), a dinner conversation with friends included a couple discussing their need to create a plan should an attack happen while they are in separate locations. These conversations occur regularly in this militarized space.

When geopolitical tensions rise, Guam residents do not need to see the news to know; military bombers start doing exercises over the island, and more ships arrive. You see and feel the tension. All these threats illustrate how islands are used to buffer external military threats from the mainland. The people of Guam live in a precarious state, knowing that their island's geopolitical positioning for the United States has made them among the United States' most vulnerable citizens. As indigenous Chamoru activist and scholar Julian Aguon (2022) clarifies, "We are in danger no matter which country is flexing its military muscle in this tense geopolitical theater. . . . When you live in a colony, you're easy meat." (26).

The residents of Guam continued to fight for increased autonomy after passage of the Organic Act. Their persistence realized notable gains, including allowances for a locally elected (instead of appointed) governor in 1968, a delegate to the U.S. Congress in 1972 (who can only vote in committees), and a Supreme Court with a direct link to the U.S. Supreme Court in 1998 (Perez 2002). Despite these victories, Guam's political relationship with the United States overall continues to be ambiguous (Perez 2002). At the same time, relationships between the people of Guam and the rest of the United States have become increasingly connected and interdependent. Guam residents typically have family scattered throughout the United States and usually have at least one family member enrolled in the U.S. military, which is one of Guam's largest employers. Evidence of this fusion is evident everywhere, from the American flags on bumper stickers to the excitement, energy, and long lines following every new opening of an American chain restaurant (Applebee's, IHOP) or big-box store (Home Depot).

When I spoke to Guam residents about their desires for decolonization, some wanted independence and some did not. This was in part due to the realities of being connected with and therefore dependent on the rest of the United States. Bonilla offered similar insights in Puerto Rico, where in this globalized era, families span far beyond the territory, and thus "independence has increasingly become a foreclosed option" (2015, xii). Another reason people are less confident about a future of independence is because they witness the poverty of neighboring islands in Micronesia that some perceive to be the result of independence from the United States. Again, Bonilla (2015) offers a comparison where those with "flag independence" in the postcolonial Caribbean are struggling, perhaps more than those without sovereignty. In reality, non-sovereign territories must contend with military occupations, are used for statecraft, and are at times medical guinea pigs, while those with independence are struggling with structural adjustment programs, imperial dictates of global trade, and general challenges of small island economies (Bonilla 2015). The circumstances are similar in Micronesia. Neither is truly a form of sovereignty.[10]

Despite the view of *some* residents that independence from the United States is undesirable or not feasible, the belief that Chamorus of Guam have the right to self-determination is nonetheless very popular; this is so even though the end goal, whether independence, statehood, or some other formalized relationship, is subject to debate. Since the first U.S. occupation, indigenous activists in Guam have organized through various means to determine their own futures, and since the mid-twentieth century, this has included constitutional conventions, commonwealth drafts and votes, and committees on decolonization and self-determination. Delegates from Guam also testify at the U.N. Special Committee on Decolonization every year, appealing for their right to self-determination. Chamoru women are at the forefront of this resistance (DeLisle 2016; Frain 2017; Mack and Na'Puti 2019).

America's Trust Territories

The American occupation of Micronesia marked a convergence of colonial histories for the people of Guam and those throughout the region, including Chuuk. During World War II peace talks, the United Nations agreed to allow U.S. administration over all of Micronesia in what was deemed a strategic trusteeship. Although eleven trusteeships were created by the United Nations following World War II, only the U.S.-Micronesia agreement was regarded as strategic, which gave the United States complete military control over the entire region (Kiste 1994a). The trusteeship included the Caroline, Mariana, and Marshall Islands, which were broken up into six districts, collectively known as the U.S. Trust Territory of the Pacific Islands (USTTPI) (Rogers 1995; Hezel 1995); Truk (now Chuuk) was one of these districts. The United Nations remained in charge of overseeing the U.S. support of the islands' eventual move toward self-government (Kiste 1994b). Guam was not included in these negotiations because the United Nations already considered it a U.S. possession.

U.S. administration of these islands in the ensuing two decades was one of "benign neglect," by which the U.S. Navy denied access to the islands from the outside world while simultaneously ignoring, or forgetting, most inhabitants (Kiste 1994b, 230).[11] The politics of benign neglect, or staying while leaving, is a common but largely invisible strategy to regulate colonies and maintain empire through slow and limited attention and resources. Henry Kissinger, national security adviser to Richard Nixon, was perhaps the most explicit in his justification of this U.S. imperial strategy when he stated of Micronesia, "There are 90,000 people out there. Who gives a damn?"[12] This continues to be the strategy in the region today.

While the United States neglected its purported role to support the independence of these territories, its military activities were assuredly not neglectful. Trust territory districts became sites for U.S. experimentation of military strategies, studies of sociocultural norms to best manage (or control) inhabitants, and, most harmfully, nuclear testing experiments. In particular, the Marshall Islands became the site of U.S. nuclear testing from 1946 to 1958, the health and economic repercussions of which still persist today for the Marshallese people (Barker 2004). Dozens of bombs were dropped on the Marshall Islands, including the now infamous atomic bomb named Bravo, which detonated in a massive explosion on Bikini atoll in 1956. Chuuk was a site for sociocultural and ecological research, led largely by anthropologists (see chapter 2).

As Guam fought for self-determination and greater autonomy in the mid-twentieth century, the Organic Act also moved USTTPI administration from the U.S. Navy to the Department of the Interior in 1951, signaling that these islands were insular, or part of, the United States.[13] Puas (2021) alternatively argues that this move was made not to signal their insular nature but rather to indicate that the United States was simply an administrator responsible for overseeing these islands' progress toward self-government. While the navy era included provision of extensive goods and services, the Department of the Interior was perceived by locals as underfunded and slow (Heine 1974). During this time, the United States slowly established island governments, but despite the agreement with the United Nations to do so, it did not move Micronesia toward independence. The United States controlled all governance, including movement in and out of Micronesia.

The Department of the Interior did not recognize the unifying strength of Micronesians seeking an alternative to the benign neglect of the current slow-development arrangement (Puas 2021). Frustrated with the lack of U.S. support for infrastructure and development on the islands, Micronesian leaders asked the United Nations to visit and assess the role of the U.S. government in decolonizing Micronesia (Heine 1974). As a result, the United Nations conducted a study and issued a report in 1961 condemning the United States for the poor state of education, health, economic and political development in the USTTPI (Kiste 1994b). With pressure from the United Nations, President Kennedy approved National Security Memorandum 145 in 1962, which made it official U.S. policy to attempt to permanently incorporate the USTTPI into the United States (Lutz 1984). Soon after, a task force was sent to investigate and make recommendations on how to implement this policy. The resulting Solomon Report recommended that the United States inspire Micronesians to remain connected by pouring large amounts of money into the region to foster long-term dependency and to promote a positive attitude toward America through education (Lutz 1984). The U.S. strategy to foster dependency in the region was advanced through ongoing negotiations with the USTTPI for a new status (Petersen 1998). Bigger budgets were approved for an increasing range of services, with the goal of delaying or lessening Micronesian desires for independence or autonomy.

Consistent with the Solomon Report's recommendation to promote positive perceptions of the United States through education, the Peace Corps entered Micronesia in 1966. With the Peace Corps came more funded projects, more schools run by volunteers, and thus more high school graduates (Hezel 1995). Many of these high school graduates began to migrate to the United States for college, particularly to Guam and Hawai'i, where they learned more about U.S. relationships with indigenous communities (Marshall 2004; Petersen 1998).

In this era, in particular under the Kennedy, Johnson, Nixon, and Ford presidencies, administration of the USTTPI included development of all sorts, particularly economic development to align these societies with American interests in capitalist expansion (Hanlon 1998). Economic development is a key strategy of empire domination; while it presents as benevolent—creating new economies for "native others"—it is as destructive as other forms of imposed change, creating unsustainable economies with inequitable distributions of resources

(Hanlon 2009; Bonilla 2013; Escobar 2011). Social development was intentionally focused on Americanization as well, as evidenced by the introduction of television and American movies (see, for example, O'Rourke 1980), English-taught high schools, and American treats (foods, technology). I elaborate on some of their development initiatives—and particularly those that have to do with gender, reproduction, and sexuality—in the chapters that follow.

Moving toward Independence

> For Micronesians, their choice in the plebiscites was as "free" as those of boat passengers who have been taken far from their shore by a pilot whose interests and itinerary are not their own and who are then given the choice of remaining on the boat or swimming the 200 miles back to shore. Micronesia was not given the choice of complete political independence combined with an assured foreign aid package that would be directed towards the repair of the damage done to their economies and social systems by the strategic colonization of that area by the United States over the last forty years. (Lutz 1986, 26–27)

As a means of complying with the U.N. requirements, the Solomon Report suggested the creation of a Micronesia-wide deliberative body that would help advance the islands of the trust territory toward independence, or at least self-determination. The resulting organization became known as the Congress of Micronesia. Puas (2021) argues that the congress was created when Micronesians decided to begin dialogue about their political futures across the islands. However, with U.S. intervention, it was designed with a U.S.-style deliberative structure at its core. The Congress of Micronesia thus further served to perpetuate U.S. hegemony and male-centric participation. Congressional appointees were mostly (male) traditional leaders and relatives. This system was so starkly different from traditional Micronesian modes of leadership and decision-making that some of these leaders quit the congress before any decisions were even made (Hanlon 1998).

According to Robert C. Kiste and Suzanne Falgout (1999), negotiations for a new political status began as early as 1969 and were certainly shaped by the ongoing Vietnam War. Recognizing that the movement toward independence was growing, the United States offered the entire USTTPI and Guam the collective status of a commonwealth, but this offer was turned down by the Congress of Micronesia (Puas 2021; Hezel 1995). Historians suggest that Guam delegates rejected the American offer because of continued resentment toward the Chamoru of the Northern Mariana Islands, who assisted the Japanese during the island's occupation in World War II.[14] Others from around greater Micronesia rejected it because they wanted more autonomy and independence for their islands. Guam was not offered another option, so it remained an unincorporated territory.

At this point, some members of the Congress of Micronesia had been educated in U.S. colleges and had learned through experiences abroad about the disenfranchisement and poor conditions that Native Americans, Native Hawaiians, and Chamorus faced as occupied U.S. territories (Puas 2021; Petersen 2004). They saw how the loss of land was a major way in which indigenous peoples lost their sovereignty across the globe and decided to fight to maintain authority over their territory (Petersen 2004). To consider their best options for self-determination, they also studied postcolonial arrangements between other islands and colonizing nations throughout the Pacific. In particular, the Cook Islands (Māori: Kūki 'Āirani), which was in a type of Free Association with New Zealand, had secured an agreement that the Micronesians perceived to offer greater autonomy, and thus they pursued a similar arrangement (Petersen 2004).

When the Northern Mariana Islands split off and agreed to commonwealth status on their own, the remaining islands of the USTTPI rejected all U.S. offers that were short of independence (Puas 2021). At that point, they began to splinter off into smaller island groups and negotiate their own deals. Some scholars have argued that the United States fostered this splintering to reduce the individual negotiating power of each territory (Puas 2021; Lutz 1984). Puas (2021) points out that this conduct was counter to the agreement of the USTTPI and the U.N. precedent on how to work with non-self-governing territories. After Palau and the Marshall Islands began negotiating their individual agreements, the remaining districts in the Caroline Islands, including Chuuk, Pohnpei, Kosrae, and Yap, were left to join and form one nation—the FSM. Although these former trust territory districts came to constitute one nation, they contain significant diversity, which continues to affect the overall cohesiveness of the FSM (Carucci and Poyer 2002).

The United States ratified COFAs for the Republic of the Marshall Islands and the FSM in 1986, and for the Republic of Palau in 1994.[15] The UN recognized the FSM in 1990, removing the USTTPI status and welcoming them as a member nation in 1991. Chuuk became one of four states in the newly formed FSM. The FSM recognizes the date of November 3, 1986, when the COFA was ratified by the United States, as the end of colonialism, celebrated as FSM Independence Day (Puas 2021).

Although each island nation negotiated with the United States and entered into a COFA, signaling that they were an independent nation with self-governing rights, the United States maintained the right to deny entry to foreigners and military powers.[16] Further, the new nations continued to be dependent on U.S. funding to support their path to full independence—including financing for education, economic and political development, and healthcare infrastructure (Hezel 1995). With this agreement, although they are technically independent countries, COFA nations have U.S. postal, weather, and aviation administration services; disaster relief; and many other U.S. federal programs.

Several criticisms have been directed at these compacts, starting with the constraints created to support their inception (Hanlon 2009). Requirements set forth within the compacts constructed oversized governments and economies that did not align with the material realities of these small island states, ultimately serving U.S. interests by maintaining a relationship of dependency with the mainland.[17] As Glenn Petersen (1998) explained, "It is difficult for Micronesians to claim simultaneously that they are fully sovereign and independent, *and* that they have no choice in the character of their relations with the United States. This is, nevertheless, precisely the nature of their ties to the US" (as cited in Smith and Castañeda 2021, 151). The limited autonomy of these new nations was even further constrained with the amended COFA agreement of 2003, which increased U.S. monitoring requirements of COFA nation budgets while decreasing U.S. congressional appropriations to their budgets each year (COFA 2003).[18] The 2003 agreement was meant to be the final compact, and for years, the unknown future was a major source of anxiety for leaders of these countries. Since 2020, however, negotiations for a new compact have been underway, and COFA nations have had more leverage due to China's increasing influence in the region.

In recent years, China has expressed interest in forming varying agreements with Pacific Island countries. China's interests include attempting a comprehensive bilateral agreement with each Pacific Island nation in which China would invest significantly but also expect adherence to the China First policy.[19] Some Pacific Island nations have aligned with China under this policy. At the same time, Guam is experiencing a military buildup and Micronesian islands are being considered for more U.S. military bases; the FSM has agreed to a military facility (Gelardi 2021; Lum 2023). FSM president David Panuelo and others have argued that they do not want to be caught between these two powerful nations or become casualties of another world war (Panuelo 2022; Perry 2023). Yet, it is clear these islands remain embedded within the broader geopolitical posturing of powerful nations. But these island nations can strategically use this geopolitical posturing to their advantage (Puas 2021).

As of March 2023, compact renewal negotiations are nearly complete, but not yet public (Lum 2023; Martina and Brunnstrom 2023). What is known is that President Biden's FY 2024 budget includes $7.1 billion for the region, which is a considerable increase from previous compact budgets (Lum 2023; Martina and Brunnstrom 2023). This increase, subject to U.S. congressional approval, is great news to the communities of the FAS nations, as it may provide a significant economic boost to the region if approved. But even this new leverage does not change the fact that the power lies with the United States in deciding the final terms of this agreement, and their relationship overall.

Indigenous scholar Gonzaga Puas (2021) offers a critique of this oppressive narrative that the United States has all the power, recognizing that Micronesians have always managed the outside world in strategic ways that are not well understood by colonial regimes or researchers. He asserts that "polite smiles of silence" were misunderstood by outsiders to be "compliance and consent" rather than strategic patience, an indigenous cultural practice used to manage disasters both natural and human-made (93, 122). While colonial powers have always tried to impose alien systems, he argues, it has never resulted in Micronesians abandoning their own systems, which are embedded in the FSM Constitution. To him, the constitution they created represents the collective identities of Micronesians in this modern state, conveying their "continuity and resilience" as a people (86). He also points out that scholars typically depict cultural loss in Micronesia without attending to the survival of cultural norms for over one hundred years of colonization.

OUTSIDERS IN GUAM: CONTROLLING MIGRATION TO MAINTAIN EMPIRE

The COFA is considered by many to be the reason for the FSM's struggling economy, crumbling health and educational infrastructure, and endemic poverty; it is a tool of the strategy of benign neglect. The COFA is a key factor in answering the questions set forth in this book, not just because of its social and economic impact on the FSM but because of its role in fostering increased migration to Guam. One of the COFA provisions is that citizens of COFA nations can travel, live, and work in the United States with the status of "nonimmigrants" who are "habitual residents." The Congress of Micronesia strategically requested this language in the agreement with the United States, based on its estimation that the government might not have the economic potential to support all citizens immediately. This provided a mechanism for the management of overpopulation on the islands and was meant to ensure Micronesia's economic and political survival (Petersen 2004). Yet with persistent shortcomings in island infrastructure, migration to the United States has primarily been in one direction. Micronesians, particularly from Chuuk, have little to no economic or educational opportunities to enable widespread return to their home islands.

Chuuk is the most populated state of the FSM. It has twenty-three inhabited island units of 45,973 people (thirty-five municipalities) divided over five regions, with a population density of 993 people per square mile. Chuuk is the poorest state, with limited sanitation, water shortages, and power outages where infrastructure exists (in Wééné). The central islands of Chuuk lagoon, particularly Wééné, are where people migrate to work, seek health care, or attend school. Wééné is a somewhat typical Pacific Island port town; it is hot, dusty from the dirt roads, and bustling with activity during the day.[20] People—especially women—walk along the roads, visiting the small local market, grocery stores, or a handful of stores selling a little of everything (fabric, plastic bins for cooking and storage, cooking gas, and other important supplies). Cars slowly zigzag their way down the pothole-marked roads, never going more than ten miles an hour, some drivers sitting on the right of their cars, some on the left, since imports come from (mostly) the United States and Japan. As traffic slowly crawls through the main center of Wééné, people joke that drunk drivers have a telltale behavior here. Those who drive straight through such a potholed street are intoxicated, those who weave back and forth are sober and protecting their cars from the deep waterlogged holes. Taxis (usually personal vehicles, such as white trucks) drive people to and from more remote villages into offices and stores each weekday, usually for one dollar or less per ride. Boat traffic is even more pronounced; small panga commuter boats line the docs central to Chuuk (see figure 9), while others land near their familial plots throughout the island. Large numbers of family members live in houses here, hosting those who come from other islands. Houses in most of the villages are on a power grid, but they must prepay for power, which not everyone can afford. It is lively, but signs of neglect are ubiquitous, with the deteriorating buildings, the unkept roads, and people from other islands struggling to pay for life there with such limited and low-paid job opportunities.

Wééné is also the first stop before migrating beyond Chuuk because it hosts the airport. On flight days, the airport is filled with observers picking up or dropping off family, or simply watching the flights land and takeoff. Chuuk is also the first stop on the only regional Island Hopper air travel with service to and from Guam. For these political-economic and geographic reasons, Chuukese people frequently migrate to Guam.

During Guam's occupation by outside forces, the island became a place where colonizers brought the colonized. The first to arrive, during Spanish rule, were the Filipinos, who were brought over to help translate, convert the Chamoru people to Catholicism, build infrastructure for the new port, and support Spanish troops (Rogers 1995). Under U.S. rule, the federal government continued to manage Guam's immigration, first through navy control and then, since 1962, through civilian U.S. immigration procedures. During the early years, Filipinos were brought through guest-worker programs, and navy families settled in this new territory. Later on and to the present, Guam has been used to process refugees, including 100,000 Vietnamese refugees and over 6,000 Kurdish refugees during the Vietnam and Gulf Wars, respectively, as well as nearly 1,000 Burmese refugees and a substantial but uncertain number of Chinese asylum seekers (Coddington et al. 2012). Not only has U.S. policy brought refugees, guest workers, and military personnel to Guam; it has also fashioned the island as a tourism site for Japanese and South Korean nationals, completely transforming Guam into a major cash economy (Diaz 2010). And since 1986, Guam's visitor logs included increasing numbers of citizens from COFA countries.

As with any military base, the demand for both physical and sexual labor brings many migrants to Guam. Pacific scholar Teresia Teaiwa called this "militourism"

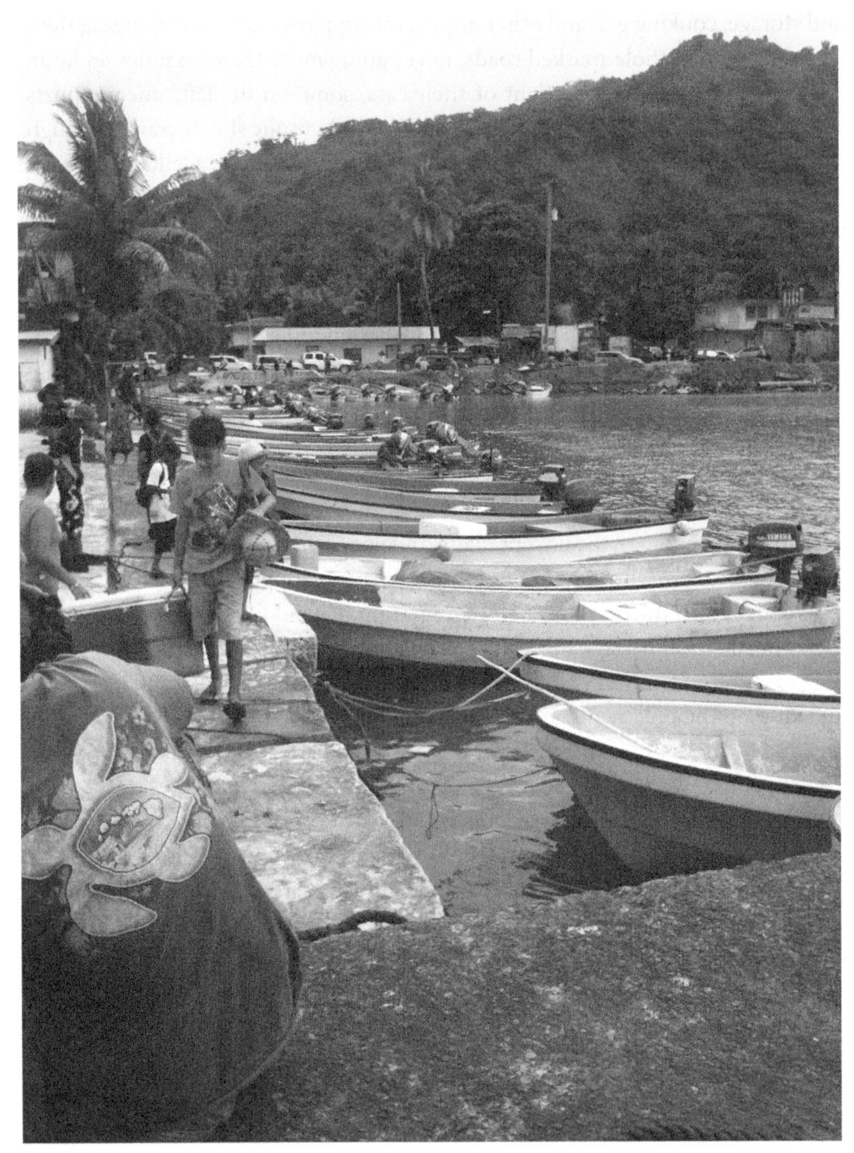

FIGURE 9. Typical Friday boat traffic in Wééné. Photo by Sarah Smith.

(1999, 249). Scholars studying islands as subnational jurisdictional territories note that the common elements of these territories exist in Guam. That is, they mix military and tourism economies that rely on authorized migration and are used to control other forms of migration, such as asylum seeking (Coddington et al. 2012; DeLisle 2016). Each is located closer to the originating countries of migrants than to their imperial holder and the migrants' final destination, as well as proximate to transnational ocean journeys where migrants are intercepted. This is the case for Chuukese migrants. While they are legally able to migrate farther than Guam, they are often constrained by economic circumstances.

Due to the conditions of mobility and migration fostered by the United States, the indigenous Chamoru of Guam represent just under one-third (33 percent) of the total island population, followed by Filipinos at 29 percent, and then white and Chuukese people each at almost 7 percent (U.S. Census Bureau 2022).[21] There are also relatively large communities of Chinese, Japanese, South Korean, Vietnamese, and other COFA-citizen residents (U.S. Census Bureau 2022). The lack of control over immigration by the people of Guam has led to tensions between Chamoru and non-Chamoru communities residing there (Diaz 1995, 2010). This continuously changing demography, particularly including reductions in indigenous communities and additions of outsiders, has increased Chamoru fears of "demographic theft"—a concern that immigration over time will completely change or steal the demography of a community, with outsiders taking over as the majority population (Castañeda 2008, 340). COFA citizens, as the most recent migrants with a large presence on the island, face anti-immigrant sentiment that is the product of this fear of their invading bodies, with implications for their sense of identity and belonging and their health.

IMPERIAL BODIES

As I have illustrated, empires claimed Micronesia since the sixteenth century. In the most recent iteration of imperialism, the U.S. empire enacted partial forms of sovereignty to maintain control of these islands, with the promise to help them develop their independence. The politics of benign neglect, manifested through the structural violence of the limited and shrinking funding that these island territories receive, continue to limit access to health care, education, and economic opportunities.

Modern empires are often perceived as unique or postcolonial because there are ambiguous levels of sovereignty and citizenship statuses, with confusing idiosyncrasies. Anthropologist Ann Stoler (2016) argues that there is no such thing as postcolonial, just different configurations of empire present in the modern world. Assuming we are in a postcolonial era can mask configurations of imperialism today. The COFA and Guam are excellent examples of these indeterminant statuses that manifest in modern empire building.

In a similar framing, Bonilla (2013) considers postcolonial sovereignty to be a fiction. Drawing from one of Michel-Rolph Trouillot's (1990) challenges to Haiti's supposed uniqueness, Bonilla argues that the history of the entire Caribbean and other postcolonial states are portrayed as special exceptions to a "normal" clear path to postcolonial sovereignty. In reality, ambivalent states with varying levels of autonomy are ordinary forms of sovereignty. Stoler (2016) and Bonilla

(2013) may be analyzing two different processes as fictions—postcolonialism and sovereignty, respectively—but these are intimately intertwined. Postcolonial sovereignty is a fiction because imperialism as a past event is a fiction. Both COFA nations and Guam portray manifestations of this fiction, or graduated sovereignty (Ong 2006).

Graduated sovereignty, indigenous scholar Michael Lujan Bevacqua (2012) has argued, must be used in order to enact sovereignty. Using Giorgio Agamben's concept of "homo sacer," or "bare life," Bevacqua posits that that which is neither entirely sovereign (i.e., sacred) or not sovereign (i.e., profane) must exist to completely understand that which is sovereign. In other words, sovereignty is formed only by exclusion of other spaces, which are semi- or non-sovereign:

> Guam . . . takes on a curious significance, as it is placed right on the edge of an edge. As the United States, America and the world are laid out, Guam represents a piece of the outside inside or the inside outside, an exceptional zone, which can conceivably be used to represent the exteriority of the interiority of the United States. . . . Guam is therefore like a distant outpost, not really part of the foreign or the domestic. It is too simplistic to say that it straddles these two ways of mapping the world or a particular nation. It is instead something . . . *that can be pulled back and forth across that line* (italics in original) (2012, 59).

The sovereignty of the United States is only constructed, recognized, and maintained when considered in juxtaposition with its ambiguous colonies.[22] Unclear borders, ambiguous access to property, legal rights, mobility, and citizenship, Stoler (2016) argues, are defining features of empires; they thrive in partial forms of exclusion. Calling them unique obscures the history of and contemporary forms of imperialism. This analysis applies not only to Guam but to Micronesian nations in a COFA with the United States.

These graduated forms of sovereignty, divided into subnational jurisdictional statuses such as unincorporated territory, commonwealth, and freely associated states, are particularly effective on islands, where remoteness and invisibility can be used to maintain exclusion (Mountz 2011; Ong 2006), supporting modes of benign neglect. Discourses of remoteness and smallness in maintaining narratives of invisibility have also been analyzed as a strategy of empire maintenance (Puas 2021; Na'puti 2019). Indigenous Scholar Tiara Na'puti (2019) labels this strategy cartographic violence. Creating the imagery of remoteness and invisibility—allowing the mainland to forget about this territory—plays an important role in maintaining strategic military control in the Marianas archipelago (Amundsen and Frain 2020; DeLisle 2016) and all of Micronesia. These strategies were common to empire maintenance throughout the twentieth century and were often employed with the assistance of anthropologists and missionaries. I consider the implications for their work in chapter 2.

2 • IMPERIAL OBSERVATIONS

Outsiders visit Chuuk for three major reasons, the first being to dive. A tour of Chuuk for visitors goes something like this: they stay at Blue Lagoon or Truk Stop, the only two hotel-dive operations in Chuuk. Once acclimated from the long travel, visitors dive or snorkel in the lagoon. These dives are magical. It is breathtaking to see the remnants of massive ships and planes sunk during World War II and submerged in crystal-clear blue lagoon water, surrounded by the reefs and sea life that have made these vessels their home for over seventy years. Above the water is amazing as well; boat rides show the vast blue lagoon, at times busy with small commuter vessels but usually an immense space of water, with lush green islands popping up in various sizes in every direction. Visitors can end each day with a sunset in hues of purple, orange, red, and pink, reflected in the lagoon's water.

Experienced divers consider this a bucket-list location; it is incredibly expensive to get to but, to most, worth every penny. When not in the water, divers typically take a tour of Wééné with an employee of their hotel. These day tours, scheduled on the last day of divers' trips,[1] are really the only time they are encouraged to leave the hotel grounds. With a local guide as an interlocutor of safety and comfort,[2] day tours include visiting a high school established and run by Jesuit Catholics, seeing wartime relics slowly deteriorating in the tropical jungle, seeing an old Japanese lighthouse, and little else. Tours on other islands usually include seeing World War II Japanese barracks and picnics on beautiful remote beaches. Thus, almost every site visited by divers is centered around Chuuk's colonial history, either through imperial occupations and the wars they brought or through the missionaries who worked alongside them. This is basically the only tourism industry for Chuuk.

Another reason for outsiders to visit Chuuk is because they work for a development agency, volunteer for a mission, or do development-adjacent work. Consultants from the CDC, UNICEF, and the Secretariat of the Pacific Community arrive regularly to observe, check on projects, consult, or provide some sort of education. The Peace Corps, Jesuits, Seventh-day Adventists, and Church of Jesus Christ of Latter-day Saints are all established in Chuuk; the Peace Corps and Jesuit missionaries are typically recent college graduates who make up a large proportion of Chuuk's high school teachers.[3] I also met physicians associated with Christian denominations who arrived regularly for healthcare missions. It is not, however, just religious mission healthcare providers who arrive; for example, I observed a floating U.S. military health center and hospital (on a huge ship) park outside the lagoon for a few months to provide specialty care. Anthropologists like me do research trips and often consult, too. We are rarer now, but people in Chuuk are much more familiar with the discipline than are most people I meet on the U.S. mainland. This is inevitably a result of the years of anthropological work during the trust territory period.

All these people are associated with developing Chuuk. This category of visitors (including me) is invited to see all the same sites as the divers but also to tour buildings and facilities that need foreign funding to survive (and are often in deteriorating shape, like the hospital) or new buildings paid for by a foreign entity (e.g., Japan or China). While long-term visitors—such as anthropologists, Peace Corps volunteers, and multiyear missionaries—have more personal relationships with Chuukese families than do tourists and short-term consultants, their relationships are still shaped by imperial histories and colonial circumstances. First, outsiders—particularly those with American passports—can come and go easily,[4] their hotel fees, paid family stays, and general spending contributing important cash to the economy. These relationships are always built with the knowledge that—like many migrating family members—outsiders will ultimately leave, with more power and resources to come and go.

The third reason for those from outside Chuuk to arrive is when other Micronesians want to go to what is considered the best high school in Micronesia. Drawing students from the entire region, Xavier High School is run by the American Jesuits in Chuuk. They are also temporary visitors, there only because of missions established during the century of colonization, which included the formation of this high school. The impact of colonization is thus visible everywhere, even when simply considering who visits and observes Chuuk, and why.

Anthropologist Catherine Lutz (2006) has advocated for more ethnographies of empire, specifically asking how U.S. imperial projects create vulnerabilities in communities and how people resist the consequences of imperialism through their bodies and social worlds. Missionaries, anthropologists, and imperial development specialists of the U.S. Trust Territory of the Pacific Islands (USTTPI), many of whom remain part of Chuuk's landscape, must all be examined in this context. In this chapter, I first briefly outline how nineteenth- and twentieth-century missionaries shaped gendered discourses of Micronesia and consider how those discourses affected Chuuk. I then describe how anthropologists worked with colonial governments in the mid-twentieth century to assist in imposing patriarchal American systems and discourses in Chuuk. I next illustrate how discourses on gender, sexuality, and reproduction were shaped by each of these outside observer groups. Finally, I consider how efforts to develop Chuuk used anthropological accounts and perpetuated these colonizing legacies in the later twentieth century and up to the present day. While missionaries typically sought to learn about sexual practices in order to change them, and imperial managers needed to understand how to prevent the spread of sexually transmitted infections (STIs) to colonial officers and workers, anthropologists often sought to discover the exotic other (Reed 1997). Each helped facilitate changes in Chuuk's gender structures, with lasting impacts for women.

MISSIONIZING MICRONESIA

While Guam is largely Catholic, a consequence of the Spanish occupation, Chuuk is split. Over 90 percent of Chuukese people identify as Christian, but about half are Protestant and half are Catholic. This means that spending time in Chuuk entails being asked regularly: Are you Protestant or Catholic? I was asked this question nearly every time I met someone new and had more than a thirty-second exchange with them. My default answer was that I was raised by a Protestant (Methodist) mother and that my husband's family was both Catholic and Protestant. What I was really doing was avoiding the question for polite, "How's the weather?" level chats. When the conversation went deeper, I explained that I was not personally religious but respected both traditions. This was met with polite silence or, with more outspoken elder women, invitations to prayer groups.

Being Catholic or Protestant and sticking with your own religion is important to Chuukese families. I heard stories that were reminiscent of Romeo and Juliet when Catholics and Protestants fell for each other. At other times, women told me they were close with both Catholic and Protestant people and made a point to say that everyone gets along. The Chuuk Women's Council, for example, had a Protestant president and a Catholic vice president (see chapter 7); these women were very close friends. Yet even though the narrative was that everyone respected both traditions, these distinctions were made regularly and were clearly as important to communities as were distinct identities related to islands and regions of Chuuk (chapter 3). Community villages and sometimes entire islands are exclusively Catholic or Protestant, following 150 years of missions' competitive proselytizing in the region.

Missionizing Chuuk occurred much later than it did on Guam and a bit later than it did on other Caroline Islands, such as Pohnpei and Palau. The American Board of Commissioners for Foreign Missions introduced Protestant Christianity to this part of Micronesia in the 1870s. This was followed by the evangelical Lutheran group the Liebenzell Mission, which took over in 1907 (soon after the German occupation) (Marshall and Marshall 1990). Today, both churches exist, and people who adhere to these churches refer to themselves as Protestants. The Catholic missions made it to Chuuk's outer islands in 1911 and to central Chuuk the next year (Hezel 1970). This first group were German Capuchin missionaries who came by way of Hawai'i, then Spanish Jesuits when Japan took control of the region. After World War II, American Jesuits ran these Catholic missions (Hezel 1970).

Christian missions throughout the Pacific transformed gender roles as they converted populations (e.g., Flinn 2010; Grimshaw 1989) and, as elsewhere, had lasting impacts on gender roles in Chuuk. The missionaries in Chuuk made conscious efforts to discourage extended-family sleeping arrangements, celebrations of female sexuality, and any exercise of power or influence by women over men (Flinn 2010). Instead, they stressed the values of Western notions of nuclear family households in which women submitted to their husbands' authority and served a role akin to that of a domestic housewife (Flinn 2010; Jolly and Macintyre 1989). Further, they discouraged divorce and the use of contraception (condoms, early birth control pills) made available through the Department of the Interior during the trust territory period (F. B. Caughey 1971). While it is impossible to fully understand gender stratification before missionaries arrived in the late nineteenth century, what we now see as Chuukese gender roles and expectations are likely largely connected to the adoption of these Christian patriarchal values. Missionaries are historically villainized by anthropologists for working to change community values (Stipe et al. 1980), but anthropologists are often complicit in efforts to reshape communities as well, largely through colonization.

COLONIZED ANTHROPOLOGY

> For Hawaiians, anthropologists in general... are part of the colonizing horde because they seek to take away from us the power to define who and what we are, and how we should behave politically and culturally. This theft testifies to the stranglehold of colonialism and explains why self-identity by Natives elicits such strenuous and sometimes vicious denials by members of the dominant culture (Trask 1991, 162–163).

> The anthropology of colonialism is also always an anthropology of anthropology, because in many methodological, organizational, and professional aspects the discipline retains the shape it received when it emerged from—if partly in opposition to—early twentieth-century colonial circumstances (Pels 1997, 164–165).

Since the early years of the profession, both American and British anthropologists have worked with government administrations (Alcalay 1992), celebrating the value of anthropology in assisting colonial regimes to understand "the natives" of occupied areas (Gough 1967; Asad 1973). Connections between anthropology and imperialism grew deeper toward the mid-twentieth century. Between

World War I and World War II, anthropology's professionalization included efforts to assert its role in reducing conflict and indigenous revolt in colonial settings (see, for example, Malinowski 1929, as cited in Pels 1997). The Society for Applied Anthropology was formed to support anthropologists working in the war effort.[5] As World War II ended, anthropologists made concerted efforts to demonstrate their utility in war; others argued the value of their expertise in postwar occupied zones. John Fischer, an anthropologist who worked in Micronesia, explicitly advocated for a sort of "anthropological missionary" to help the "inferior cultures" of postcolonial sites (J. L. Fischer 1951, 134).

In the initial post–World War II era, advertisements for anthropology jobs in the military and various intelligence communities appeared in American Anthropological Association (AAA) publications (Price 2016). Reports advocating the strategic advantages of integrating social sciences into intelligence work flourished in the discipline and in government agencies. The primary funding mechanism in the United States for social science projects became these U.S. military and intelligence agencies (Price 2016; Solovey 2001). The Human Relations Area Files, for example, outsourced a contract for writing army handbooks, and the Central Intelligence Agency funded bogus research institutes and used anthropological research for training manuals (Price 2016). The main role of the discipline in this era was, again, the study of the "changing native," predominantly meant to serve the planning efforts of colonial governments in their new territories (Pels 1997).

As the Cold War progressed, members of the discipline began to challenge anthropology's role in wartime and postwar occupation work. Challenges to this type of work grew as military-sponsored research programs like Project Camelot came to light (Solovey 2001; Horowitz 1966). Project Camelot was an army research program created through the Special Operations Research Office to study revolutions and counterinsurgency tactics in conflict zones (starting with Chile) (Solovey 2001). While it was canceled before it even began because of the public controversy,[6] the project remained an important example of what social science and defense marriages could do. Reacting to Camelot, a contentious debate over anthropology's role in this kind of work ensued at the AAA annual meeting that year. Afterward, the AAA council revised its ethics statement, reflecting the growing sentiment that anthropologists should resist participating in the advancement of imperialism and instead help indigenous communities with their struggles under the legacy of colonialism (Pels 1997; Council of the American Anthropological Association 1967). However, more scandals of anthropologists working in clandestine research followed Camelot. The Thailand Controversy, which included the public outing of both American and Australian anthropologists who worked with military operations in Thailand, reignited the debate and led to more contentious AAA meetings and another revision of the code of ethics (Petersen 2015; Wolf and Jorgensen 1970). These controversies revealed a shift in most anthropologists' perspectives on working with governments. Anthropologists were more actively questioning their role in colonial rule more broadly,[7] including some recognizing their own past work as complicit in imperialist domination (see, for example, Rosaldo 1989).

The crisis in representation and ethnographic writing that followed in the late twentieth century generally occurred as a response to these questions around colonial rule and the need to decolonize the discipline (Rosaldo 1989). The postmodern turn and efforts at decolonization in the late twentieth century led the discipline to better examine its positioning in colonial history, inequity, and power, with particular attention to the ease of anthropologists from colonizing countries to enter many communities colonized by their homelands, and their power and privilege to represent those communities.[8] But while much work for at least the last thirty years has called for efforts to decolonize the discipline,[9] some scholars contend that decolonization has yet to happen. Anthropologists Jonathan Rosa and Yarimar Bonilla (2017) pointedly argue that the conditions ripe for an epistemic shift around the postmodern turn were lost when scholars of this moment began focusing on ways of writing and representation rather than radically reassessing the discipline's foundations and resulting assumptions. In one example of this missed opportunity, concerns about representation have often led anthropologists to focus on using the voices of participants, but engaging with, debating, standing alongside, and taking seriously the analysis of participants remains minimal (Bonilla 2015). Further, while anthropologists have largely stopped working for imperial governments to assist in colonial rule,[10] anthropological work in development agencies has proliferated (Pels 1997). For some, this turn to development meant a barely masked reappropriation of those from colonizing countries studying those from the former colonies to remake new nation-states into the image of the previous colonizer (Adams 2016a; Rosa and Bonilla 2017). Instead of officially being the colonizers, however, the work happens through international aid, funded through donor nations (Adams 2016a).[11]

After years of debate, much is not resolved. Decolonizing anthropology means enacting different strategies for different people. For me, it means acknowledging that my own power as a white person with an American passport in formerly (Chuuk) and currently (Guam) colonized communities shapes the relationships and conversations I have with people in these spaces. It also means engaging in strategies to reduce that power to the extent that I can. To do so, I shared drafts of chapters with Chuukese women and sought their feedback. When they were not interested in reading or did not have the time to do so, I shared my ideas to get their verbal input. I privilege the *analysis* (not just voices) of these participants and Chuukese and Chamoru colleagues and engage with their perspectives, whether through personal conversations or their published work. I tell personal stories to keep the process a truly collaborative project, make my presence clear, and demonstrate my power to decide what to include and exclude from the book. I am cognizant that representing myself as simply an ally is insufficient. Ruth Gomberg-Muñoz (2018) argued that the popular ally role perpetuates the myth of the innocent ethnographer observing (with little action); instead, we should be accomplices to decolonization. My focus on imperial domination and colonization in this book reflects my efforts to be an accomplice to decolonization work for the region and the discipline. Decolonizing anthropology includes exposing, challenging, and revising the narratives that influenced and shaped imperial policies in places like Micronesia (see also Petersen 2015).

Observing Micronesia

> And I came to realize that the Micronesia of the oral tradition and the Micronesia of the written literature are not the same and that, although the assessment of the "outside observer" was nice to have, most of the time it was not a true reflection of the real Micronesia I thought I knew (Heine 1974, ix).

American anthropologists began work in Micronesia before World War II was over, even before the United States occupied the region, to help the U.S. military prepare for occupation. The Yale University Cross-Cultural Survey, led by anthropologist George Murdock (who became an official naval officer), began data collection and analysis on Micronesia soon after Pearl Harbor (1942). He created a list of anthropologists and sociologists with local experience for the army and navy (Mason 1983; Alcalay 1992). Anthropologist Douglas Oliver of Harvard University was then enlisted to survey the Micronesian islands for future assistance in naval administration of them (Alcalay 1992; Oliver 1951). By 1943, Murdock, then a commander, distributed military handbooks on postwar naval administration of Japanese Micronesia (Kiste and Falgout 1999).

This work inspired the navy to sponsor what is often recognized as the largest natural and social science project ever undertaken by the U.S. government in Micronesia. It began after World War II ended and Micronesia became the U.N.-designated USTTPI. First, the National Science Foundation created a Pacific Science Board to assist the navy in better understanding this new de facto possession and created the Coordinated Investigation of Micronesian Anthropology (CIMA), headed by George Murdock (Kroll 2003; Price 2016; Kiste and Marshall 1999). This project was modeled after earlier (pre–World War II) studies, such as the Philippine Ethnology Survey, in which the colonial administration was informed by ethnographic work (Price 2016).

Considered by scholars to be an "ethnographic zoo," forty-one field researchers (of whom twenty-five were anthropologists) were sent to study the territories from 1947 to 1949 to better understand local communities and inform naval administration and development planning.[12] Using the language of "zoo" and "museum" denotes who were authorized to access and observe (usually anthropologists), and who were kept in the boundaries of their islands (Micronesians) (Heine 1974, 21, 57).[13] This project was followed by the Scientific Investigation of Micronesia (SIM), which continued anthropological and ecological studies in the region (Kiste and Marshall 1999). These studies resulted in training handbooks for Micronesian administrators of the USTTPI (Price 2016). The handbooks included suggestions to be followed by administrators and contributed to policy and administrative decisions for how to manage development in the islands before, during, and after the COFA negotiations.

Studies published during anthropologists' academic careers form the basis for the history of American anthropological work in the region.[14] These are considered important applied projects (Kiste and Marshall 1999). But much like others from this era, the scholars often glossed over the role of World War II and its aftereffects, demonstrating what they perceived as an objective point of view (Price 2016). In reality, findings were quite subjective, as they were censored by the navy, which dictated what could be published and what needed to be suppressed to protect national security (Kroll 2003). Further, early researchers supported the navy's argument that there was little room for industry or capitalist expansion, reinforcing Micronesia as an opportune space for military expansion (Kroll 2003). In other words, they reported what the navy wanted to hear. Scholars like Douglas Oliver (1951) resisted this narrative and instead demonstrated the devastation caused by the war; he advocated for restoration of the indigenous communities. But even those who resisted were funded by the U.S. Navy's projects (Kiste and Falgout 1999). As Glenn Alcalay argues, "Anthropologists—some naively caught up in the cold war and others more consciously all-too-willing collaborators—helped to lubricate the machinery for American's immediate post-war colonial enterprise in the remote and strategic reaches of Micronesia and the Western Pacific" (1992, 174).

Observing Gender, Sexuality, and Reproduction

Populations were surveilled and controlled through discourses of sexuality and reproduction;, considered key to the project of colonization.[15] Ideologies about sexuality, reproduction, and the family were central to the U.S. imperial project, and studying them in a colonized space reveals how knowledge and discourses about colonized sexuality and reproduction work as a tool of empire (Briggs 2003; Stoler 1995).

As a conceptual bridge between the making of race and sexuality, one way in which the imperial "other" was formed was through discourses of sexuality and reproduction. Connections between scientific knowledge, sexuality, and concepts of race are ubiquitous in early studies of colonies (Manderson 1996; Stoler 1995). This is portrayed in scientific studies of gynecological differences in the "different races" of new colonies and concerns about their bodies, which connect the tropics to their reproductive and sexual selves. These discourses produce taxonomies of power that align with the intersecting hierarchies of nation, gender, race, and class (Stoler 1995). Colonial knowledge and power predictably attend to genitalia and sexuality in the making of race, confirming the role of sex in the making of racial power, and all of this is contingent on a discourse about native women as objects of the white male gaze (Manderson 2018; Stoler 1995). Further, imperial surveillance of sexuality and reproduction often presents itself through studies of "traditional" sexuality and reproduction, attempts to control or enhance women's rights (by way of their reproduction), and organizing the rules of reproduction and sexuality around colonial narratives (Manderson and Jolly 1997; Manderson 1996; Anderson 2006). Within these narratives of the colonized "other," oxymorons emerge whereby imperial subjects are described as both childlike and underdeveloped, and oversexed and seductive (Stoler 1995; Anderson 2006).

For anthropologists, the fascination with exoticizing the sexuality of occupied peoples is clear from the birth of the discipline and throughout the early to mid-twentieth century (see, for example, Malinowski 1929; Mead 1923). Early anthropologists often claimed their interest was to develop a comparative lens to challenge the idea that Western heteronormative practices were innate or biological; Margaret Mead's portrayal of Samoan adolescent sexual practices is probably the most famous example (Manderson and Jolly 1997; Manderson 2018; Reed 1997). Critics have pointed to the ways in which sexuality was considered, always putting Western heterosexual practices at the center for comparison (Manderson and Jolly 1997). Additionally, early researchers conflated gender and sexuality without recognizing their separate but intimately intertwined roles in communities (Manderson and Jolly 1997; Vance 1991).

With specific attention to the U.S. project, Laura Briggs suggests that these considerations are not simply a *part* of colonialism; rather, "discourses of domesticity and science, reproduction and sexuality organized US colonialism" (2003, 197). Briggs examined studies of sexualization in the non-sovereign territory of Puerto Rico, where women are at times portrayed as threatening, sexually available, and diseased; at other times as victims, endangered and sick. Both portraits are useful to the imperial project. Micronesia's experience with anthropologists in the period of post–World War II nation-building mirrored these trends. Anthropologists racialized Chuukese women by exoticizing their sexual and reproductive practices vis-à-vis their own Euro-American Christian patriarchal values. Micronesian anthropologists' attention to gender, sexuality, and reproduction informed U.S. colonial and, later, development initiatives in the region.[16]

Discourses of Sexuality in Micronesian Anthropology

In one of his many publications on mid-twentieth-century Chuuk, the trust-territory-era anthropologist Ward Goodenough (1949) described how people were expected to have several sexual partners prior to marriage and that, while clandestine, those sexual encounters were acceptable (see also A. Fischer 1963; Gladwin and Sarason 1953). Anthropological interest in night crawling (described below) in Chuuk and other parts of Micronesia mirrored Mead (1923) and her portrait of Samoan adolescents. These scholars claimed that sweethearts were said to give women more orgasms than spouses (A. Fischer 1963; Goodenough 1949); some described sexual positions in which Chuukese couples succeeded in this feat (Mahony 1969; Swartz 1958). Scholars depicted sex as a fight to get to orgasm, embarrassing men who lose the fight (J. L. Caughey 1977; Gladwin and Sarason 1953; Moral 2002), which produced anxiety for men (Mahony 1969). The importance of the size and shape of women's vulvas were illustrated, as were fights between women in which they displayed their vulvas to demonstrate their beauty (Gladwin and Sarason 1953; Moral 2002). Love magic was also a topic of great interest,[17] described as an exotic and playful tool through which people pursued the person they loved, with no attention paid to it as an issue of gender and power (except Mahony 1969; see Dernbach 2005 for a pointed critique).

In this nearly all-male field, USTTPI-era anthropologists were clearly fascinated by Chuukese sexual "freedom," and their voyeuristic accounts were laden with American misogynistic ideas about female sexuality. Not only were they exoticizing, but at the same time they portrayed women as somehow both stupid and manipulative. Further, USTTPI scholars focused on pleasure and the sexual acts themselves, overlooking or failing to see the gendered inequities embedded in heterosexual relationships. They were obsessed with the more exotic elements of sexual activity.[18]

These studies and the connections between empire and sexuality are not lost on Chuukese communities. When I told people I was an anthropologist studying sexual health, reproductive health, women's health, or any other related topic, a common question was whether I had heard of love sticks (a special stick made by a lover for late night tactile identification when sneaking out of the home to meet up, known as night crawling). Some people who were more open would ask if I had heard of fights between women showing their vulvas, or whether I had heard of Chuukese hammers (a sexual practice). It was as if they were expecting my interest in anything that could be perceived as exotic. I had not brought these topics up; the association with my colonizing homeland and interest in these practices were assumed.

Although sexual freedom and desire were standard themes for USTTPI-era anthropologists, there was some acknowledgment of the unequal standards between men and women (Goodenough 2002; Swartz 1958). Women needed to keep their premarital sexual liaisons secret and intimated that failure to do so might reduce women's chances of finding a marital partner (J. L. Caughey 1977). Older men and women would reportedly have sex with adolescents to "teach" them how to have sex (Goodenough 2002; Swartz 1958). Further, young girls were said to be "offered" to chiefs or special visitors for company (Goodenough 2002; Swartz 1958). Men were also reported to sneak into houses to have sex with women or look at their genitals, and to blackmail women into having sex when caught doing something perceived as embarrassing (e.g., masturbating) (Swartz 1958).

Two women, both wives of the original hires for the post–World War II CIMA program, also published in this area. This was not uncommon; women often did as much or more work than their husbands, though many received little credit (Lewin 2009). In Micronesia, Ann Fischer (1956, 1963) and Frances Caughey (1971) both published work on mothering and reproduction under their own names. Fischer (1963) reported that Chuukese communities had a clan-based matrilineal structure with significant importance attributed to land. She argued that women gained respect and power through mothering. Caughey (1971) focused on the Chuukese island of Uman and reported that it was patrilineal, contradicting much of the work on Chuuk but also reflecting the vast differences in traditions for these twenty-three inhabited islands. She also explained the importance of pregnancy and childbirth, particularly of the first child, and described many pregnancy and postpartum taboos. Both Fischer and Caughey avoided the tropes of Chuukese sexuality. On the other hand, they paid little attention to the shame associated with sexuality and first pregnancies and the importance of women avoiding conversations about their sexual bodies.

Post-COFA-Era Research on Sexuality and Reproduction

> Through the lens of foreign visitors, Chuukese women's public silence appeared to be a sign of their inferiority. Thus, anthropological writings and other scholarly literature mostly continue to describe Chuukese women as submissive, quiet, and inferior—an image that has become visibly predominant in writings about Chuuk and embodied by more recent generations (Kim 2020, 150).

Since the USTTPI research programs, few scholars have attended to Chuukese reproduction or heterosexual experiences, but those who did focused on gender inequalities in ways absent during the USTTPI research programs. These include studies of mothering (Fitzgerald 2001), sexuality (Moral 1996, 1998a, 1998b, 2002), and masculine sexual violence (Rauchholz 2016). Several other researchers focused on different aspects of Chuukese life but included parts of their sexual and reproductive lives.[19] This compilation of work demonstrated late twentieth-century and early twenty-first-century scholars' increased notice of gender inequities in sexuality and reproduction. But while this work is less exoticizing and at times acknowledges imperialism, some paint Chuukese women as lacking agency to challenge cultural narratives or to resist masculine violence; in other words, they are often portrayed as merely victims. Indigenous scholar

Myjolynne Kim, quoted at the top of this section, offers a critique of what these oppressive and one-dimensional descriptions can do to women in her community as they embody such narratives. Anthropologists' work had a lasting impact on discourses over Chuukese women both within and outside of these communities. Their work informed modern-day narratives about Chuukese gender and sexuality and contributed to ideologies of the "savage" Micronesian who needed to be developed.

DEVELOPING WOMEN

In 2012, I traveled to a National Women's Conference in Chuuk, hosted by women's groups and attended by female leaders from all over Micronesia, with particularly high attendance by women from Chuuk and other federated states (Kosrae, Pohnpei, and Yap). Women leaders flew in from surrounding Micronesian islands, and around two hundred Chuukese women came by boat to Wééné from all over Chuuk. On the plane from Guam, I sat next to a woman from Guam who was also attending the conference. She told me how "traditional" and "low" Chuukese women were, and how she anticipated pushback or angry silence for any discussions around equal rights for women or standing up to sexual violence. I did not take these assertions very seriously, but I did make a mental note of how her sentiments so precisely echoed stereotypes about Chuukese women in the region. I wondered how many other attendees shared these views.

As I sweated through the opening ceremony in this large covered outdoor space, using a handmade fan left on each guest's seat, I saw a sea of mwárámwár (head coverings or necklaces/leis of flowers). The sweet, vibrant smell of ylang-ylang from all the mwárámwár wafted through the air, mixed with the salty smell of sweat on this predictably hot, humid day. This is a powerful olfactory memory I share from so many special occasions in Chuuk and Guam thereafter. The attendees were mostly middle-aged or elderly women. Children were relatively absent, except for a few toddlers in their grandmother's laps; most were presumably left behind with elder children and younger women, for this was an important adult event. Women in this crowd wore colorful Chuukese dresses, as it was a mostly Chuukese audience and too special of an occasion for a casual cotton skirt and T-shirt. Some groups wore uniforms: dresses made of the same island-style, colorful polyester-blend fabric bought at one of Wééné's general stores and sewn for the occasion. Coolers upon coolers of food were lined up, ready to be plated in Styrofoam to-go containers wrapped in plastic for the guests—just like at funerals—except the food, like the head coverings and attendee gifts (fans, handicrafts), were not sourced from the family of a deceased person but from women's groups from all over Chuuk. The level of preparation was impressive and signaled the importance of this event.

At one point we had a powerful rainstorm. Rain pounded on the metal roof and came in sideways, spraying everyone and giving us a little relief from the heat. And then, it was gone, just like that. The conference schedule was delayed, however, because the power went out and thus the microphones would not work. As we waited for the power to turn on and the official conference to start, Chuukese women in the crowd began singing, encouraging the entire space with well over one hundred people to join in. Some elder women started dancing and laughing in the middle of the space—a few stood up on chairs—drawing everyone's attention.

This conference, organized by women, with this spontaneous entertainment and a panel of leading women (alongside men), led me to question the accuracy of what I had read of significant and stark inequities by gender in Chuuk. The existence of this conference suggested to me that Chuukese women possessed some level of institutional power within society. However, I also learned that the male political leaders of Chuuk did not consider this conference a threat to their power and standing; they dismissed it as nonserious.

When the electricity was restored, the official conference began. Female presenters stooped when walking up to the stage, ensuring, as a gesture of respect, that they remained physically lower than the seated men.[20] Each offered thanks to the leaders who attended and proceeded to outline the conference program. Some quoted from Christian bibles about the importance of women's roles; others noted their appreciation to the many traditional (male) leaders in the audience and then introduced the next speaker. Women's rights were not explicitly on the agenda. But about halfway through the opening ceremony, a new speaker from a different Micronesian island stepped onstage. At first, I noticed this woman because she was dressed in a local dress but with a Western-style suit jacket. She walked onstage standing upright and tall. She omitted the routine ceremonial prayers and polite greetings and opened by saying, "Welcome to Chuuk, where traditional women had greater roles, but in the constitution of the [19]80s, men took over" (Smith and Katzman 2020, 1152). I was shocked by her very different and direct manner of speaking. She went on to talk about traditional roles of women being more valuable than those in the present day and spoke of the significance of women. She talked also about the importance of getting women into the legislatures of all the Micronesian states. While I was surprised, the audience remained moderately attentive, as they had with all other speakers. It did not appear to anyone else that this person represented a different perspective. However, later, Chuukese women's group members talked privately about the tones of women from other island states, explaining to me that these women were "more assertive and equal to men," so they could say these truths aloud. It was not that her perspectives were different, just that she felt she could safely and assertively state them. As I would learn over time, the preceding speakers also effectively critiqued and sought to elevate the status and power of

Micronesian women, but they did so through more subtle approaches that respected the local norms of public engagement. They tied much of their oppression and many of their lost rights to the role of the U.S. government, beginning during the USTTPI years (see also Kim 2020).

Informed by anthropologists' consultative work, the USTTPI agendas included efforts to support equal rights for Micronesian women, arguing that traditional patterns placed women in subordinate positions in society (Hanlon 1998). This agenda of emancipation of women was common in colonial agendas and discourses of the mid- to late twentieth century (Pels 1997). Yet women lost power through the synergy of Micronesian traditions and the imposition of American patriarchal values on a government and economy built to mirror those of the United States.

The naval administration and then the Department of the Interior primarily employed men, mirroring broader U.S. patriarchal and capitalist systems. Further, development of the government conferred occupational roles to women along gendered lines, directing them to work in lower-compensated positions associated with women in the United States (e.g., as nurses, secretaries, and teachers). Additionally, land ownership in Chuuk was typically inherited through matrilineal relations, and women were traditionally expected to stay near their property. Yet secondary schools were built by the USTTPI on only a few islands, requiring most students to travel to continue their education. This discouraged some parents from sending daughters off-island for school. Further, some families began passing land down through men. Additionally, women were traditionally expected to remain silent in public debate, offering their concerns before and after public discussions to their male familial counterparts (uncle, brother) for consideration. The new governments in Micronesia, mirroring U.S. political structures, included politicians and government officials publicly debating and discussing issues and actions. This structure further discouraged Micronesian women's participation. These foreign articulations of rule did not give women equality, as the USTTPI administration and, later, the new constitutions claimed to address. Instead, they reconfigured power. Hence, a new patriarchal infrastructure was imposed that nonetheless derided traditional Micronesian gender structures.

USTTPI rule gave women the right to vote, institutionalized equal pay for equal work, and, in theory, ensured equal access to education and the right to land ownership (Hanlon 1998).[21] These were common strategies of nation-building in former colonies at the time, an approach in which governmentality focused on saving the "third world woman" (Escobar 2011).[22] In reality, this form of governmentality—a Foucauldian concept reflecting the biopolitical control that manages populations through the production of knowledge and the funding of programs—imposes ideologies from the dominant powers that finance them (Hanlon 1998). What these efforts resulted in were the imposition of a new patriarchy—in this case U.S. patriarchy—and the adoption of a "home economics" approach to women's issues (Hanlon 1998; Escobar 2011, 173).

However, the USTTPI administration encouraged the formation of women's groups, which have grown significantly in power over time. Members of women's groups in Chuuk recognized that the development of a U.S.-structured economy and political system reshaped their power, largely keeping them in the domestic sphere. Cathy, an active women's group leader, critiqued her self-described lower status in politics by remarking, "This politics is not our culture. So why do we have to respect it? It's not ours" (Smith and Katzman 2020, 1152). Given that many Micronesian communities have matrilineal inheritance, some have argued that women should be involved in government, and a bill was unsuccessfully introduced in 2010 to reserve seats for women in Congress. Despite this bill's failure, women are starting to be appointed and elected to key positions in government. The state government—as of this writing—has a woman serving as chief of staff, and some women have been appointed directors of government agencies. In 2017, the first woman was elected as Chuuk state senator (Bryce 2017), and in November 2021, the first woman—a Chuukese woman—was elected to the FSM Congress (Congress of the Federated States of Micronesia 2021). Despite these advances, the gender inequities that women experience remain imprinted on their bodies. As the following chapters will illustrate, such inequities stratify their reproduction.

3 • IMPERIAL MIGRATIONS

Rosie was forty-eight, from the Northern Nómwoneyas region of Chuuk lagoon. We sat side by side on a bench outside an empty school courtyard in central Wééné. It was a beautiful warm evening, and we watched the sun go down over the lagoon, sharing this quiet space, rarely a passerby greeting us. We talked about her upbringing and migration experiences. She had spent her early years in grade school on her home island, living with her grandmother, then moved in with her parents to attend early high school in Wééné. She remembers her early days as fun filled: "OK, my childhood is, I remembered that um, my family really spoiled me. . . . You know in a Chuukese way like when you're the eldest in the family, they do everything for you, like [you're] the queen or the king." Rosie elaborated on how the firstborn woman in the family (finniichi) becomes the keeper of the family and the land when she grows up.[1] Because of this, Rosie was told by her mother that she was supposed to focus on school while her younger sisters did all the cooking and cleaning. To that end, Rosie relocated to Pohnpei (the national capital of the FSM) to complete high school, and then she began her college studies at the main campus of the College of Micronesia. After a few years in Pohnpei, she returned to Chuuk to visit her family; shortly after, she moved to Saipan, Commonwealth of the Northern Mariana Islands (CNMI), to attend Northern Marianas College and finish her degree.

Rosie graduated and stayed in Saipan to work and send money home. She met a Chamoru man there, and her mother somehow learned she was openly dating. Rosie told me her mother was "not happy, she just came up and said, 'We go back to Chuuk.' . . . I'll never forget that time. We went up to the airport and that guy came, he said, 'Are you going to Chuuk?' I said, 'Yeah.' [He said] 'So what about me?' I said, 'What about you?' He said, 'You listen to your mom?' I said, 'Of course I listen to my mom, my parents come first.' He was like, not understanding, thinking that I will be going with him." Rosie was then twenty-one years old. Even when we spoke and Rosie was in her forties, and a grandmother herself, she said that her mother was still her boss.

Rosie lived on her home island near Wééné for two years before she began a secret relationship with a new young man, resulting in an unintended pregnancy.

Her parents were initially angry and ashamed that she was sexually active out of wedlock, but they soon curbed their anger and supported an engagement. Shortly after, Rosie's partner decided they should move to Guam to find work. Although she did not want to leave Chuuk again, her new partner insisted this was the right decision for their livelihood. Her parents agreed.

Rosie moved to Guam while still early in her pregnancy, and she was miserable. This was her first pregnancy, and she wished she were home near her mother and other women relatives for support and guidance. She returned to Chuuk to spend the last months of her pregnancy with her mother, and there, she gave birth to her first daughter. After recovering from the birth, Rosie reluctantly moved back to Guam to join her new husband, along with her parents. She lived in Guam for ten years and had four children; her parents stayed for a year. Her relatives back in Chuuk—particularly her mother—cared for some of her infants in their early years to help Rosie balance work and family obligations, returning them to her before grade school. During this decade, Rosie worked in a few banks on the island and regularly encountered customers who questioned how she—a Chuukese woman—could get a job at a bank. Instead of assuming she was educated, they told her that she did not belong there or that she was lucky to have the job. She told me, "I feel very offended when people ask me, 'Where are you from?' When I tell them Chuuk, they're like, 'You're so lucky you work here.' And I'll be like, 'There are eight of us working here.'" Rosie told me she felt unlucky; she worked very hard and barely made ends meet while facing this type of discrimination regularly: "They [Guamanians] really look down on us." These experiences contributed to her desire to move back to Chuuk: "I'll be honest; I really don't like it there. It's like a force for me to stay there. . . . To me it's like, there's no relaxing time for me. I have to think, think, work, work, work. No time to relax."

Rosie's household also made for difficult times in Guam. First, she constantly had different family members staying with her. Sisters, daughters, nieces, and nephews, both young and grown up, were always present and needed care as they moved in and out of her house, either headed back to Chuuk or on to Hawai'i. Some stayed longer for school or work. Her husband did not hold a steady job and spent freely on alcohol, staying out all night with friends and other women. He was also physically and emotionally abusive; thus, despite her modest income, Rosie visited her family in Chuuk as much as she could.

What ultimately brought Rosie back to Chuuk for good was again a family decision: following her parents' advice, she took her children back to Chuuk when her oldest daughter was in high school to ensure that her daughters would learn Chuukese culture. Her extended family challenged this choice. "Everybody was really like, 'Why do you have to move your kids back to Chuuk? . . . They're going to miss the good school,' and I said, 'Well I want them to learn my beautiful culture, sorry.'" Her family moved back, and with the support of her parents, she separated from her spouse.

As darkness set in, Rosie got to her favorite part of her life story. Her ride had arrived. Rosie told me the man in the car was her new partner—she gushed over him as we spoke. She said he was everything her first husband was not: kind, loving, great with the kids. Her children are enjoying Chuuk, and her oldest is now a mother, too. Rosie lives and works in Wééné, returns to her home island every other weekend or so, and is truly happy to be back. She has everything she imagined she wanted and is where she wants to be—in Chuuk. Rosie maintains steady work, so she can afford to travel to Guam for private health care and other needs about twice a year.[2] This flexibility to go back and forth for Rosie and other Chuukese women is possible because of the migration clause in the Compact of Free Association (COFA) agreement.

THE MICRONESIAN EXODUS

Prior to the COFA, obtaining an I-9 visa to pursue further education was the primary mechanism by which Micronesians entered the United States. The COFA allows citizens with FSM passports to enter Guam or any other U.S. jurisdiction simply by arriving and completing an I-94 form (Arrival/Departure Record). The COFA allows unprecedented access to the United States and (inadequate) development funding to COFA nations in exchange for exclusive U.S. military access to Micronesian waters. After the 1986 agreement, COFA nonimmigrants began moving into the United States in large numbers, creating a distinct diaspora (Hezel and McGrath 1989; Kihleng 2015). As of 2012, a modest estimate places roughly one-third (49,840) of the FSM population as living abroad, predominantly in places like Guam, Saipan, and Hawai'i (Hezel and Levin 2012; Hezel 2013); as noted earlier, the Chuukese represent nearly three-quarters of Micronesians in Guam. Education, health care, and available employment were initially primary pull factors contributing to intense migration following the COFA, and due to ongoing U.S. developmental neglect of COFA nations, people often remain in U.S. jurisdictions for far longer than originally planned.[3]

While the 1986 COFA agreement led to the exponential growth of FSM migrants, Chuukese and other Micronesian communities were mobile long before European colonization. The late indigenous scholar Joakim Peter (2000) argued that the Chuukese people—especially Chuukese men—have always been travelers, with a history of significant exploration and movement.[4] He reasoned that what was new about this movement was the power that defined how it occurred. Since the end of World War II, that power was the United States.

GENDER AND MIGRATION

> Like, that's the custom. Men [are] always gone, but the women have to stay home.
>
> —Jessica, forty-six-year-old woman from the Fááyichuuk region

Most Chuukese communities have a clan-based matrilineal structure wherein inheritance of the land is passed through the female line, and the eldest females of families oversee the land (Kim 2020).[5] Consequently, women are perceived as less able than men to leave Chuuk.[6] Like Rosie, some women's earliest experiences with migration were much closer moves: they attended regional schools on other islands or went to Wééné for high school. Since they had to move to go beyond elementary school, education initiated their migratory lives. But as more and more men migrated out of the FSM, they began bringing their families; eventually women also began migrating to more distant destinations in large numbers for education, employment, and health care (Grieco 2003).

Guam is particularly attractive to women because of its close proximity to Chuuk. Since a direct flight from Wééné takes less than two hours, some women believe they can easily and regularly move between the two islands. The possibility of traveling home to attend funerals and other important clan events is what makes Guam attractive. Indeed, the airport is always packed with people of all ages before a flight to and from Guam, as residents of Wééné arrive to watch the landing or greet their relatives coming and going. For many, Guam is also a compromise between the ideal scenario of living on Hawaiʻi or the U.S. mainland—where there is greater health care, education, and economic opportunities and perceivably less xenophobia than on Guam[7]—and staying in Chuuk. Siera, a boisterous and jovial forty-seven-year-old woman from the outer Mortlock Islands of Chuuk, always found the money to get back to Chuuk and to frequently bring or send her children, siblings, and parents back and forth between Chuuk and Guam. This is despite having very little money for bills, often not enough to cover essential expenses. Siera is one of many women who really wanted to move to the mainland, but her uncle forbade it, wanting her to stay in Chuuk. She negotiated, and they compromised; he allowed her to move to Guam. She reflected on her dreams to move farther away: "Maybe if I go to the States, I will like it, yeah? But it's OK. Guam's closer to home." While obtaining education and work abroad can appear to give women more power than was traditionally relegated at home, others continue to dictate their movement: parents, uncles, or spouses decide when and where women should migrate and when they should return.

In accordance with their connections to the land, women return home on average twice as often as men and are more consistent remitters (Bautista 2010). Siera's familial home in the Mortlock Islands was not frequently visited, as it was very difficult to get there, typically by boat, and she got seasick. But she regularly flew directly to Wééné to see her mother and other family members there: "So [at] that time [in the late 1980s and early 1990s] I can travel every weekend. I go to Chuuk, come back. 'Cause the tickets [are] very cheap then. . . . When I get paid from work, 'OK I'm going!'" Women like Rosie and Siera moved back and forth regularly, so much that Micronesians have been labeled "commuters" rather than migrants (Grieco 2003, 81; Rubinstein and Levin 1992). While the increased price of plane tickets has made commuting less possible in the last two decades than in the 1990s, even those women who cannot easily afford to travel back and forth contribute funds for family members to visit them or send additional remittances for events.

This circular flow is not just between Guam and Chuuk. Every Chuukese migrant I spoke with had extended family members spread throughout the United States and the FSM. Women have siblings and close cousins in Pohnpei, the Republic of Palau, Guam, the CNMI, and many states, including but not limited to Hawaiʻi, California, Oregon, Washington, Alaska, Colorado, Kansas, Texas, and Florida. These are not simply connections; women perceive these places in which they have relatives as an extension of their home. If they can raise the funds to get a plane ticket, they can live in any of these places with their relatives. Kaylyn—a thirty-five-year-old woman who moved from Chuuk to Guam while in grade school—explained the importance of her extended network when she moved back to Guam two years prior to our conversations: "You know, the doors are always open. . . . It's interesting how, like, 'cause in all there's probably like close to sixty-some first cousins. . . . We are so close it's like we are sisters, you know?" Young women are sent out regularly to assist family members (e.g., new mothers and elders) and attend better schools. Toddlers like Rosie's children are often sent back to Chuuk to be raised by grandmothers and aunts, then sent back to their parents abroad at some point for better schooling. These migration patterns allow for the continuity of historical extended family households in new spaces (Marshall 2004). They also allow us to reconsider home less as a physical space and more as a conceptual connection to kin. Indigenous scholar Gonzaga Puas (2021) sees these connections as simply the latest manifestation of the ainang, or extended family clan system:

> Since Micronesian people are historically mobile, they naturally continue to transplant themselves further afield. This is made possible by the global transportation system and political links with former colonial powers. . . . This new diaspora will continue to expand as a result of the globalised world and the inherent urge of the Micronesian people to travel to join their families now searching for opportunities outside Micronesia. It is argued that a consequence of this process is the exportation of Micronesian ideologies to the new spaces in order to facilitate Micronesians' transition to their adopted environment while maintaining a connection to their island homes. The ainang system is the glue that links geographically dispersed clan members to each other and their nation state (Puas 2021, 172).

Maintaining this glue is a particularly important way of being for Chuukese futures, as people's physical homes are increasingly threatened by climate change.

Loss of land by the encroaching sea, loss of freshwater sources for crops due to saltwater intrusion, and increasingly dangerous typhoons have all been reported by Micronesians as ways in which climate change is pushing them out of their home islands (Puas 2021; Hofmann 2018). Yet while climate change is perceived as a major threat for Micronesians, migration or temporary relocation due to natural disasters has deep traditions using the ainang system, in which communities sought resources or help elsewhere after storms or other natural disasters (Puas 2021; Marshall 2004). What has changed is the extent and permanence of the damage resulting from climate change, including loss of coastlines, corals, fisheries, and food sources, and the ever-expanding global reach of the ainang system (Puas 2021). While the ainang system continues to expand, Guam remains the first stop. But—as Rosie said—it is hard to live there.

Living in Guam can be exhausting. Women perceive it as a frenetic metropolis from which they sometimes desire to escape back to the quieter, slower-paced life on Chuuk, or rather a romanticized version of home where one has the time and ability to relax (Eria, Hofmann, and Smith 2022). In their imagination, Chuuk is full of people of all generations, supporting one another and enjoying the everyday life they remember as youth, a time when only the privileged were leaving and most everything felt the same. They told me how they miss the nights when a dozen female relatives would sit around and tell stories, make food, and watch the little ones. These versions of Chuuk leave out the reasons for leaving and do not reflect what Chuuk looks like after years of outmigration.

Early in my fieldwork, a good Chuukese friend who lived in Guam invited me to join her when she traveled back home to Chuuk. She was there to organize a gathering to commemorate the first anniversary of her father's passing. She flew into Chuuk from Guam and picked up supplies in Wééné, then we took a small motorboat to her family island. We arrived at night after riding through a storm that left us cold and tired. We quickly fried some Spam and turkey tails (bought in Wééné) over a small camp-stove-sized butane burner (a staple kitchen tool in Chuuk), put these fatty meats on rice, and ate. We then went to sleep on mats in a small house that barely fit the four women and three children in our group. The next day, as the sun lit my surroundings, I saw that this concrete house was one of four on a larger family compound. These concrete houses had large porches with decorative concrete posts originally painted bright colors, the colors now faded after years of sun exposure. The houses sat in a circle of a compound of mostly cleared land, along with shower-bathroom houses, cook houses, a family burial plot, and a few breadfruit and coconut trees peppered throughout. A communal space (concrete floor, thatched roof) was at the center of this compound and where the events of the first anniversary funeral would take place. Behind the compound the land sloped up into the mountain, and a pipe bringing water in was sticking out of the side of it, where water was collected for washing, cleaning, and bathing. This was a setup I would witness repeatedly as I visited different

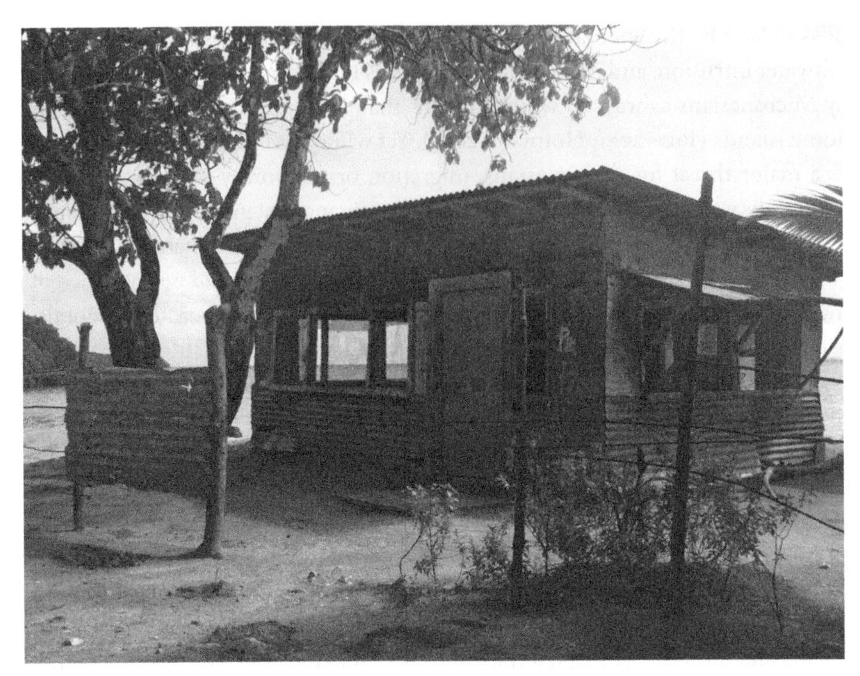

FIGURE 10. Empty house maintained by remaining family members in Chuuk, FSM. Photo by Sarah Smith.

islands in Chuuk. But the place in which we slept was the only inhabited house there. The rest were empty, kept clean by the few remaining family members but otherwise slowly deteriorating in the island's tropical conditions. Their owners all resided in U.S. jurisdictions. While empty, they proved useful; plating food for guests that day happened in their empty spaces.

I walked through the village and saw very few people or houses that looked lived in. Some were similarly faded concrete buildings; others were more make-shift, composed of plywood, corrugated metal, and other easy-to-access materials (see figure 10). These houses were not surviving quite as well as the concrete in their owner's absences, with elements of the tropics taking over and making them a green space again. In time, I learned that this island was not uniquely empty; on most of Chuuk's islands, except for the busy central island of Wééné, there are only a few elderly inhabitants per family compound,[8] and a similarly small number of infants and young adults. My guide that day—a teenage girl left behind in Chuuk to care for her grandparents when most of her family moved to the United States—told me she was bored because there were so few people around who were her age. Local families explained to me that it was relatively common for a few adolescents to be sent home to aid or be raised by their grand-parents, who did not desire to live abroad. Nelly, a fifty-year-old woman from the Southern Nómwoneyas who had lived in Guam for over twenty years, reflected:

"My generation, they always came [back], always every year, [but now] no more people. . . . Now they move to Guam, Hawai'i, the States and that's it." My friend was privileged enough to come to Chuuk for both her father's funeral and the one-year anniversary of his death because she lived in nearby Guam and had a steady income; her siblings in Hawai'i could not afford to return for both.

The exodus of Chuukese people from Chuuk has increased, as even those with few resources find relatives abroad to help them migrate out of Chuuk. Therefore, the concept of home is a space thought of very differently by those abroad and those who remain in Chuuk. The women who return regularly sometimes concede that their view of Chuuk is romanticized, but those who have not returned in years have a harder time imagining the increasing difficulties of living on the islands that inspired their movement in the first place (Eria, Hofmann, and Smith 2022). Their dreams keep them firmly in a transnational space—living in Guam but committed to Chuuk. Some, like Rosie, happily return. Maureen, a sixty-year-old woman from Fááyichuuk, also returned. She complained to me that she returned because Guam is too focused on money for survival: "I just didn't want to stay [in Guam]. Yeah, I like [it] here [in Chuuk], very quiet. Things are easygoing. . . . Guam, you have to rush all the time. You must work to live. Yeah, here [in Chuuk] you can sleep because you have taro, and [there is] breadfruit hanging free. [In Chuuk] I can get sick and rest, peacefully. In Guam I have to go to work to have money to pay for rent and food and water and toilet paper. . . . Everything is money. Here [in Chuuk] if you don't have money, you still can survive."

When migrating to Guam, women imagine a life where their children can get a good education and they can quickly find a well-paying job and thus send money back to their kin in Chuuk. However, once the women arrive, they realize that jobs are challenging to find. Women lack childcare, have to care for other relatives, some lack English proficiency, struggle with transportation access, or have spouses who insist they stay home. Jessica explained: "For us [Chuukese, Guam is] hard. Especially everything [costs] is raised up. That's why sometimes I say, 'Oh I wish I would go back to Chuuk.' [In Chuuk] You don't pay rent. We have our own house, our own land to stay [on]. Only in Moen [Wééné] we pay . . . but, in our island, no. We sleep together, we don't care if plenty people, 'cause we don't pay rent, and we have our own water from our [freshwater sources], you know? Very hard in Guam." In Guam, landlords impose limits on the number of people in any apartment or house, water and electricity bills add up, rents are high, and women struggle to find jobs.

When women do get jobs, they often make much less than they imagined, resulting in them barely making ends meet. These women are often dismayed to find that life on Guam will not allow them to achieve their dreams of supporting family or having a commuter lifestyle. Laurence Carucci (2012) similarly depicted Marshallese migrants in Hawai'i. They had moved with visions of a life of "abundance" ahead but came to feel as though they would not survive if they ever just chose to "remain still." Increasingly they saw themselves as "powerless" and "deficient" (Carucci 2012, 205–206).

The disappointing realities and feelings of deficiency and powerlessness are also related to the discrimination Chuukese people face in Guam. Rosie told me she never grew to love Guam, partly because she did not feel Guam loved her, or any Chuukese people: "Guam is very different from Saipan. Saipanese love Chuukese. They treat us very nice.... Guam, they... treat us really bad."[9] Discrimination is embedded in all life processes in Guam, in part a result of the circumstances of their citizenship status in juxtaposition with the struggle between the United States and Guam to control the borders.

EXCLUDING IMPERIAL BODIES

COFA-citizen access to the United States is unique in its ease of entry, but as I argued in chapter 1, this does not put COFA migrants on any path toward permanent U.S. residency. They are deemed outsiders who, while they can move with great ease, never fully belong in the United States. Emily Mitchell-Eaton (2016) has called this a form of "imperial citizenship," an example of graduated citizenship created by nation-states like the United States to maintain empires (Ong 2006). Imperial citizenship is typically characterized by its "provisional, partial and revocable nature," as it enables mobility while maintaining outsider status (Mitchell-Eaton 2016, 12). This status contributes to a liminal sense of belonging and precarious status, which promotes exclusionary discourse in the sites of migration (see also Smith and Castañeda 2021). Rosie and others struggled with the ways in which their precarious status excludes them from resources, communities, and friendships in Guam. The ambiguous outsider status of COFA migrants allows for exclusion at structural, social, and individual levels.

Excluding the Body Politic

At the structural level, important U.S. federal resources have been lost due to the ambiguous status of nonimmigrants, leaving Guam responsible for meeting the needs of the COFA community. COFA citizens originally had access to the same safety-net services as U.S. citizens,[10] but federal legislation changed this access a decade after the COFA was enacted. Specifically, the Personal Responsibility and Work Opportunity Reconciliation Act of 1996 (PRWORA) stipulated that only legal resident-alien migrants could access these services. Nonimmigrants, also known as habitual residents, were never considered resident aliens, so they lost access to all these programs. This legislative oversight demonstrates how the imperial citizenship status of nonimmigrants is ambiguous enough to be forgotten in the U.S. federal legal landscape, a strategy and consequence of benign neglect. Removing access to Medicaid severely affected access to health care for migrants.

In more recent years, the Affordable Care Act could have alleviated the problem of health insurance access. However, the federal insurance mandate excluded territories of the United States, including Guam, illustrating again how the structural violence of benign neglect is enacted in zones of empire. Medicaid access to COFA residents was reestablished as part of Congress's 2020 end-of-year spending bill after several stories about the impact of COVID on COFA communities inspired broader support for fixing part of this mistake of nearly twenty-five years (Diamond 2021). This one correction, however, did not change the imperial citizenship status or alleviate the social conditions of liminality it creates, which continues to render bodies vulnerable to poor health outcomes.

Since the removal of COFA migrants from most federal services after 1996, Hawai'i and Guam continued to provide some services for this population, such as insuring them through their own local programs. Affected jurisdictions filled this coverage gap with the expectation that they would be reimbursed by the U.S. federal government as expressed under the COFA agreement (Pobutsky et al. 2005). However, for decades now they have received a fraction of what they believe they are owed, labeling the cost of hosting COFA migrants in their community the "Compact Impact" (Calvo 2014; Hezel and Levin 2012, Leon Guerrero 2019). Compact Impact reports from the affected jurisdictions consistently demonstrate insufficient U.S. reimbursement, which the U.S. government disputes as inflated and incorrect. When counting costs to public services, these reports often include both COFA citizens who migrate to Guam and people with COFA-nation ancestry who *are* U.S. citizens born in U.S. jurisdictions (e.g., COFA migrants' children born in Guam) (Levin 2010). Conversely, the U.S. federal government only counts COFA citizens; those born in Guam are excluded from the federal government's responsibility for compact reimbursement. In this context, COFA bodies are either strategically used, counted, or forgotten in order to advantage the priorities of the empire or the colony, a productive consequence of their ambiguous citizenship (Smith and Castañeda 2021). Tension arises through these disagreements of policy between the United States and Guam on caring for Micronesians, and this spills over into local communities on the island. The resulting hostility from local communities further shapes the complicated experiences of Chuukese women when they migrate to Guam.

Excluding the Social Body

While each affected jurisdiction has had some negative reaction to COFA migrants, the Chuukese are the focus of these sentiments in Guam.[11] As Chuukese people migrated to Guam in large numbers, they entered an environment already tense with a long history of colonizer-sanctioned guests, and this increased in the years after the COFA. Anti-immigrant sentiment increased dramatically after the economic slowdown in the 1990s throughout the United States (and consequently Guam). Concerns about the Chuukese coming to

Guam only to give birth for U.S. citizenship, food stamps, and welfare were widespread, embedded in and reflecting larger fears about Guam's economic problems. This sentiment was exacerbated after the 1996 federal legislative oversight removing COFA migrants' access to federal programs, and is being stoked by and reflected in public discourses in Guam about Chuukese migrants.

Guam newspaper articles regularly focus on the various iterations of the Compact Impact but never on the larger COFA agreement and the rights and obligations set forth in it by COFA countries and the United States.[12] As a result, many Guam residents appear to have a very limited understanding of the COFA except for the perceived aspects that directly affect Guam: migrants invading their land and costing money—costs that are not adequately reimbursed by the United States. A large proportion of residents equate the entirety of COFA with the Compact Impact. This false equivalence is so persistent that I witnessed local politicians mistakenly describing the official compact using these words. From an anthropological perspective, language is both a reflection and a reinforcement of community discourses, and it is telling that policy makers referred to these communities in ways that specifically emphasized their negative impact.

In February 2015, Guam's governor at the time, Eddie Calvo, claimed that Guam was at a breaking point financially due to caring for COFA migrants, whom he described as sick and uneducated (Daleno 2015). More recently, Governor Lou Leon Guerrero reflected similar sentiments about costs of the compacts in her 2019 state of the island address, but with more welcoming language:

> In order to fully address GovGuam's financial situation, we must be strong in addressing the unfunded federal mandates that create a huge hole in our pockets—including the Compacts of Free Association Act. . . . The people of the Micronesian islands have always been united through, and not separated by the Pacific Ocean. So we welcome our fellow brothers and sisters from our "Blue Continent" to our home. Yet the Compacts of Free Association Act has led to an increased demand on our local services and infrastructure, and Congress has refused to cover the costs of this burden on our government.

The pandemic exacerbated these sentiments, as the FSM shut down its borders, stranding many FSM citizens who were simply visiting relatives and did not live in Guam (Daleno 2020). Governor Leon Guerrero wrote to the U.S. government in April 2020 stating that Guam could not afford to quarantine or support COFA citizens during this time. These community sentiments only heightened as the first publicly known hot spots for high positivity rates were in well-known Micronesian migrant neighborhoods (Salinas 2020).

Reflecting and reinforcing community sentiments, the Guam legislature has attempted through several bills to enact discriminatory legislation to alleviate this impact, including efforts to cut insurance coverage, remove or reduce access to the Guam Housing and Urban Renewal Authority (GHURA), and deport FSM citizens.[13] Some local legislators resisted these attempts and advocated for the rights of Chuukese people, but the sentiment remains part of the narrative of many leaders in Guam.

Deportation of felons was advocated by local leadership for years, despite the lack of response from the federal government that ultimately regulates immigration in Guam. In 2016, then governor Calvo and his administration unilaterally commenced deportations using an unorthodox legal strategy: commuting sentences for convicted felons in Guam's prisons and buying plane tickets to send them to their country of origin (Stole 2016).[14] Governor Leon Guerrero (2020) signaled similar support in her 2020 State of the Island address: "While Guam must be a place of opportunity for everyone—regardless of their race or creed—there can be no reward without accountability. Those who habitually avoid responsibility, those who do not seek to better themselves through education, violate the spirit of the Compact Agreements. And those who commit crimes against our community will be subject to deportation." Yet FSM citizens ensnared within the criminal justice system are not the only focus for some leaders. Although it has yet to occur, some legislators, including the past vice speaker of Guam, suggested that the administration not stop with just deporting those convicted of a crime, but request U.S. authorization to deport those who are unable to support themselves (Miculka 2014). This request is based on the COFA and the Immigration and Nationality Act, both of which state that any nonimmigrant alien who "cannot show that they have sufficient means of support in the United States" is deportable (USCIS 2018). This form of deportability is another manifestation of their imperial citizenship (Smith and Castañeda 2021). These sentiments reflect the idea that not "all Micronesians" (including Chamorus) can work together, as former Governor Calvo argued (see chapter 1); instead, they are inherently different peoples.

Throughout the Guam community, Chuukese women are perceived as backward and "too cultural," with their Chuukese combs and ethnic skirts and dresses (see figures 11 and 12), perceived hyperfertility, and subsequent overuse of social services. Stereotypes about men include that they drink alcohol excessively and break the laws.[15] This rhetoric closely mirrors anti-immigrant sentiment toward many migrant groups throughout the United States and demonstrates the hegemonic power of the colonizer in shaping local social environments.[16]

Anti-immigrant sentiment, deportation efforts, and the constant negative public rhetoric surrounding the Compact Impact are some ways in which COFA migrants are affected by larger struggles between Guam and the United States. As Guam and the United States position COFA migrants precariously in the middle of control over autonomy, managing migration takes center stage. Imperial citizenship manifests not just in social and political exclusion but in everyday exclusion.

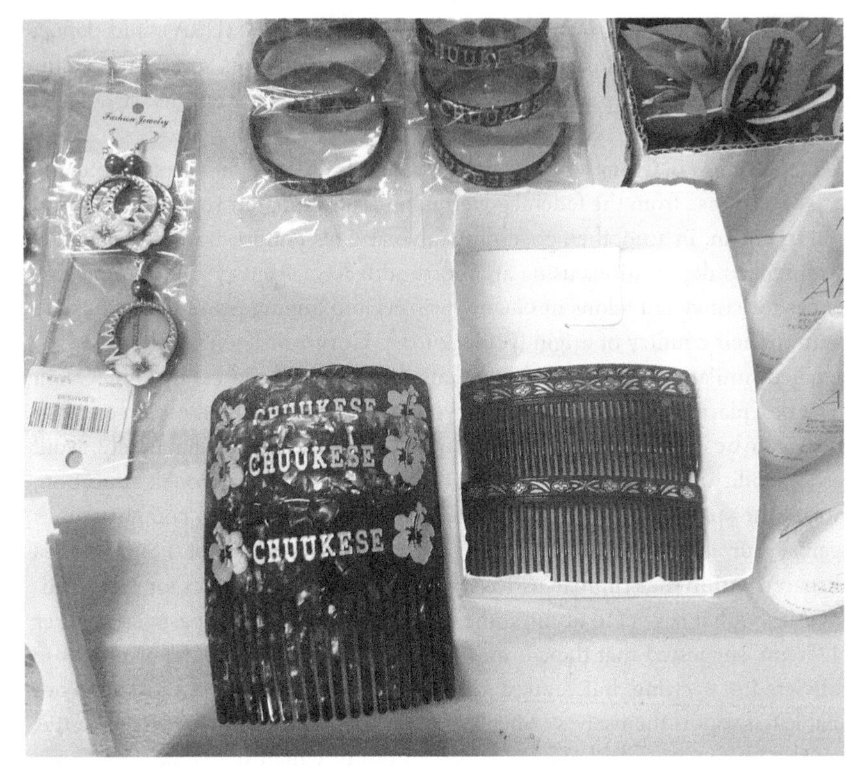

FIGURE 11. Plastic Chuukese combs sold at Chuukese store in Guam. Photo by Sarah Smith.

Everyday Exclusion

Kaylyn was thirty-five when we first met in 2013; she had moved to Guam with her parents when she was in elementary school, a few years after the COFA was enacted.[17] Her parents knew what to expect, having already lived in Hawai'i in the 1970s on I-9 student visas. They were part of a small cohort of students encouraged to attend college and return to help develop Chuuk, and they did just that. Yet Kaylyn's parents were keenly aware of the dramatic differences in economic opportunity and the quality of education between the FSM and U.S. jurisdictions. After the enactment of COFA, they decided to move from their home in Chuuk and settle in Guam to give their children greater opportunities. However, the COFA made this move a far different experience from the one they had as young college students. Instead of a small group of students sent for college, there was a mass exodus of FSM citizens into U.S. jurisdictions. While Kaylyn's parents felt welcome and safe in Hawai'i as part of a tiny cohort of Pacific Islanders from a then unknown and faraway U.S. trust territory, Kaylyn was one of many new students arriving to Guam in large numbers in the late 1980s. Some of her first memories in Guam were of local boys taunting her at

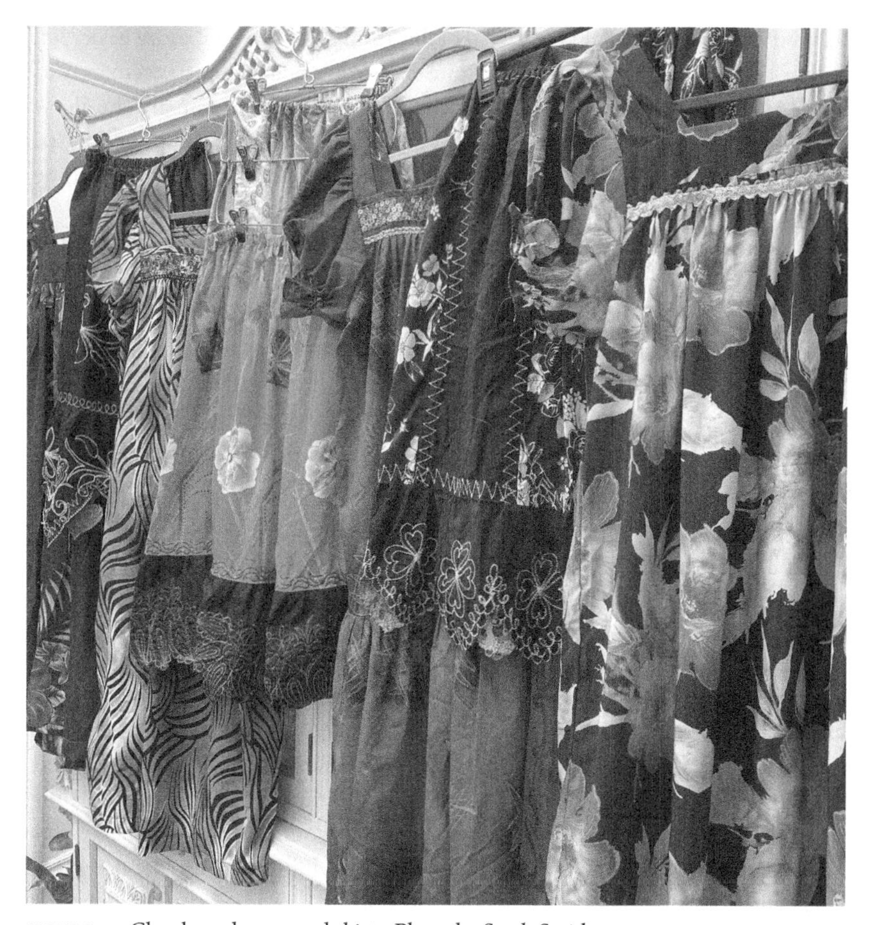

FIGURE 12. Chuukese dresses and skirts. Photo by Sarah Smith.

school, calling her a "dumb Chuukese" and telling her to go back to Chuuk. By the time Kaylyn was in middle school, her family had left this increasingly hostile environment and moved to Hawai'i, which—with the influx of new arrivals from the FSM—was also more hostile than it had been the previous decade, although still friendlier than Guam.

Kaylyn spent the rest of her middle and high school years in Hawai'i. Her family had enough money to visit Chuuk every few years, so Kaylyn still felt connected to home, but given the limited job opportunities, she knew she could not make a life there. After graduating high school, she joined the U.S. military and periodically moved to assignments across the United States over the next decade. During these years abroad, her parents moved back to Chuuk, feeling the strong pull of home after they finished raising their children. When I first met Kaylyn, she had recently moved back to Guam. She had considered settling in Chuuk but decided against it given the continuing lack of opportunities. Specifically, she decided her children would get a better education and she could more easily finish her college degree in Guam. Despite harboring bad memories, Guam was close to Chuuk, and many of her relatives still lived there. Additionally, she chose Guam over Chuuk because in some ways she felt more at home in the United States, as she had spent most of her life in U.S. jurisdictions. For Kaylyn, settling in Guam allowed her to reach a compromise between her identity as a Chuukese woman and her desire to expand her education and career opportunities and to keep her children in U.S. schools, despite the racism she had encountered and imagined her children would also face.

Young people face discrimination often, as Kaylyn did when she first moved to Guam. Young adult Chuukese women told me their earliest experiences in Guam were of Chamoru and Filipina girls teasing them at school for their clothes. Some also expressed the frustration of routinely being met with suspicion of theft and of ongoing overt surveillance by employees in retail markets. When they walked into a nice store, they were immediately told, "We don't need any help here," and were then followed around the store, implying that work and theft were the only possible reasons for Chuukese people to browse their stores.[18] Women fear for their children, especially their boys, facing these forms of discrimination.

As we sat on the floor of her living room–kitchen space in her small dark apartment in Hagåtña, Guam, Siera told me a story of her son's experiences of discrimination at high school: "One day they [Chamoru and Chuukese boys] had a fight. The [teacher] aides were taking care of the local, Chamoru. . . . They say, 'You Chuukese, you go back home, this is not your island.'" She shared this story as we sat on woven pandanus mats, relaxing while Siera's middle daughter, Erica, stood in the kitchenette making us a snack. As Erica cooked over the butane camp stove, which sat on top of the actual (but unused) apartment stove (a common setup in Chuukese apartments), she chimed in that this kind of stuff happened all the time at her high school. She complained that teachers never believe Chuukese students. She and others also told me about the segregated "wings" at school in which people socialized, each denoting a different ethnic group.

Pamela, a thirty-nine-year-old Chuukese migrant from the Northwest Islands, told me a similar story of the police responding to a scene of Chamoru boys surrounding Chuukese boys (including her son) and taunting them. According to Pamela, the police—instead of questioning the local boys or breaking up the confrontation—agreed with the Chamoru boys' taunts: "Well, boys, that's true, this isn't your island." Jevlyn, a forty-three-year-old woman from the Mortlock Islands, described fights that broke out in her neighborhood between Chamoru and Chuukese boys, in which the police were called and only the Chuukese boys were arrested. These experiences demonstrate the explicitly unwelcome messaging they received and, from a gendered lens, begin to contextualize the disproportionate arrest rates of Chuukese men and boys in Guam. While people with FSM origins make up less than 10 percent of Guam's population, they accounted for nearly one-third (32.1 percent) of Guam Police Department arrests in 2021 (Guam Police Department 2023). As I noted previously, nearly three-quarters of FSM residents in Guam are Chuukese.

Each woman I spoke with experienced some sort of racism in Guam. For Kaylyn, this started in elementary school. For Rosie, it was when she worked at the bank. Maureen also told me she was questioned by bank employees as to why she was allowed to make deposits for her employer. Rosie complained that people in Guam say, "'Oh you Chuukese, you have more kids cause you want the food stamp. You want food stamp!' They say that!" This harsh treatment also played out in their attempts to access public services. When seeking help with housing through the GHURA, they were often denied; when they were awarded housing, they were surveilled regularly: agents would arrive unannounced to check for the number of people living in the household. In social services and healthcare contexts, Chuukese women experienced rude encounters, longer wait times, and refusal of service, as further described in chapter 6.

These exclusionary narratives, perpetuated at individual, social, and political levels, affect the stability of Chuukese people in the community. Nearly four decades after the COFA agreement, Micronesians still occupy the lowest levels of the job sector in Guam. The COFA average household size in Guam is 5.4 persons, but the average household income is only $24,832.00 (Hezel and Levin 2012). This low household income is insufficient given the cost of living on Guam, which is inflated due to the significant U.S. military presence (and military personnel's significantly higher salaries) on the island (Hezel 2013; Vine 2015). These forms of exclusion affect not only Chuukese migrants' economic vulnerability but also their sense of identity and notions of belonging.[19]

EXCLUSION AND IDENTITY

Kaylyn told me she ultimately felt too American for Chuuk and too Chuukese for America: "My mother and father's generation . . . all of them, they had to migrate out to get an education, but most of them, eighty percent went back. You know, they had this pride, this love of Micronesia. Whereas our generation, we're just gone and that's it. We don't go back. We don't belong anywhere because we are Compact migrants" (Smith and Castañeda 2021, 138). As Kaylyn described, many Chuukese community members—particularly those born around or after the COFA—explained feeling in-between; not welcome in Guam, not completely connected to Chuuk. Kaylyn said growing up in-between was nice in some ways, "almost like having two lives here: growing up in Guam and going down [to Chuuk in the summers], we weren't expected to . . . do as much [chores as the other kids]." While that part was easier, young people who were deported or sent back by families to Chuuk were taunted for being culturally too American (chon Merika, or "people from America") and told they spoke Chuukese like children. Glorida, age fifty-three, an animated native of Wééné who went to college in the mainland United States, told me it was difficult when she returned: "Yeah . . . when I came back from school, I realized that I was very high minded. I was very Americanized. I couldn't get along with anybody in Chuuk." Glorida did not subscribe to gendered rules of wearing skirts and remaining silent, and this led to many arguments between she and her cousins. She eventually settled in Guam.

Similarly, those who remained in Guam—many born or raised in Guam—never felt that they belonged there; they were constantly told this was not their island. They were perceived as outsiders because of their COFA ancestry. Many, like Kaylyn, felt as if they did not belong anywhere. Older women who were raised in Chuuk and migrated later in life had fewer struggles with their identities and sense of belonging, but they also felt frustrated at being discriminated against because of their culture. Siera said succinctly, "People don't like us when we come here because we bring our culture with us."

Tensions between Chamoru and non-Chamoru populations in Guam are inevitably connected to constructions of culture and the ways in which these two communities have negotiated their identities in relation to the dominant United States. The Chamoru of Guam are often described as having an identity distinct from the rest of Micronesia due to the colonial separatism imposed on them by each imperial power (Bautista 2010; Kiste 1999). The divergence in colonial histories meant centuries of limited contact between these geographically close communities. Chamoru communities in Guam have been depicted as being more Westernized (Kiste 1999) or as having "lost their culture" (Diaz 1994; Guerrero and Salas 1995). Of course, indigenous rights scholars contest these problematic notions of lost culture among Chamorus (Diaz 1994), as do I. Nevertheless, colonial separatism did have an impact on the relationship between Chamorus and non-Chamorus (Diaz 1995). These separate identities contribute to the discrimination toward COFA migrants, in their eyes, because of their culture.

One highly publicized example was when the larger Guam community learned of Micronesians living on large swaths of land in the northern part of Guam, which did not have plumbing and sometimes lacked electricity and phone lines as well. When I first visited one of these subdivisions, Zero Down,[20] I felt like I was driving down dirt roads in parts of Chuuk. Much like in Chuuk, there were some established one-story mid-century concrete houses peppered in between more makeshift spaces, where people used plywood, tin, corrugated metal, tarps, and other materials to build homes. Breadfruit, mango, and coconut trees swung in the breeze here in this windy part of the northern island. Several household complexes had outdoor cookhouses like in Chuuk, and grills and water containers made from old shipping barrels. I remember feeling particularly struck by the large luscious gardens people planted in these spaces. Families took getting this land as a win, as it gave them property they could build on instead of living in public housing and small unkempt apartments. However, since the land was not developed according to Guam (or U.S.) standards, particularly in the Gil Baza subdivision, the larger Guam community expressed outrage that these spaces were unfit for human habitation. Some of the larger Guam community expressed concern over the victimization of these families in light of the developer selling land that was not in fact developed; others expressed distaste for the COFA migrants' "choice" to live in "backward" ways without plumbing.[21] Their ways of living and being were a constant source of attention, further differentiating them from other Guamanians.

Politicians, community leaders, government social and health service workers, university students, and newspapers argued that Chuukese or Micronesian migrants simply needed to learn how to live and behave in ways reflecting U.S. hegemonic cultural ideals. In other words, they believed that these migrants were too cultural and must assimilate, and that their problems lay not with imperialism, poverty, and racism but rather in the simple fact that they did not understand Guam's U.S.-imposed culture and laws. Bridges (2011) calls this narrative a form of "culturalist racism," wherein the concept of culture has replaced race but continues to do the work that the concept of race did historically: separating and marginalizing communities. Similarly, Trouillot (2003) argued that the concept of culture was an accessory to racism.

Discrimination toward COFA migrants from community leaders, newspapers, and residents typically lump COFA migrants from all Micronesian islands (including three countries, dozens of distinct island identities, and over a dozen languages) together as a singular group. Micronesians are lumped into one category in discriminatory exchanges, which contradicts how they feel about their own unique island identities. Discrimination also contributes to how they view one another. While all COFA migrants in Guam experience discrimination by non-COFA residents, the Chuukese also experience discrimination from other COFA communities (see also Falgout 2012). Chuukese migrants' behavior in Guam is blamed by many in the larger COFA network for the discrimination they all face.

Reinforcing their own island or regional identities, Chuukese people often explain how many different Chuukese communities exist, telling me, for example: "People here don't like people from Chuuk, and they don't realize we are all from different islands." Juliana Flinn (1990) argues that these identities date back to divisions between communities prior to imperial occupations. Since the state of Chuuk was not a collective nation-state or community before the occupations, it was created not based on alliances but on geography and UN decisions about what constituted trust territories. Being Chuukese is only an identity outside Chuuk, constructed for all people from the twenty-three inhabited islands forming the state. Within the state, regional, island, and village identities are primary (Marshall 2004).

Women often compared regions of Chuuk for me, differentiating the communities in each region and island. At each level, a region or island is distinguished from their own and blamed for the stereotypes they face abroad (although some women distinguished their own communities as the ones to blame). Even within an island or a region, people tend to set up boundaries and consider specific villages as more well-behaved (or not). Many claim that where culture is stronger, such as in the Mortlock and Western Islands, people "behave" (i.e., do not fight, steal, or drink alcohol), while in Chuuk lagoon, culture has broken down, and thus people drink alcohol to excess and exhibit violence. In this way, Chuukese communities credit culture for good behavior, contradicting Guamanians' and other COFA migrants' tendencies to blame culture for bad behavior among Chuukese migrants.

These regional identities shape villages in each migration center, from the Chuuk state capital of Wééné to Guam and to every U.S. state in which a large population has settled (Flinn 1990; Marshall and Marshall 1990; Marshall 2004; Bautista 2010, 2011). Neighborhoods and apartment complexes are often occupied by people primarily from one island or region (see also Bautista 2011). When conducting outreach to Chuukese migrants in Guam, service providers recognize that multiple community leaders must be approached from different communities/regions. But the segregation of different Chuukese communities from one another presents a barrier to unifying them in Guam, preventing them from collectively asserting their rights with the level of power assumed as representatives of nearly 7 percent of the island's population.[22] Yet while island and regional rivalries are reflected in migration destinations, they are not fixed. Chuukese migrants from different regions often find one another in Guam, particularly the youth. Those who grow up in or move to Guam as children or young adults connect through their greater identity formations as Chuukese people and their (often lacking) sense of belonging in Guam.

While youth often connect through a sense of lost identity or not belonging, many older women I interviewed held firmly to what they considered their culture or their customs. Transnational and global studies have contributed to the deconstruction of bounded communities and cultural specificity in anthropological theory.[23] But while anthropologists broke down these bounded notions, communities frequently built them up, further constructing and claiming cultural identities. Chuukese women often purposely demonstrate these identities through physical and social expressions, using the social body as a representation of society (Douglas 1973). Wearing distinctive combs (figure 11) and colorful skirts and dresses (figure 12), getting gold teeth, and expressing humble, respectful behavior are some of the ways in which they actively embody their Chuukese

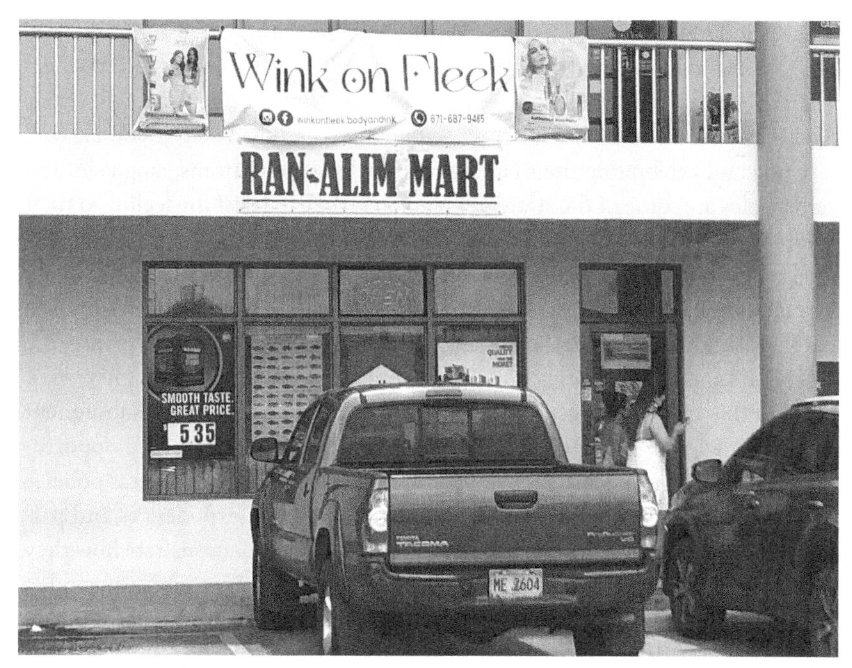

FIGURE 13. Ran-Alim Mart, Guam (Ran-Alim means "hello" or "good day" in Chuukese). Photo by Sarah Smith.

identities. Women share a pride in these symbols despite the experiences with racism attached to them, as these symbols connect them to home and strengthen notions of who they are, reflecting a form of bodily praxis (Bourdieu 1977). These symbols may also be a form of resistance to assimilation.

This concept of cultural pride was invoked when women told me about their food, language, and customs. Eating local food is always a topic of conversation, and coolers arrive on every flight from Chuuk full of kón (pounded breadfruit), puna (pounded taro), iik (fish), núú (coconuts), and other island delights. Chuukese stores are scattered throughout Guam to sell these desired food staples, along with skirts, combs, and other popular items (see figure 13). Teaching children born or raised in Guam cultural expectations of Chuukese behavior—such as how to show respect (suufén), show humility (mósónósón), and reflect appropriate gender-role behaviors—is also important to many women. Some send their children home to Chuuk out of fear they do not understand what it means to be Chuukese, complaining that McDonald's, Domino's Pizza, television, and other Guamanian (and U.S.) influences are getting in the way. Rosie took her whole family home and was proud of how much more respectful her children were when compared to her sister's children (who were entirely raised in Guam). Praise, a fifty-year-old woman from the Southern Nómwoneyas region, also credited strict cultural rules with her children's better behavior compared with other Chuukese children in Guam: "We teach them about our custom, and they eat . . . local food. . . . They['d] rather eat the breadfruit [than rice]. And they eat fish, they eat mackerel, whatever we eat in Chuuk." Praise continued, telling me, "And they listen. For those th[at] work they help us [financially], you know?" Teaching and celebrating their children's knowledge of customs, language, and gender roles are some of the strategies women invoke to resist the feeling in their children—like Kaylyn had—that they do not belong anywhere. Others, like Jasmine, a fifty-year-old woman from the Southern Nómwoneyas, complained that their children had no interest in returning to Chuuk. Some expressed frustration that their children barely understood the Chuukese dialect of their region.

Kaylyn's and Rosie's stories, and the sentiments of several other women introduced in this chapter, reflect the ways in which the COFA and the subsequent migration to Guam reshaped Chuukese women's lives, identities, and opportunities. Their stories are instructive in understanding how U.S. federal policies and local forms of discrimination form their immigration experiences and particular vulnerabilities in Guam. These women's narratives demonstrate how they negotiate their transnational lives at home and abroad in the context of gender, their imperial citizenship status, and the consequent precariousness of their residency in Guam. These experiences also shape reproductive and sexual health outcomes.

4 • REPRODUCING IMPERIALISM IN THE BODY

Praise is a thoughtful introspective grandmother from the Southern Nómwoneyas region of Chuuk and an advocate for Chuukese communities in Guam. She is also a masterful storyteller and is intimately invested in Chuukese women's health. We would sit and talk for hours when we got going, sometimes relaxing on the Chuukese sleeping mats behind closed doors in an air-conditioned room at her home. Here we found respite not only from the heat but from the children running around the rest of her cinderblock home in the northern Guam village of Dededo. If too many people were going to be at her house, we would instead meet at my apartment and would inevitably end up sitting on the porch, enjoying the breeze and sunset, with the wild chickens—ubiquitous on Guam—entertaining us from below. Chickens are really the only birds you hear on Guam, since invasive brown tree snakes were introduced by colonizer ships, killing off many other birds typical in this region.

Praise's smile was reserved, with just a hint of a gold tooth gleaming as she recounted her younger years; but when laughter came, that smile widened, infectious to all around. She loved sharing stories from her childhood and young adult years, often laughing about the absurdity of youthful adventures. She also thought about how imperial influences on religion, medicine, gender roles, and transnational movement shaped Chuukese women's health, and she enjoyed sharing her analysis with me. I begin here with her experience of menarche.

Praise woke up one morning and saw she had blood on her underwear. She knew this meant that she was a woman, and it scared her: "You know, when I saw blood, I was so scared because I heard that if a lady already, you know, slept with a guy, you know, she will have blood.... I hid it from my mom." Like many women, Praise understood menarche to be an indication that a young woman had had intercourse with a man; she feared her mother would accuse her of doing so. She ran to a stream on the mountain pathways behind her house and cleaned her underwear, padded it with some cloth, and tried to hide this new development. As a novice at menstrual hygiene, Praise's padding was insufficient;

her mother noticed a stain on her skirt later that day. When the family was outside, she called Praise inside for a private conversation. Praise was terrified, slowly approaching the doorway to their two-room concrete house, her eyes facing the floor. Her mother asked her directly if she had started to menstruate. Praise nodded yes, and her mother insisted she sit down. Rather than being mad or accusatory, as Praise expected, she seemed proud of her daughter's new status and shared with her what this meant: Praise was growing into a woman and had to start acting like a woman. She was instructed to always practice good hygiene, to stop wearing shorts or pants, and to only wear long skirts and dresses.

Praise received no lessons on sex or sexual and reproductive health aside from warnings about avoiding gifts or spending time alone with boys and men, and the importance of respecting brothers and other males. She ignored some of this advice: "I read the letters. But I was advised from my mom that the reason for not taking things from the boys [is that] they may use magic and then I will go crazy. I was told from my mom to give [gifts and letters] away." Praise's mother also told her to never go anywhere alone: "Don't stop if the boy talks to you. Just keep going." Her cousins snuck away with boys: "They can go disappear after they go into the jungle.... They're so like, more open?... They go out, you know, meet up with their boyfriends.... But me, I feel scared." Praise did not have a boyfriend until she went to college because of this fear.

While Praise did not have much by way of sex education lessons, she did learn about reproduction earlier than many women because her mother assisted women with prenatal care and birthing, and Praise would accompany her. Her mother and other local[1] practitioners provided women with prenatal medicines and massage; provided steam and fire treatments during pregnancy and labor or for healing after birth; stripped the membranes to get labor going; moved breeched presentation through internal and external massage; fixed spiritual and medical afflictions of pregnant or birthing women; and provided medicine to bring the milk and to make the postpartum mother strong and healthy, as well as to prevent miscarriages, stillbirths, and infant mortality. She was in awe of their expertise and celebrated home births and local practitioners in a way that was rare among the women I interviewed, all of whom grew up in an era in which biomedicine was growing in prominence.

When Praise finished high school—taught mostly by Peace Corps volunteers—she was sent to college in Oregon, where she could live with relatives. Going to college in the United States was one of the only legal pathways for visiting the U.S. mainland during the trust territory period. But not everyone could be educated. For Praise, this was a great honor and reflected the faith her parents had in her success at a time when families had to pick and choose who among their children were worthy of the investment. When she was in Oregon, she focused on school, but she also met her first sexual partner. Praise was raped. She fought and cried through the experience, and when it was over, he cried and apologized, excusing his behavior because he misunderstood her to already be sexually active; this, he claimed, justified his actions. Praise accepted his apology and forgave him. They began a relationship, and she became pregnant. She had to reveal this to her uncle and his wife, who were hosting her, and they supported her during her pregnancy. Her uncle's wife took her to the hospital when she was in labor and stayed with her throughout the birth. She told Praise they were not in Chuuk, so if she needed to cry or scream, it was OK. The hospital staff was also very helpful. Praise felt safe and well cared for in this environment. This first birth shaped her perceptions and expectations of future births.

Praise felt great shame for having a baby when she was supposed to be finishing her studies: "I was crying, [thinking] what am I gonna do? What am I gonna tell my parents?" She wrote letters home to her parents apologizing for the shame she had brought on them by getting pregnant. Praise stayed to finish school so that she would not completely disappoint them, though she would ultimately drop out. She tried for two years, taking the baby with her to classes. Praise had limited support, however; her partner was abusive. Two years into their relationship, she sought the help of her brother to buy a plane ticket back home to Chuuk. When her partner was at work, she escaped the house with her baby and headed to the airport. She succeeded and moved back to Chuuk, where she would stay for several years.

Upon arrival back in Chuuk, Praise moved to her home island with her family and eventually met the man who was still her spouse when we met decades later. They had a loving relationship and six children together. Two were born on her home island with assistance from her mother, local medicine practitioners, and biomedically trained birth attendants, all working together to ensure that Praise was safe and comfortable. Praise also birthed in Chuuk State Hospital, Saipan's Commonwealth Health Center, and Guam Memorial Hospital (GMH). Each of these choices was the product of circumstance, as she happened to be working in those locations when she was ready to deliver.

Because Praise experienced pregnancy and birth in numerous locations, she had much to compare. She had few opinions about prenatal care, except that she was shy about seeking care in Chuuk, reluctant that other Chuukese people might see her private body parts: "In Chuuk, you know, the people. I feel so, like, not like in Saipan. I don't care if they see my privates, but in Chuuk, you know, like, I'm kind of hesitant." She preferred blending local and biomedical traditions, and in Guam, her biomedical prenatal care was supplemented by care from a local practitioner who visited regularly. But she vacillated in terms of her preferred place of birth. Oregon had merit due to the high technology and respect of the healthcare workers; home was her preferred place, because she felt safe and supported, surrounded by experienced female kin. Next in rank was the Saipan health center; there she thought that the nurses and nurse-midwives, whom she believed came from the South Pacific (she presumed Fiji), were very well trained and respectful. Next was Chuuk State Hospital; while she was able to have her mother and husband accompany her, and the care was fine, she knew that women were more recently forced to birth alone and that the care was barely adequate. Still, even with less adequate care, she much preferred this option to GMH, where women were subject to disrespectful treatment and were ignored by nurses. GMH was a clear last place.

Praise raised her children in all the places she birthed them, but she spent the most time in Chuuk. When she left for Saipan or Guam to earn higher wages, she always felt compelled to return. When I met her in Guam in 2012, she was making plans to retire to Chuuk, having spent the better part of the last decade in Guam. Her older children were beginning to have children of their own, and she was settling comfortably into the role of grandmother.

Praise's reproductive life story exemplifies many of the themes in this chapter, reflecting how gender inequalities and migration histories are imprinted on women's reproductive bodies. Reproductive life experiences elucidate the ways in which gender, kinship, and migration are produced and reproduced through Chuukese women's bodies. Using the framework of stratified reproduction, I relay women's experiences and analysis of reproduction from their perspectives in a linear fashion, starting with their childhood memories and continuing through pregnancy and childbirth, in Chuuk and abroad. Pollution and shame (seu) about their sexual bodies was inherent in all the lessons they received, but so was a certain pride at their ability to reproduce the clan. Women's bodies are symbolic of the entire clan, with considerable pressure on women to maintain honor. The ensuing surveillance and control of their bodies is a consistent theme throughout their lives.

EARLY LESSONS ON SEX AND REPRODUCTION

Some of women's earliest memories—like Praise's—included playing with all their cousins, although many reported that they would be scolded or spanked if they were seen playing in mixed-gender groups or stepping over their brothers, a symbolic marker of disrespect shown when someone is considered higher in status. They did not completely understand these gendered rules at the time, especially because they were also being taught not to step over adults. I witnessed many occasions when toddlers still learning these rules were lightly scolded for stepping over me as I played with them. But as women reflected on their memories as adults, they interpreted the rule related to brothers as an early lesson on the separation of gender in larger Chuukese society, where avoidance serves to reduce any sexual desires in men. It was the only common lesson on sexuality prior to menarche.

Like Praise, several women told me that as young girls, they believed that menstruation came after having sex and feared they would be suspected of sexual activity if their mothers found out.[2] Other women did not know to expect menstruation at all. Yet when mothers were told about their daughters' menarche, they rarely reacted poorly. Most reported that their mothers lectured them about being a woman but did not provide any sex education (see also McMillan et al. 2020). Their mothers explained that being a woman meant that they could not speak harshly to or challenge their brothers (including male cousins) and that generally, they should avoid them.[3]

Beatriz Moral (1996), an anthropologist who studied Chuukese sexuality in the 1990s, theorized that the rules and norms surrounding sexuality in Chuuk are structured around an incest taboo between brothers and sisters (including male cousins) (see also Goodenough 1978). She argued that the taboo guides most symbolic and structural thought on behavior in Chuukese social life. Incest taboos between brothers and sisters are one of the most common taboos across all human communities, but Moral believed that the Chuukese taboo was uniquely powerful. Indigenous scholar Myjolynne Kim (2020) agreed with Moral's assessment. When women reached menarche, the rules around this taboo intensified.

Women were expected to inhabit a silent, subdued habitus upon menarche wherever male relatives were present (Moral 1996, 1998a, 1998b). A woman merely talking aloud shows off her sexuality, they learned. These lessons were not just about the taboo but to prevent them from facing sexual violence. Norita—a thirty-six-year-old woman from the Southern Nómwoneyas—was told by her mother that it was her responsibility to avoid sexual assault by being modest around male family members because "[we] women, we have to protect it. We have to protect our own selves not to start them [male family members] thinking those bad thoughts." Some women reported that in Chuuk, boys move out of the family house to other homes on the family compound when their sisters reach menarche. Girls were also told not to go into their uncle's homes alone or be alone with any male relative.

In 2014, the FSM government conducted a national study of violence against women; 17 percent of Chuukese women reported that they experienced sexual abuse by a non-intimate partner before the age of fifteen. The most common perpetrators were male family members (Leon and Mori 2014).[4] The Chuuk Women's Council promotes health education campaigns to prevent sexual violence, further indicating that family sexual violence is common. Women explained to me that while this is never acceptable, responses to it vary, and mothers sometimes ignore assaults on their adolescent daughters because of their reliance on the perpetrator for housing and food. Others send their daughters to live with a distant relative to separate them from the perpetrator. Some, however, blame the girls. Keeping the cases private is common; announcing it or accusing the perpetrator openly will bring shame to the clan (see also Rauchholz 2016; Goodenough 2002).

Migration, including moving in with family in Wéénè, Guam, Hawai'i, or beyond, may have additional risks. According to Guam's 2018 Youth Risk Behavioral Surveillance System—a national U.S. survey conducted in high schools—17.7 percent of "other Micronesian" (i.e., not Chamoru) students in Guam reported forced sex at least once in the past year (David 2018). These data did not distinguish between family and nonfamily violence, but family sexual violence has been documented in *all* of Guam's larger communities at high rates. In 2020 alone, 303 cases of sexual abuse of a minor were referred by Child Protective Services for investigation (Government of Guam 2021). Chuukese women and Guam's violence prevention advocates from Healing Hearts Rape Crisis Center and the Guam Coalition against Sexual Assault and Family Violence both contended that young women are often assaulted by a male elder when they move in with distant relatives to attend Guam's high schools or colleges, or to help around the house with a new baby or elderly family member. Women could no longer adopt the practice of moving away from a male relative when family compounds in Chuuk changed to small shared apartments in Guam. There were also cases in which extended family members trafficked adolescent women from Chuuk to Guam (DOJ 2012; Aguon 2017, 2013).

Kesapw tupu ngeni aat (Do not pay attention to boys)

Lessons to stay away from boys and men were not limited to kin. Mary, who was thirty-six years old when we first met, was a warm, polite, and playful firstborn daughter of a firstborn mother, a powerful status position for a woman in a Chuukese family. When Mary experienced menarche, her mother told her, "Kesapw tupu ngeni aat," not to listen to or fall for boys.[5] Talking to members of the other sex might imply a sexual relationship to onlookers or at least interest in a sexual relationship toward the person to whom she was speaking, and so this injunction extended to include sex. This lesson made women like Rosie and Siera, who both went to high school in Wéénè, scared of boys until they were in college. Siera explained, laughing, that when girls told her a boy had a crush on her in high school, she would go out of her way to avoid him so he could not use love magic on her. Rosie told me she admired guys in high school, but she would just ignore them because she was scared of her mom. Most women, like Praise, were taught love magic could be imparted through food, touch, an object (like a letter), or even a stare.[6] Some, however, thought these ideas were silly old myths, but they still needed to avoid boys in their youth so that no assumptions about sexual interest were made.

Women were also warned as adolescents to avoid being alone outside at night; often, their mothers made them sleep right next to them in order to prevent them from sneaking out. "If we were playing in the mangroves or on the beach with boys who are not relatives and it's getting late," Glorida explained, "we would come home, and they would say, 'Man you want those guys to step on you?'" Glorida told me that she never understood that saying as a child. Glorida was the youngest child, and she challenged everything, including gender roles; she was neither quiet nor demure. She told me she had recently asked her aunt why the elders always said "Ke mwochen pwuuri nuukomw?" (You want them to step on your stomach?) when they meant rape.

Some women, like Praise, were sexually assaulted in their first encounters with boys, and they understood or believed that women were at fault. Norita's mother told her that girls were assaulted by boys inside and outside the family because they brought unwanted attention to their bodies. "That's what my mom said, she said it's not the boy's fault, it's the girl's fault. Because, the way she dresses, it makes the boy . . . start thinking of having you know sex? When he sees her body" (Smith 2019b, 151). Glorida—speaking with great frustration over this perception—described her grandmother's lessons succinctly: "If he forced me, it's my fault. It's not his fault, it's my fault" (Smith 2019b, 152). Some women resisted the shaming narratives. Gloria did not believe that blaming women was fair or reasonable.

Despite the warnings of violence and coercion, several women still recounted the fun and exciting memories of young heterosexual romance. A common theme in their stories is when a young man pursued a young woman to demonstrate his love for her, going to great lengths to prove his dedication, including leaving Chuuk to find her after she migrates with her family. Many women shared love songs their suitors sang to them. One woman told me how her first sweetheart committed suicide because she migrated; another had a cousin whose love interest coerced her into sex by threat of suicide.[7] These women typically refused to meet or have sex with boys until they were pursued by one who they thought was marriage material. Several women divulged how they eventually broke the rules to meet the lovers they thought worthy. These relationships continued in secret, either at night or by day, when a girl is completing a chore (e.g., laundry) far away from the family.[8] Women found this easier when they migrated, attributing their absence from home to work or school obligations. No family members knew they had partners except perhaps a cousin or sister who was a confidant. These women believed that relationships could not be made public until couples were committed to marriage or experienced unintended pregnancy.

Chuukese women thus begin learning about gendered expectations for their behavior early on, when they are taught to act modestly through quiet, submissive behavior, dress discreetly, and avoid being alone with men. These women are taught to value virginity in their youth and to avoid bringing shame to their family when they choose to engage in vaginal sexual intercourse. No public demonstrations of relationships prior to marriage are acceptable, so secret meetings are how young people got to know each other. Women are taught that all these rules are important for maintaining not just their own honor but the honor of the clan, as their bodies are the physical and social reproducers of the matrilineage.[9]

Indigenous scholar Myjolynne Kim explained: "The environment bears life just as a woman bears life. In Chuukese ontology and structures of feeling, we are all connected through maternal creation. As mothers, women embody the environment, making visible in human domains its broader role in giving birth to all living things, human and nonhuman, spirits and nonspirits" (2020, 147).

This symbolic manifestation of the important role of women contributes to coercion and control of these bodies, but these narratives also mirror those of the cult of virginity and shame embedded in Euro-American Christian traditions and brought to the islands through missions and U.S. patriarchal values (Valenti 2010; Kim 2020). In analyzing these practices, I asked an indigenous colleague to read my analysis of these norms. As was common with Chuukese women, she shared her feedback through a story:

> Before I came out here [to the United States] I went down to Chuuk for two weeks. I knew it would be a long time before I will see my (extended) family again, so I made it a point to visit my home island and see the two remaining elders—my grandfather's two sisters. Both in their 80s, calling the shots on our mostly empty lands. One of them regaled me with stories about their mother. She called her a loose woman who slept with many, many men because it was like a competition between the women back then to have many lovers. My grandfather (he has passed on already) and his sisters were the only ones remaining when I was growing up, but there were about 10 of them, and many of them did not share the same father. My grandaunt stressed the fact that her mother was a "wanted" woman (that is, a sexually active woman), but even as she said that she was kind of in awe of this mother who did what she wanted and literally shared her conquests in love with the other women of the village. This is so different from my upbringing where my own sister was shamed for getting pregnant out of wedlock.[10]

As I depicted in chapter 2, missionaries sought to demonize sex outside marriage, reduce women's power and authority over men, limit divorce and contraception use, and reduce the importance of extended family relationships while heightening the importance of male-headed nuclear families.[11] As Josealyn implied, women were once celebrated for their sexual success; now, they are shamed.

Alternatively, young men are expected to experiment with sex and pursue girls and women their entire lives. The assumption that men need to seek additional sexual partners exists on a continuum of behaviors that boys are socialized to engage in to prove themselves as men; sexual success is part of the masculine framework (see also Rauchholz 2016). If boys and men rape, impregnate, or elope with girls, they do not face the same shame as girls. In this environment, men are perceived as unable to control their sexual desires, and it is women's responsibility to control all heterosexual behavior inside and outside their family.

These lessons and early experiences reinforce *global* patriarchal discourses that men are aggressive and need sex, and women need to control them or submit (Gavey 2013; Torres and Yllö 2020). Yet, Micronesian "culture" has been publicly blamed for sexual assault by at least one of Guam's leaders (Flores 2019). Her perspective is not isolated; I heard this narrative from service providers and community members in Guam regularly. Anthropologists are not innocent; the discipline has also contributed to culture-blaming for sexual violence in various communities (Baxi 2014). This blaming of some idea of a bounded, unchanged and monolithic "culture" for such violence is just another example of "culturalist racism" (Bridges 2011, 132). Blaming culture ignores the colonial foundations and global reach of such patriarchal discourses. Still, these lessons and discourses shape the vulnerability women face, beginning in adolescence and continuing into their marriage.

Sexual Initiation, Shame, and Marriage

Women explained to me that there are three typical ways in which marriage was initiated when they were young.[12] The ideal version is when a young man visits her home with his entire family and brings gifts, and the eldest male of the family, as well as the man himself, ask permission for him to marry the woman. Jessica explained that the suitor is expected to return repeatedly until the male leaders of the woman's family agree. Jessica kept her relationship secret until her boyfriend and his family participated in this ritual. The more typical but less ideal versions still include formal requests and gifts, but only after a couple runs away together for a few days or a young woman becomes pregnant.[13] I knew several young and adolescent women who had unintended pregnancies, reflecting this pattern. Kaylyn explained how running away works, although it is not always planned:

> Like you know, running away? That's a marriage contract right there, unless the boy doesn't really want to, yeah [if] he was just doing it for fun. . . . Those are usually the things that lead to marriages, like sometimes 'cause if a girl sneaks out, of course you know, and then someone happens to be up at the same time and discovers her missing, she's gonna run away with the guy, 'cause she's not going to risk coming back in the house. . . . They come back like a week or two later and then she gets beaten up, and then they, then it's OK for them to get married, or he'll get beaten up by the family, you know. . . . I heard all my mom's sisters actually they got beaten up. . . . Yeah, they each went through the process.

Running away and unintended pregnancy are more shameful ways to get married, but since a young woman is publicly identified as sexually active in both scenarios, the family usually acquiesces to her request. Yet as Kaylyn expressed, family violence may be part of the process for many women. Once families accept the relationship—shameful or not—a couple moves in together; this constitutes marriage.[14] At some point, they also have a church ceremony, but the community considers them married as soon as they cohabitate. Women remembered their first pregnancy and marriage stories with contradictory combinations of joy and shame because of the circumstances in which they happened. Siera met her husband when she was a college student at the University of Guam (UOG). Soon after they met, they became intimate, and Siera got pregnant. She laughed, uncomfortable as she sat on my old brown couch in Guam, drinking sugary black tea bought at the local mom-and-pop store down the street. Looking around the tiny apartment to confirm again that we were alone, she continued her story of this unintended pregnancy. She told me she was really scared and did not want the relatives she was staying with to know because she was not married. To hide the pregnancy, Siera wore larger and larger skirts and waited. When she felt she was in labor, she revealed her secret and asked them to take her to the hospital. Soon after the birth of her oldest daughter, elder male cousins from Chuuk came to visit and heard the baby crying. Her grandmother told them the baby was Siera's: "You have to forgive her. There's nothing we . . . can do. But, we just hope she finishes her school." They told the Chuuk side of the family upon returning home, including Siera's mother. Siera's mother wrote her a letter stating that she wanted to kill her, but soon after, she wrote another letter telling her to come home to raise the baby if she was dropping out of school. Siera replied that she did not want to leave school, so her mother came to Guam to help with childcare. Siera married the man and had three more children, but that did not dim the shame of her first pregnancy, which she still embodied as she recounted the story from nearly two decades prior. Rosie had a similar experience, hiding her first pregnancy from her parents as long as possible by wearing large clothes. She told me she was too scared to announce it; when she did, her mother told her she was a disrespectful daughter.

According to Ann Fischer (1963), the concept of illegitimacy was not relevant in Chuuk because children and motherhood were much more valuable than marriage. She argued that all Chuukese women desired to be mothers; it was synonymous with being a woman (see also Flinn 2010). However, women like Siera and Rosie hid their pregnancies because they were outside marriage, contradicting the older reports. Fischer may have essentialized women's experiences with pregnancy, ignoring circumstances bringing shame, or this shame has increased since the trust territory period.

Since the trust territory days, there was an established pattern of girls migrating out, getting pregnant, and returning home (Flinn 1987). All the women I interviewed told me relatives had warned them not to do this when they migrated. Glorida, Mary, Norita, and Jasmine were very conscious of this pressure and the need to succeed. Glorida explained: "Micronesian students were starting to move, go to school in the U.S., and all they do is party, get pregnant, come back home.

That was really prominent in my brain, just don't want to screw it up." Even so, four women experienced unintended pregnancy while attending college in the United States.[15] They also advised their own daughters not to repeat their mistakes. Siera sent her oldest daughter to the U.S. mainland for school and told her to make sure she did not bring home a "talking diploma." We laughed at the playful banter she used to impart wisdom, as her girls smirked at these jokes, listening in on our conversation in her apartment that day.

In total, seven of the fifteen life history participants experienced unintended pregnancy before marriage, whether abroad or at home, and all participants had sisters, cousins, or daughters who experienced unintended pregnancy and faced familial shame. Several told me they went to great lengths to hide their pregnancy for as long as possible, wearing skirts higher and higher, like Siera, with extra layers of skirts and dresses to hide the bump. Once discovered, a woman is expected to formally apologize, wait out the anger of her elders, and then move on to her next phase of life: marriage and motherhood. Moreover, most babies are welcomed immediately; their arrival often signals the end of hostility toward the new mother.

My findings came from older women who had experienced unintended pregnancy in the 1980s and 1990s, but the same Chuukese friend and colleague whom I asked to read and critique my analysis had a reflection on these expectations for young women. She reported:

> I feel like I'm reading my life story as I read further and further. I can relate to every single story, the sexual abuse from a relative, the clandestine meetups between lovers, the hiding of pregnancies. Chuukese women go through so many hoops and twists and turns . . . so much expectations on their shoulders, one could almost say that they single-handedly carry their family's reputations . . . perhaps they do. When my youngest sister found out she was pregnant, she hid it from everyone until her belly couldn't be hidden anymore. I absolutely concur that the shame of it was because it was out of wedlock, a totally western concept, but the journey of motherhood and childbirth and eventual child rearing is so accepted in our family that the initial shame seems ridiculous in hindsight. Yet now, as a single woman, my parents encourage me to get pregnant even though they know I have no boyfriend; it's the desire for the continuation of our family as well as the future security that a child would bring me that makes them wish childbirth on me.[16]

Similarly, Kim (2020) recounted her own experiences of shame with a pregnancy outside marriage but also noted that the shame dissipated and turned to joy once the baby was born. A more recent study in Wééné confirmed that this remains the case to the present (McMillan et al. 2020): young women continue to disguise their pregnancies, sometimes with the help of their mother, who is often blamed for the unintended pregnancy. The shame directed to young women has implications for reproductive health access and outcomes, such as delayed or no access to prenatal care. These experiences are distinct from those who have intended first pregnancies. For those with sanctioned pregnancies, the celebration of new motherhood and fear of maternal and infant mortality are elucidated in rituals and practices associated with maintaining safe pregnancy and childbirth experiences and general familial support. They enjoy special treatment by spouses, mothers, and other kin, and are encouraged to relax, care for their bodies, and prepare for the approaching birth and motherhood role.

INTENDED PREGNANCIES, CELEBRATING MOTHERHOOD, AND BIRTHING THE CLAN

I first met Mary in Chuuk, where she had spent the last several years following the birth of her first child. She was making plans to move back to Guam, however, and when we finally talked about her pregnancy experiences, it was in Guam. Mary was excited to host me once she was settled in her one-story, three-bedroom concrete house in the northern Guam subdivision near Gil Baza, a settlement with many Micronesian families in both established and makeshift homes. When I approached this house for the first time, I saw the jungle taking over broken-down cars, an old, rusted shipping container emerged in the green foliage of the tropics, and piles of old tires and trash right outside her property line. She had a chain link fence around her property, however, and within that enclosed space was a manicured lawn, hanging laundry, large Ti plants outlining the front of the house, and a few outdoor boonie dogs that came to greet you as you entered.[17] As I walked in, I recognized a (typical) very clean, junk-free Chuukese home. Jesus was framed on the wall, with the Virgin Mary right next to him, and these framed pictures were above a shelf full of religious icons, with necklaces and plastic lei flowers strewn about them, a sort of home altar. Mary had a couch, a coffee table, and an old tube TV, much like a typical American home, but also mats off to the side for family members to sleep in the living room when visiting. The kitchen—part of the greater living room—was packed with typical supplies: a five-gallon orange water dispenser; a rice cooker; several large colorful plastic bowls for mixing or cleaning food; large clear bins for marinating meat, taking food to gatherings, and simply storing food; and a small butane-burner camping stove, used instead of the standard oven-stove in the house. She made us some instant coffee, and we caught up for a bit. Then when others had settled back into their rooms and we were alone, the air-conditioning window unit blocking our voices, we began to talk about Mary's first pregnancy experience.

Having finished her college degree, Mary was living in Guam with her husband and working at a local bank when she became pregnant for the first time; she had been trying for quite a while. Soon after learning she was pregnant, Mary told me she began to feel very sick and angry; she thought this was because she was stuck in Guam when she really wanted to be with her mom in Chuuk as she transitioned to motherhood. About two months into her pregnancy, she decided to fly back to Chuuk. She immediately felt more at ease, and her relatives practiced various massage and local medical techniques to help her manage her symptoms. Mary explained: "Some pregnant women are treated a special way depending on how they get pregnant and depending on their families. For my village, if it's like second, third pregnancy they don't really pay attention with like whatever [but] . . . the first pregnancy we have, it's like culturally it's very important and you give the attention, you give the help. You get food from families. Families take care of you very much. The first one. But after the first one . . . it's ordinary." Praise, in contrast, was treated well with every pregnancy except the first one (because she kept it secret); she reminisced of people's accommodation of her cravings and their willingness to do her chores. Some families hold ceremonies when women reach their second trimester to celebrate and protect the mother.

Mary stayed in her quiet village for the remainder of her pregnancy, traveling to the central island of Wééné only for prenatal care and the birth. Her husband visited occasionally, but most of her time was spent with the women in her family. Mary complained, graciously, that her female relatives were full of annoying advice for her to ensure a safe pregnancy. She and other women told me about a vast and diverse range of taboos, behaviors, and local medical practices to protect them from vulnerabilities such as spiritual attacks. Families find it particularly important to protect pregnant and nursing mothers from the spirit of a woman who had died in childbirth, as she is known for trying to collect more women to stay with her on her canoe so that she is not alone (Dernbach 2005). Mary was advised to be active but to lighten her load; to avoid the ocean, the night air, and various locations because of the bad spirits; to avoid salt, greasy food, and angry feelings about her physical health; to avoid sex; and to use coconut oil regularly in her vagina and on her perineum and stomach to assist with skin stretching (see also F. B. Caughey 1971). The consequences for alerting the spirits about the pregnancy by breaking these rules include slow delivery, breech babies, umbilical cord wrapping, and vaginal tearing. Mary listened to her relatives' advice but also told them to stop pestering her with their ideas when they encouraged home birthing.

When Mary began to have contractions, she went to the main island and birthed at the hospital. While she always planned to deliver there, she first took local medicine her relatives gave her to speed up the labor process. Complications led to a cesarean section. Her physicians later blamed the local medicine on her need for a cesarean section, indicating it had almost caused her uterus to rupture. Yet she also told me she was treated well because she had family members who worked at the hospital; knowing people was key.

Mary's choice to go home where she was embraced with familial care and special treatment reflected an old tradition of returning home for pregnancy and childbirth. In early-to-mid-twentieth-century Chuuk, pregnant women would go to their home compound if they were living away, such as if they were on their husband's family land or another island.[18] Being close to kin was vital for both spiritual and emotional support for birthing women like Mary and Rosie. But after the U.S. occupation and the building of a hospital, women were increasingly encouraged to seek care in biomedical spaces. By the mid-twentieth century, colonial medical care was a regular part of Chuukese life.

Biomedicine and public health surveillance were common tools of empire-building in the twentieth century. Biomedicine was introduced in Chuuk during the German and Japanese colonial eras (1899–1914 and 1914–1944, respectively), and the focus remained on keeping colonizers healthy. After World War II, however, nation-building regimes (including the United States) concentrated on keeping the colonized healthy as a mechanism for capitalist expansion through adding healthy workers to the empire.[19] For Chuuk, this happened largely after the United States took over. During the trust territory era, U.S. officials built a modern hospital and public health clinic (in 1969) in the central island of Wééné.[20] Concurrently, the United States encouraged the delegitimating of local practitioners in Micronesia (Hattori 2004, 2006; Rubinstein 1999),[21] a practice carried out in other colonized spaces since before World War II, such as in the Philippines (Anderson 2006).

As birth outcomes became a measure of healthy nations and colonies, the biomedicalization of reproduction expanded throughout imperial zones.[22] Maternity services were denigrated, and Pacific women were seen as deficient in their birthing and nurturing practices; bringing communities to modernity meant the medicalization of reproduction. Surveillance of midwives and provision of pre- and postnatal services were part of how colonizers began taking on maternity services with the assumption that they were morally and technologically superior (Manderson 1998; Hattori 2006). Training ensued to restrict and constrain certain midwife practices and often involved teaching traditional birth attendants to encourage hospital and clinic use. At first, Chuukese women just utilized prenatal care (F. B. Caughey 1971), but caught in the biotechnical embrace of biomedicine, women and their families began wanting hospital births in case something bad happened (Good 2001). Thinking that more technology meant better care became common; Melissa Cheyney (2015) describes this belief as the "obstetric imaginary."

Glorida, who grew up in Wééné, could not imagine a time in which obstetrics were not the best choice: "I don't know anybody, any of my family, that have baby outside the hospital. Yeah. I'm glad I was born this era. Hospital" (Smith 2019a, 347). Jessica, from an island farther out in Chuuk lagoon, knew people who did not go to the hospital, but she thought it was a bad decision to stay home: "It's not good to stay [on home islands]. Some, they are really brave to deliver a baby on their island, you know? . . . But me, I'm scared of delivering in my house. That's why I always go to the hospital" (Smith 2019a, 347). Rosie, from a lagoon island close to Wééné, told me her grandparents encouraged home birth, and she responded with "Ahhh, just stop your nonsense. I'll go to the hospital!" (Smith 2019a, 347). This shift in the use of biomedicine is why, of the fifteen women who recounted their birthing stories, only four birthed at least once on their home islands, and then with the assistance of both local and biomedically trained midwives. The rest delivered at a hospital.

While women embraced obstetric technology in Chuuk, Guam, and other U.S. jurisdictions, they still learned and practiced traditions that supported their symbolic maternal role in their communities. First, women and their midwives were pragmatic about what obstetric medicine they adopted and what did not suit their needs, rejecting and accepting it as they saw fit.[23] Even the four women who birthed at home all used local medicine in conjunction with biomedical prenatal, postpartum, and newborn checkups at the state public health department. Those who birthed at the hospital told me they received local massages and teas made with special plants or roots, while they also went to the clinic for prenatal vitamins and testing, often at the insistence of the same family members who were giving them local medicine. While both systems of care were valued, women told me they kept this pluralistic practice a secret from their biomedical providers. Women found biomedicine to be important—perhaps more important than local medicine—and wanted to maintain access to that care. Ultimately, Chuukese women adopt and reject what they consider traditional and biomedical beliefs and practices based on their own perspectives, negotiating cultural norms and their everyday lives in the context of the last century of imperial occupation, missionization, imposition of biomedicine, and migration in their communities (see also Kim 2020). And though women clearly negotiate pluralistic medical systems, the imposition of biomedical structures in Chuuk and Guam delegitimizes local medicine.[24] At the same time, however, biomedical facilities and equipment deteriorated as well, stratifying women's reproduction.

While women imagined safer births with increased access to biomedical technology, their expectations were often not achieved. Because biomedicine is expensive and colonial budgets are never sufficient to support high-technology infrastructure, places like Chuuk's hospital degraded over time. This included both the deterioration of the physical space and equipment, and the lack of a skilled workforce far too expensive for the FSM infrastructure (Benjamin 2000; Ekeroma et al. 2019; Palafox and Hixon 2011). The hospital became a place better known for death than healing. This is not limited to Chuuk (see, for example, Jolly 1998; Manderson 1998). Hospitals and clinics built throughout former colonies were often too costly to maintain (Lock and Nguyen 2010). These symptoms of benign neglect in the context of reproduction have recently been

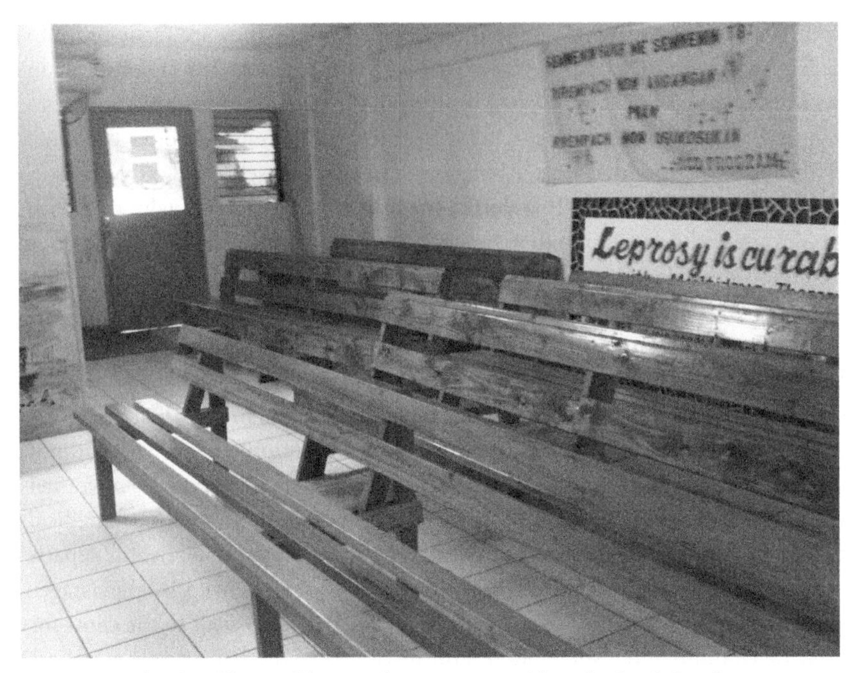

FIGURE 14. Chuuk Public Health general waiting room. Photo by Sarah Smith.

conceptualized as "reproductive abandonment" (Munro and Widmer 2022, 301). Specifically considering the case of post- and neocolonial Pacific islands, reproductive abandonment references the meeting of "settler colonialism and frontier obstetrics" resulting in "a broad failure to see the importance of birth sovereignty and reproductive autonomy for people subjected to dispossession and erasure" (Munro, Katmo, and Wetipo 2022, 402). Chuuk is one example in which reproductive abandonment occurred.

The spaces in which women receive biomedical prenatal care reflect this inadequacy of resources and funding. The building in which Chuuk's Public Health Department is housed is an old concrete structure that floods regularly. Its benches, resembling basic church pews, are lined up around the hospital's white but dirty walls, some of which host tattered old public health messaging posters (see figure 14). When women check in, they are allowed back in another waiting area where three couches sit—all donated and in varying levels of deterioration, floral covers hiding some of the mice activity, holes in the leather revealing others. Adjacent to the couches are a few offices—including two exam rooms and a testing room for sexually transmitted infections. Each has an exam table covered with a dirty sheet—which I never saw cleaned or replaced—on which the women sit (see figure 15). Given these conditions, women like Serena keep their skirts on as their own layer of protection.

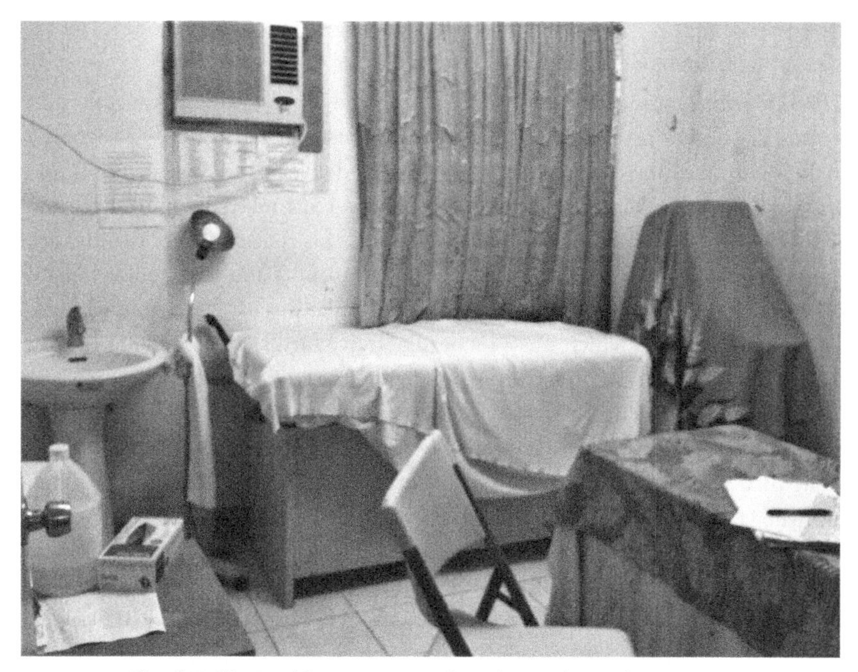

FIGURE 15. Chuuk Public Health exam room. Photo by Sarah Smith.

When they do make it to Chuuk's hospital, across a parking lot from this public health building, they encounter similarly deteriorating walls, minimal equipment and staff, and rodent and cat residents that are so plentiful, they are even visible in the daytime. Razors must be brought by the family to shave a woman's pubic or stomach area (depending on vaginal versus cesarean birth), and food and water must be provided daily by family members; otherwise, a woman who just gave birth will have no sustenance. Equipment is old and often stops working, medicine supplies ebb and flow, and limited, overworked providers are left in what amounts to a makeshift, understaffed, and underfunded field hospital (except less sanitary, because it is an old moldy building). Access to adequate biomedical reproductive health care is thus limited due to funding, staff, and supplies; these limitations are manifestations of reproductive abandonment.

Further, women's ability to travel to the main island of Wééné for prenatal care is constrained by the need for money to get on a boat (or the ability to take a very long walk or catch a ride from parts of Wééné). Despite these squalid conditions and travel difficulties, women with socially sanctioned pregnancies typically seek prenatal care by visiting the clinic every time they come to Wééné, and often try to seek care at the hospital for their births. The couches in the inner waiting room and the benches in the outside waiting room are always full of pregnant women seeking prenatal care, and the laboring room in the hospital is also quite busy.

Measuring Chuuk's Reproductive Outcomes

Chuuk's deteriorating infrastructure is reflected in reproductive health outcomes. As noted in the introduction, major causes of death for FSM women include complications during pregnancy, during delivery, and postpartum (Government of the FSM 2012a). The most updated FSM maternal mortality ratio (MMR) was 121 per 100,000 live births in 2021; this reflected only two deaths, both of which were in Chuuk; Guam's 2020 ratio was 34 and reflected one death (Government of the FSM 2022b; Gay 2020). Similar disparities exist in Chuuk's infant mortality rate, which was 24.2 per 1,000 live births (in 2021)—more than double Guam's 7.8 (in 2020). Chuuk's neonatal mortality rate was 14.8 per 1,000 live births in 2021, compared to Guam's 5.1 (Government of the FSM 2022b; Gay 2022). The only (outdated) data available on the rate of hospital births demonstrate that 45 percent continue to occur outside the hospital without a qualified midwife (i.e., a biomedically trained birth attendant) (Government of the FSM 2004).[25] The data, however, do not fully capture the extent of mortality in Chuuk.

Beyond the secondary waiting room in Chuuk's public health building, with its donated leather couches, is a conference room with several folding tables and chairs, a bathroom for employees, and a small office. This is where the public health meetings occur and where the surveillance and outreach teams sit when they are not in the field. It is always a place with laptops open, snacks shared from home, and conversation. Practitioners or employees from the Public Health Department's satellite clinics would stop in to say hello, as would friends of the employees or healthcare workers seeking a quick break from patients. I shadowed a woman in a leadership position for the department, writing grants and reports and analyzing data as requested in between my observations of women seeking health care. Because of this, I spent much of my downtime in this room. It felt like almost daily a person would stop by to tell a story of someone who went into labor or experienced miscarriage on an outer island and could not get to Wééné in time; babies and mothers often died in these stories. They were stories of suffering, but not official reports. The person who was the leader of this group would typically respond with condolences and then ask, "Did anyone report that?" As the contact for whom such deaths might be reported, she already knew the likely answer (no) and was frequently too overworked to follow up.

The imposition of biomedicine was the first tool of colonial control, and public health surveillance soon followed. As colonial medicine transitioned to (postcolonial) international health and, more recently, global health, the language of metrics became ubiquitous (Adams 2016a). Much of the work of colonizers included collecting data and surveilling maternal and child health, particularly after it was recognized how important reproduction was to labor and capitalist accumulation in the colonies (Anderson 2006; Manderson 1996; Wendland 2016).

Despite adopting metric-based goals, data collection systems in aid-dependent countries like the FSM are notoriously under-resourced, allowing for questionable data collection at best (Hoy et al. 2017; Aitaoto and Ichiho 2013; Cash et al. 2021). Young nation-states are required to meet targets with little attention to the histories of colonial and capitalist exploitation leading to the fiscal realities of meeting such targets (Adams 2016a).

My observations in that back room mirror concerns within the FSM that data cannot be consistently reported due to a lack of infrastructure at every level.[26] A recent study in Wééné further confirmed this issue. A team of researchers went to remote villages and interviewed women who either had experienced unplanned adolescent pregnancies or were mothers of these young women. They learned that many of them had birthed in their home village and never reported it, nor did they register the baby (McMillan et al. 2020). Thus, if this large proportion of women are not included in reproductive health data, then true maternal, infant, and neonatal mortality measures for the FSM—including Chuuk—may be much higher.

Problematic data are not the only issue. These metrics are the hallmark of epidemiological practices and yet can be exploitative through the silence in numbers, hiding anything (e.g., colonial history, enslavement, capitalist exploitation) that cannot be easily quantified (Richardson 2020; Reubi 2020). Further, numbers can create narratives through epidemiology. When people evaluate the numbers, it creates a story about how and who is suffering, without attending to regional differences and community dynamics (Reubi 2020). The numbers are too simplified to understand the complexity of community needs (Yamin and Boulanger 2013; Richardson 2020; Adams 2016b). And yet funding is tied to these metrics, though they often subvert coloniality (Richardson 2020) and inequalities more generally (Adams 2016c), instead focusing on neoliberal economic strategies and their efficacy.

Considering reproductive health metrics specifically, a focus on maternal health is also problematic because it often concentrates on the care women receive when birthing (or contraception) and the role of biomedicine, or its failure, in that care (e.g., births in a hospital, births with skilled attendants, contraceptive acceptance rates). For these reasons, our understanding of women's sexual and reproductive health in Chuuk is essentially reduced to a focus on the reproductive body, perpetuating the old dominant concern with reproduction of the colonies.

These data are also unreliable because they do not account for migration. The indicators are created in a way that imagines postcolonial, semi-sovereign nations like the FSM as communities in which people stay in their home spaces. Thus, the reproductive health of Chuukese women who migrate to Guam may suffer because of poverty, inadequate health care, and gender inequalities they endured in Chuuk first. However, if they get to Guam before birthing, they are not included in any standard Chuuk-based measures.

MIGRATING TO SAFETY

Mary was very grateful for the biomedicine she had access to in Chuuk, but she also told me she would not do it again. Since her daughters had been born in the early 2000s, the hospital had deteriorated significantly. She said that if she were in Chuuk while pregnant again, she would go to Guam or Hawai'i to give birth. Pamela, a thirty-nine-year-old woman from the western islands, gave birth in Chuuk State Hospital for her first baby thirteen years before we spoke and told me she would not do so again by choice: "Yeah in Chuuk it's just like, they're just like, I don't know." She laughed, paused, and then continued: "In Chuuk it's scary. . . . In Chuuk they really [do] not know anything" (Smith 2019a, 349). Maureen, a sixty-year-old woman from Fááyichuuk, told me she was admitted to the hospital recently and was disgusted by the place, asking to go home. She and I commiserated over the cats meowing and fighting in the walls and ceilings as they sought out the rats that were all over the place. I told her about my first experience in the room where women labored collectively before they were moved into the active labor room, and the very large rats running around the barrels of water (used for flushing and cleaning when the tap water was shut off, which was most of the day). Some women complained about the tired and unhelpful medical staff, although Kaylyn was sympathetic: "I'm guessing it's, you know, without the resources, really, what the hell can you do? You know? . . . I mean you can only do so much. I mean who is going to take pride in working in an environment like that?" Other women had heard too many stories of mothers and babies who died in Chuuk State Hospital. They did not know or care to hear about the metrics of development agencies; they heard enough stories to know not to trust biomedicine in Chuuk.

This did not mean that most women thought home was a better choice for birthing.[27] While adolescents hiding their pregnancies often birthed in remote villages (McMillan et al. 2020), the women I interviewed were usually privileged enough to migrate, and their concerns about the hospital meant they wanted to leave Chuuk for care. Although biomedicine had deteriorated in Chuuk, the women did not lose faith in biotechnology and biomedical clinical skills; they just sought more advanced versions of them in Guam and farther abroad. Women perceived safe birthing as getting out of Chuuk, and only those too poor to get out suffered births there—a manifestation of stratified reproduction.

When I worked in the Guam clinics, I regularly met women who first came to the clinic toward the end of their pregnancy because their spouse, parents, or extended family insisted they leave Chuuk to birth someplace safer. Typically, other women I met, like Serena, had collected funds for a one-way ticket and stayed with family. As we would sit in the sterile waiting rooms with nice metal benches, clean floors, white walls, and rows of overhead fluorescent lighting, some told me they planned to leave as soon as the baby's documents were ready for travel; this was simply a birthing trip. Many, however, ended up staying longer than they imagined because, for example, their spouses had gotten jobs and wanted to stay. Other women were already working or schooling abroad when they became pregnant, and most of them felt safer and decided to stay put for prenatal and birth care. Mary's and Rosie's returns to Chuuk when pregnant were exceptions to the norm.

Reproducing the Symbolic Body: Maintaining Traditions in Guam

As more and more women go to Guam and other parts of the United States for birth, they find ways to sustain their traditions. While they cannot be surrounded by kin on familial land, family often come to them. If financially possible, a mother, an aunt, or a sibling or cousin will come to help the mother with the new baby wherever she is living. Further, they continue to practice lessons learned, such as the importance of birthing without expressing pain through facial expressions or yelling and screaming. Screaming out or demonstrating pain during childbirth is said to bring great shame and potentially harm the child.[28] I frequently encountered young women in the clinics who told me about their mothers' advice (or pressure) to be brave (through silence) with every discomfort while coaching them about their first birth. Siera described her experiences at GMH and how her grandmother lectured her as she was in labor:

> I was breathing hard and complaining of the pain and my grandmother said, "I don't want to see your face like [that], crying. Be strong!" . . . In the morning, the nurse checked on me and I was fully dilated. She said: "How come we didn't hear you screaming?" I told her, "Well I'm not supposed to scream, because I'm a lady." Back home, I remember when ladies would scream out, people would say, "Oh, don't, don't be like them," and people with the woman would scold her, saying things like, "Who told you to open your legs?" The nurse at GMH was surprised by me being quiet, but I was surprised all the other ladies [giving birth in GMH that night] were screaming like that.

Praise's mother told her screaming is shameful and shows weakness. Women are also told that if they can handle sex, then they can handle the pain of childbirth. Essentially, they are taught that the pain of childbirth is a punishment for their sexual activity, likely reflecting Christian missionary teachings about Eve's punishment for eating from the tree of knowledge, combined with earlier values of endurance and fortitude. Women like Siera who did not scream during labor were very proud of themselves. Those who did were scolded in the moment and were mocked by family members.

Siera and several other women lived in Guam long enough to recognize the cultural differences in birth experiences by the time we spoke, including the observation that some women from other cultural backgrounds express their pain loudly. They explained to me that silence is a Chuukese thing. Alternatively, younger Chuukese women who had recently migrated for college were bemused by the American movies they saw in which women screamed or cried out during pregnancy. We discussed this difference in gender studies courses I taught at UOG.

Healthcare workers told me they are aware of and bewildered by this practice. Many asked me why women stayed silent and complained to me that they could not gauge Chuukese women's needs as a result. When birthing at GMH, several women reported that the nurses often did not know how bad their pain was because they were silent. Kaylyn and Glorida explained that they were quiet for hours and felt ignored at GMH. They learned that the screamers got attention, and thereafter, they followed suit.

Silence was not the only thing Chuukese women are known for in Guam. Despite their attempts to keep it secret, providers know and complain about Chuukese women in Guam delaying clinic care while using local medicine (Hattori-Uchima 2017). They are also regarded as late arrivals to the hospital. One healthcare worker told me Chuukese women have "amazing pelvises." She said, "They just wiggle their toes and oh! There's a baby." My initial reaction to this comment was how racialized their pregnant bodies are to these healthcare workers, as if their pelvises are unique. As I spoke to more and more Chuukese women in the clinics, I started to learn how proud they are of being good at giving birth, particularly in knowing when it is time to seek care, which to them is when they are ready to push. Several women, like Pamela, proudly told me they knew by baby three or four exactly when to get to GMH to push out the baby. She told me about her second and third births: "The second time, I just went to GMH, maybe just one hour. But my third one? Just go there, 8:05, 8:10 and then out. Just go straight." I clarified what she meant by "straight": "But you had the pains [early contractions] at home?" "Yeah, I just waited at home," she said, "and, like, just only five minutes apart, that's when I asked my cousin to drive me." Laughing, she told me, "That's why we just . . . We go into the emergency room, and I just push like this." She imitated how she was breathing and pushing and told me, "And they are like, 'What's your birthday?' and I'm pushing!" Imitating her breathing exercises at the time, she yelled, "February 12!" Pamela and I laughed at the absurdity of birthing while completing paperwork, and she concluded, "That's why we really need to go register, before."

Pamela intentionally arrived just in time to push the baby out for her third birth. She explained that GMH expected pregnant people to register long before the due date, but registration is complicated. Registration is not too difficult for those with insurance if they can find the time and transportation to be present at the hospital. But people who are uninsured are expected to make a down payment of over $2,000 to register. If they have bills due from previous care, these bills must be paid before registering. When women are uninsured, lack the cash, and may be indebted to GMH already, they cannot register before and must check in while in labor, delaying access to prenatal records and imminent medical needs, thus increasing their vulnerability for poor outcomes.

Surveilling Reproductive Bodies in the Affected Jurisdictions

Guam and other U.S. territories are expected to maintain metrics on reproductive health outcomes. What they reveal is that while women migrate to seek better care, their reproductive health outcomes remain stratified. As described in the introduction, Chuukese women have almost double the rate of cesarean sections and suffer more pregnancies with untreated gestational diabetes when compared to the rest of Guam's residents (Alur et al. 2002).[29] A retrospective study of maternal mortality in Guam from 1968 to 2018 through a review of death certificates revealed that Chuukese women represented 16 percent of all maternal deaths during that period (Gay 2020). This is despite the fact that they did not make up a substantive proportion of the population until after 1986, and even today, they represent only about 7 percent of Guam residents. Further, even with lower overall rates in Guam, infant mortalities are disproportionately high in the Chuukese community: in 2014, Chuukese women suffered 21.4 percent of the islands' infant mortalities and 60 percent of all fetal deaths (Government of Guam 2017). A study measuring births from 2013 to 2019 in Guam found that Chuukese women accounted for more than 39 percent of all fetal deaths (Gay 2020).

Researchers and clinicians report similar outcomes in Chuukese communities of the Commonwealth of the Northern Mariana Islands (CNMI) and Hawai'i. Fox and Parker (2005) found that Micronesian women are more likely to have stillbirths than the rest of the CNMI. Researchers in Hawai'i report concerns about pregnancy complications, low birth weight, high infant mortality rates, and low immunization rates (Pobutsky, Krupitsky, and Yamada 2009), all of which demonstrate limited access to care and follow-up. One study demonstrated that Chuukese women had the highest rate of cesarean sections in Hawai'i; other Pacific Islander groups have higher rates of unmanaged gestational diabetes and hypertension yet fewer cesarean sections (Chang et al. 2015).[30] Another study found an increased risk for cesarean in non-English speakers—43 percent of whom spoke a Micronesian language—when compared to English speakers (Sentell et al. 2016). An in-depth examination of why these disparities exist revealed the perspectives of obstetricians in Hawai'i, which indicated that communication barriers, stoicism while birthing (which led to missed signs of complications), familial involvement in decision-making, and racism were likely factors contributing to the disproportionate rate of cesarean sections (Delafield et al. 2020). A chart review revealed the ways in which obstetricians react to these dynamics; Micronesian women are more likely than white women to have cesarean sections for what are deemed subjective indicators (Delafield et al. 2021).[31] Thus, women are not always safer when they migrate for higher-technology care.

Researchers and clinicians often blame Chuukese women for these poor outcomes, citing their lack of prenatal care.[32] Many women do delay prenatal care until late in their pregnancy (e.g., the second or third trimester). Some Chuukese women told me they feel like they already know how to manage pregnancy and birth after the first time and thus do not see the need for care. But others—many of whom I followed in clinics—were getting care. Moreover, some women who had just migrated received prenatal care in Chuuk, but the records do not easily transfer from Chuuk to Guam. Finally, some want prenatal care and struggle to get into the healthcare system. Rarely do healthcare workers discuss how Chuukese women face anti-immigrant sentiment and the structural factors influencing their access to care.[33] As I discuss further in chapter 6, several barriers to care, such as language proficiency, transportation, and limited insurance, plus poor treatment in obstetric settings, contribute to their delayed care seeking and thus poor maternal health outcomes. These effects present themselves not just in maternal and infant morbidity and mortality but in women's other sexual health outcomes, such as contraceptive decision-making and access, sexual and bodily autonomy in heterosexual marriages, and sexually transmitted infections. I turn to these issues in chapter 5.

5 • DISCOURSES OF IMPERIAL SEXUALITY

> Yeah. I didn't wanna have a baby, I was just trying to find a way to get out.... Either come back here [Chuuk] or go to school. It was late. I was trying all possible ways. They said if you drink a lot of soy sauce then it will kill them. Or if you take medication that will. I tried both. They didn't work. And I was thinking God won't allow me to do bad things.... I couldn't take soy sauce for how many months after that. The smell... (Maureen)

Maureen scrunched her face and shifted in her chair as she told me this story, remembering the nausea she associated with soy sauce, and the pain of having to manage an unwanted pregnancy. We were sitting at the kitchenette in my temporary apartment in Chuuk, cooling off in the air conditioning I was privileged to have in this dark, dank efficiency space typically reserved for Truk Stop Hotel contract workers from the Philippines. I got up to make us instant coffee, a staple in Chuuk, giving her a minute to process her feelings. After boiling the water and spooning in the dark powder, I brought the cups over to the little table. She shifted in her chair and thanked me for the coffee, stirring in the Carnation milk and sugar. I also brought over Chuukese donuts, a semisweet doughy delight fried daily by families all over Chuuk, some of which are sold on the main street in the mornings. I like to dip them in my coffee instead of using sweetener; she laughed at my odd choice, and then tried it herself. Maureen rarely laughed; she was a reserved, serious, and strong-minded woman. Educated in the United States and very confident and powerful in her age (sixty) and education levels, Maureen preferred to make eye contact as she told me her life story, contradicting stereotypes about Chuukese women as submissive or quiet. After finishing our donuts, she continued, coffee cup in hand, to tell me of her painful experience of reluctantly becoming a new mother; she knew that her husband was already cheating in that first year of their marriage.

Maureen identified staunchly as Catholic. She attended church every week and cited religion as the guiding force in all her decisions, but that did not stop her from attempting to terminate an unwanted pregnancy when she found herself in a bad relationship. Like so many women in the world, she did everything she could to abort her fetus. Abortions at clinics or hospitals were not accessible in Chuuk at the time (nor are they now), so her only options were to try methods she had heard about from other women, like drinking a bottle of soy sauce or swallowing an entire bottle of antibiotics or ibuprofen—essentially taking whatever was available. None worked, and she felt she had no choice but to accept the pregnancy. Her story, and those of other women, are typical throughout the world, but as described in chapter 2, they are not consistent with anthropological narratives about women and reproduction in Chuuk.

CONTROL OVER PLANNING THE FAMILY

Older anthropological accounts and my more recent conversations with clinicians reveal a common assumption that all Chuukese women desire many children. But not every pregnancy is intended or desired. When I interviewed women in the clinics about planning their families, most wanted two to four well-spaced-out children (although some wanted more or less).

To prevent pregnancies, women were advised by elders and local practitioners not to have sex during the first year of the baby's life because spirits could make the baby sick (with diarrhea or sluggishness). Women told me they clearly understood that this rule was also a good family planning measure. While complete sex avoidance was what older female kin conventionally recommended, it was rarely practiced for the full period, partly to reduce the chances of their husbands' infidelity. Several women tried the calendar method, avoiding sex on certain days of the month after learning of this from family planning professionals and Catholic leaders in Chuuk and Guam. This, of course, depended on husbands agreeing to not have sex on the days when they were ovulating. Women told me stories of relatives with husbands who got angry and forced sex on their partners. Jessica, for example, told me about her aunt's husband ripping up the actual calendar and demanding sex. When she told Jessica the next day, they both laughed.

Women also recognized that breastfeeding offers some protective benefits. Historically, women breastfeed for about a year, or when babies begin to walk.[1] Most women told me they breastfed all their children, but not exclusively; those who used formula—accessible through the Women, Infants and Children supplemental nutrition program in Guam—typically did so because they had to return to work. Working and formula needs were much less common in Chuuk, but when breastfeeding was not an option, some babies were fed with canned milk (which was discouraged by public health practitioners), and others were breastfed by alternative nursing family members. In Guam, healthcare and STI prevention workers discouraged the practice, often citing concerns about HIV, but they also conveyed disdain over what they saw as a "backward" cultural practice.

BIOMEDICAL CONTRACEPTION

According to UNICEF, the 2015 contraceptive prevalence rate in Chuuk was 55 percent, somewhat higher than elsewhere in Micronesia. More recent attempts to assess this rate and the unmet need for family planning by the Centers for Disease Control and Prevention (CDC) were unsuccessful because the data were not reported consistently or uniformly, and even if these data had been available in this study (as in other COFA nations), researchers note that these data were for married women only (Green et al. 2020). These measures indicate the existence of contraceptive devices at Chuuk's public health office but not how they are accessed. Green and colleagues (2020) interviewed leaders across the U.S.-associated Pacific Islands about contraception access and found that transportation, limited contraceptive provision sites, and a small number of providers trained to provide contraception were all barriers to access. I found these also to be barriers in Chuuk and Guam, related to gender inequities and stereotypes fostered by healthcare workers. This is another reason why metrics like "contraceptive prevalence" or "unmet need for family planning" do not reflect reality in smaller under-resourced countries such as the FSM, or in non-sovereign territories like Guam.

Healthcare workers often perceived Chuukese women as not wanting to use family planning methods and choosing to have several children;[2] because of these perceptions, some did not bother to provide family planning education. The discussion of high fertility was noticeable at every level of the clinics, as healthcare workers talked about their frequent "repeat customers," whom they "just saw in here nine months ago!"[3] Margot, a Guam healthcare worker who would regularly seek me out to tell me more of her (racist) perspectives of Chuukese women, told me: "We need to educate them that family planning is important. . . . That's why, you see, right after they give birth after three months, they are pregnant again. . . . It's like come on, seven kids already? Probably sometimes at three or four [kids], we try to put it in their mind that OK, life now is very hard, you need to plan." Her perceptions of Chuukese women colored her treatment. I watched her speak to patients with a dismissive tone and lecture them in ways that were demeaning or inappropriate for her role as a health provider. In one example, I witnessed Margot complete a standard intake form. She had a clipboard and did not look up once as she asked the patient questions from the form. She started with "Did you want this pregnancy?" and the patient replied, "Oh, yes." Then Margot asked, "Who lives with you?" The woman started to say her sister, and then before she could list other household members, Margot interrupted and said, "You've got plenty [of] kids there, right? And you get food stamps?"

In another example, Margot lectured a young woman about how she should mother her child. First, she asked the patient about her own childhood, and the woman indicated that she quit school and started working around the house at eleven to help her mom. Margot then said, "So what are you going to do to make your baby's life better?" The patient hesitated, then responded: "Well, I'm going to work two jobs, work very hard." Margot replied, "That's good. . . . Well, keep working. Just because you are pregnant doesn't mean you don't work." She then began lecturing the woman about using birth control to prevent having another baby. These kinds of encounters influenced how comfortable Chuukese women were when speaking with providers about family planning; some told me of bad experiences that made them fearful of discussing it even with those who did treat them with respect.

Healthcare workers' perceptions of Chuukese women in Chuuk and Guam contradicted women's own stories of seeking to plan their families. Some told me about local herbal remedies they heard of from elders, but these stories were rare. Most women used biomedical methods of birth control, such as hormonal contraception. Jevlyn used the injectable depot medroxyprogesterone acetate, and Jessica, Norita, and Glorida used birth control pills at one point, although not for more than a few years. Glorida and Kaylyn used arm implants, and Mary had an IUD. These methods were available in clinics in Chuuk and Guam, some since the navy-installed clinics in the USTTPI days (see also Caughey 1971). Now the CDC provides technical assistance and funding to support family planning methods in both places, revealing the continued non-sovereign circumstances of their health systems. However, while Guam is limited to FDA-approved family planning methods because of its official status as part of the United States, Chuuk is not and is thus able to source some methods through international aid networks instead.

The women using pills and the shot often stopped rather quickly because of side effects. Those who did not use them chose not to because of stories of relatives who had had bad experiences. One woman told me, "They say it's not good, the shot . . . because [it] makes them . . . fat, and they're, like, dark, their skin, and their hair, oily or lost." Women were especially hesitant to use long-acting methods such as implants and IUDs, which they could not control themselves, after hearing stories of healthcare workers in Chuuk refusing to remove them upon request. And I did witness a woman request to have one out a few months after insertion due to bad side effects; she was told to wait longer to see if it got better. The provider then walked away and told me it made her angry that these women wanted to waste state funds removing the devices so soon after getting them. When healthcare providers in Chuuk and Guam pressured women to use a method over which they had control, like pills or the patch, some would accept it but then not use it.

While some told me they avoided contraception in the past for these reasons, I regularly met pregnant women who were reconsidering their stance. Women visiting the clinics for an unintended pregnancy complained to me about their lack of success using abstinence as family planning, like Sheila, a twenty-two-year-old mother: "When I gave birth to my first daughter, my first baby, the doctor asked me if I wanted to take birth control, but I told him I can control myself . . . and then I get pregnant again. I wasn't planning on taking it, but now." Women would reluctantly look at their swollen bellies, telling me they were done having babies and frustrated they were back at the clinic for a new pregnancy. While we sat in a sterile patient room and chatted, waiting for a nurse midwife, nurse practitioner, or physician, women often asked me to help them make plans to prevent future pregnancies—that is, if they had not already decided on sterilization (typically via postpartum tubal ligation), the most common family planning practice. Pregnant women in the clinics asked daily for the consent forms that need to be signed sixty days before the procedure so that they could have it done when they gave birth.

At the same time, women were not always able to make decisions about whether to use contraception. Some told me their husbands wanted even more children, and they "had to respect his decision"; they did not feel they had a choice. One woman told me, as we waited for her prenatal provider, "He wants to have lots of children. I mean, I raised like two of my nephews and I never planned on having children . . . but my boyfriend wants [them], so I'm like, 'OK, one is good,' and he's like, 'Maybe five?' I'm like, 'Oh my goodness.'" She had not yet figured out how to negotiate him down but hoped to come to a smaller number. Some women reported that husbands say, "As many as God wants"; other men, and women, aim for a few more males or females before considering their family complete.

Mothers and mothers-in-law play a very active role in family planning decision-making. Jasmine told me her mother would yell at her to get pregnant again right after she recovered from her previous pregnancy; in contrast, Praise's mother would be frustrated with her if she got pregnant too quickly, adamant that she should practice abstinence to space her pregnancies. Both women, however, had mothers dictating their reproductive practices. When I talked about this to the more attentive healthcare workers, like Mike, they recognized the role of others in a woman's decision to plan her family. "Not even, not even just their spouse; I have grown women in their thirties come back and say they quit taking birth control because their mother told them to stop."[4] One woman told me her mother said she "needs to get something to stop having babies. Not so fast." Another woman told me, "I talked to my mom about it, but she said if I cannot control it by, like, myself, then I should take the medicine, birth control."

English proficiency gives others the opportunity to make decisions for women, as partners and other family members providing translation for a woman at a clinic may sometimes simply make the choice. I saw women refusing birth control their family negotiated for them—thus, some did have agency—but I also watched as many observed the conversation and waited to be told what to do.

Women who may consider birth control secretly could be inhibited by their lack of English proficiency, and translation at the clinics is fraught with difficulties (see chapter 6). However, some women who understand English use this to their advantage, getting or refusing birth control and hiding this from mothers and husbands.

English proficiency is an issue in both Chuuk and Guam, as in both places, healthcare providers are not typically Chuukese language speakers. While the prenatal provider in Chuuk did not speak fluent Chuukese at the time of my research, the family planning director did, and this could have been advantageous. However, I was told that the family planning office informally requires a husband's permission to give women birth control. The office staff felt this was necessary after a few incidents when husbands learned their wives were using contraception and threatened the healthcare workers who prescribed it.

These access and decision-making issues apply to married women. Adolescent and other unmarried women are typically given no sex education beyond being told to abstain from sex. They are often too scared to seek advice from public clinics; the sight of them walking into the family planning room of Chuuk's or Guam's public health office is bound to get back to their families (see also McMillan et al. 2020). Many unintended pregnancies among adolescent women occur before they learn about contraceptives, but even if they are aware, they do not seek them out (McMillan et al. 2020). Condoms are free and always available in Chuuk's and Guam's STI clinics, but again, being seen getting them is more than a woman can risk; condoms are associated with sex before or outside marriage. Thus, surveillance of women's bodies is a key barrier to access to family planning care.

Because women often do not have control over preventing pregnancies, some, like Maureen, attempt abortions. Ann Fischer (1963) argued that abortion and infanticide are absent as concepts in Chuukese communities.[5] This is still a common stereotype of Pacific societies. Trust territory anthropologists Thomas Gladwin and Seymour B. Sarason (1953) indicated that abortions used to happen, but at the time of their writing (and from the perspective of their male-centered research), this was no longer the case. However, every woman I spoke with had either attempted or knew someone who had attempted an abortion. Most of the stories I heard from women (about others) involved girls who were pregnant when they were not married. Some sought out older women in the community who knew of local medicine and specific plants that are said to be effective in terminating an early pregnancy. Massage often plays a big role in the local remedies, and women explained that this included the application of a very hot cloth, sand, or other materials to the woman's abdomen. Other women said that they had never heard of local medicines to do this; rather, they had heard of attempting to overdose on medicine accessible to them, like ampicillin, Motrin, and aspirin, as Maureen described. Karen McMillan and colleagues

(2020) found that most adolescent women in Chuuk did not know there were biomedical methods of abortion.

Desperate women and girls go to great lengths to avoid the shame directed at them from their families and communities for unintended pregnancies, including attempting unsafe abortions, and some women told me stories of girls dying as a result. Praise shared one story of a college student who came home pregnant. Her mother did not want her to be pregnant; they attempted an abortion, and the young woman died. Mothers are often held responsible for their adolescent daughters' unintended pregnancies, and both the pregnant daughter and her mother may risk verbal and physical abuse if her father learns of the pregnancy (McMillan et al. 2020). It is often in the best interest of mothers to help their daughters seek an abortion or, at times, to practice infanticide (McMillan et al. 2020). Every few years, a newborn is found, sometimes dead, sometimes still alive, born and left somewhere in the jungle, the lagoon, or a dumpster.

The easier and safer option would be biomedical abortion, but it is not legal in Chuuk and is constantly being contested in heavily Catholic Guam. Guam was one of the first U.S. jurisdictions to try to challenge *Roe v. Wade*.[6] Those introducing anti-abortion legislation in Guam did so in the name of protecting Chamoru-Catholic values, often standing on the opposite side of their own family members, who were fighting to protect the right to an abortion in Guam using Chamoru anticolonial narratives (Dames 2003). While the challenge failed and *Roe v. Wade* ultimately protected access to abortion in Guam from 1973 to 2022, only one or two abortion providers were present on the island at any given time. In 2018, the only abortion provider retired, and so it was impossible to get an abortion until September 2021, when telehealth medication abortion appointments became available (J. Taitano 2022a).[7] It is thus difficult to procure a biomedical abortion in Guam, and only one woman I spoke with had had one, and that was in the 1990s. Since the *Dobbs* decision came down in June 2022, the Guam Senate has already tried to outlaw abortion. In December 2022, it passed the Guam Heartbeat Act, which was vetoed by the governor (J. Taitano 2022c).[8] A local group called Famalao'an Rights (https://www.famalaoanrights.org/) has organized extensively in recent years, working with local and national partners to protect abortion rights, but the future of abortion access in Guam remains in flux (Hofschneider 2022). These U.S. Supreme Court decisions—both to uphold the right to abortion in 1973 and to strike it down in 2022—demonstrate another manifestation of Guam's non-sovereign status: the people of Guam are forced to adhere to whatever decisions are made for U.S. soil, whether they improve or stratify women's health.

Another common family planning practice is adoption and fosterage, which is described extensively in the anthropological literature for Chuuk and greater Micronesia. Adoption is used to help women who experience infertility, to bring together two families, and to care for children of young mothers who are not ready to raise children or who have two children very close together (Marshall

1976; Rauchholz 2008, 2012). Older women in the family, such as grandmothers and aunts, or cousins without their own children, are most likely to adopt. Fostering can last for a few years or for their entire lives (Marshall 1976). Several women I interviewed were adopted (or fostered) and raised by grandmothers or aunts, returning later in life to live with their birth parents. For some, it worked very well; for others, like Jevlyn, it led to a tumultuous relationship between her birth parents and her adoptive parents.

As mentioned in chapter 3, several women told me they had left their toddlers with their mothers in Chuuk (at their mother's insistence) for a few years while they worked, went to school, or became accustomed to a newer baby in Guam. For most women, mothers and husbands control their offspring as much as they control their decisions about family planning. Some, however, successfully resist their mothers' demands to care for their children if they live in a different state or territory than their mothers.

The lack of decision-making power over family planning these women experience leaves them vulnerable to unintended pregnancies and unsafe abortions. This means that more unintended pregnancies happen, and some are hidden for months, delaying or inhibiting access to safe abortion or prenatal care. Delayed access to care has implications for treating various health conditions, including pre-eclampsia, gestational diabetes, and untreated STIs that harm women and their pregnancies, further stratifying their reproduction and rendering their bodies vulnerable to poor outcomes. Control over family planning is not the only way in which women are made vulnerable to poor health outcomes, nor is it the only way in which they are coerced and controlled by their mothers and spouses. Heterosexual marriages also contribute to women's vulnerabilities to poor reproductive and sexual health outcomes through assault, coercion, and husbands' extramarital sexual relationships.

MARRIAGE AS A DETERMINANT OF REPRODUCTIVE AND SEXUAL HEALTH

Nelly was a fifty-eight-year-old Chuukese woman who had lived in Guam since the 1990s; she contracted an STI many years ago when still living in Chuuk with her husband. She told me this story as we found some privacy on her porch—the carport of her concrete home in the village of Dededo. Her husband was napping inside, enjoying his newfound retirement, and her grandkids—who also lived with them—were off at school. As we sweated on this hot and humid Guam day, listening to the constant daily buzz of weed-trimmer engines in the distance, Nelly told me with frustrated laughter about the incident. She was experiencing back pain and difficulty with her bowel movements, so she went to the doctor. After some testing, the doctor told Nelly she had contracted an STI (she could not remember the name). The doctor did not ask Nelly if she had other sexual partners. Instead, he asked her if her husband did and instructed her to bring her husband in to get medicine and provide a list of sexual partners. Her husband complied, and she read through his list, shocked. She knew he had extramarital sexual relations, but she did not think it was so frequent or so close to home. Some of her extended relatives were on the list. Nelly told me she scolded him and implored him to stop because he was now bringing home STIs. Nelly felt that he was ashamed and really did stop for a while. But when he moved to Guam to set things up for the two of them, Nelly explained, he had a whole new group of women to pursue. Some of the women I interviewed told me their husbands never stopped pursuing romance; once married, several of these men focused on other women, including their wives' family members.

A common way that relatives are pursued in Guam is when a younger woman flies in from Chuuk to assist with childcare or some other need, and sexual relations occur between this relative and the woman's husband. Jasmine explained: "Sometimes, when the family is here [Guam], the older sister buys the ticket for the younger sister to come and take care of her children because she's going to work, and the sister will stay with the children. The husband makes the younger sister pregnant. So now the [older] sister, she's really having [a] hard time trying to, find ways to remove her sister but the husband is the one who keeps holding on to the sister. So the wife, I can tell [you] that, she's really suffering, but she has no choice." This was the case for Jevlyn, Siera, and Maureen. For Jevlyn, the first time this happened, her husband left her for her sister (the visiting relative); the second time (with her second husband), the young woman was her cousin and was asked to leave when she became pregnant. Siera's and Maureen's partners had affairs with their sisters and cousins at different points when they stayed in their house, but it did not end the marriages. It is unclear how often these new housemates—primarily younger women relatives—consent or are coerced into sexual relations.

Women acknowledged that this happens in Chuuk too. Migration does not create this practice; it only shifts the power relations and spaces in which it occurs. Many women pointed to historical circumstances in which siblings shared sex partners.[9] These practices may still occur in some families. Glorida explained: "I grew [up] with that knowledge that it's permissible. It's disgusting, but we just allow it, 'cause what can we do? The Chuukese woman [would] rather share the husband with a sister than a stranger. The pain is less." Jasmine explained her mother's and uncle's lessons about this: "She keep saying, it's you, it's part of the norm of the man to keep sneaking from one woman to another to another to another. At the same time, in our culture, it's also allowed . . . to sneak into the sister of his wife, the cousin of his wife. . . . My uncle [said] . . . you know they call it 'spare.'" Several women, including Jasmine, reported that they do not approve of this and reject some men's use of culture as an excuse to engage in this practice. Cases clearly outline the gendered element of who can pursue extramarital liaisons in the family—men.

Other affairs happened outside families. Siera's husband had multiple affairs; some upset her—particularly when they were members of her family—but most were not in the family and unimportant to her. She thought of these as silly male pursuits. Siera told me her husband and his male cousins would sit around and gossip about boastful or arrogant women,[10] and her husband would ask her if he could have sex with such women. He would say: "Can I go and just take her out so she can shut her mouth?" Siera explained that in this case, "boastful" means that the woman had been gossiping about her husband liking her or had said bad things about their family. If a woman is perceived to be gossiping about a man or his wife, such as talking about how much a man wants her, the goal is to have sex with her so that everyone is clear about who wants whom. She further explained that a husband would have sex with such a woman and then come home and report his sexual activities to his wife. The wife then has power over this woman because her husband's description of the woman's body and sexual practices are in her masowen na sàngà (basket of things). Having this knowledge gives the wife power over a woman's secrets, to be used against her were she ever to disrespect the wife. This practice centers on shame as a goal—not a consequence—of the sexual encounter, and places women, as wives, as complicit in controlling and shaming other women's sexuality. Kaylyn grew up among many aunties who enjoyed the power it gave them: "Those women they take pride of the masowen na sàngà? Sàngà is that sack, you know? The ugly truth about how ugly your vagina is." She laughed and continued: "Or how stinky you are in that woman's sack." She and several younger women see how this practice reflects a woman's place: how she is expected to behave, and how she will be treated if she falls out of line. They do not approve of or support it in their marriages, reflecting again the complexity and fluidity of any practices within a community.

Shaming women into silence through sex does not just include collusion with wives but often the use of love magic, and several women told me they had become victims of love magic after talking back to a man, which concluded in the woman and this man having an affair.[11] Women rarely had extramarital affairs, and few knew of other women who had consensual affairs. Only two married women admitted to having affairs without blaming love magic. When I asked why, they pointed to shame. Praise said, "Maybe they're ashamed. But I think . . . it happens you know. Even especially when there's problems . . . just to, you know, ease . . . the pain [of the husband's affairs] I think. . . . But a lot [have affairs for] revenge [too]." Others said they were advised not to do so by their mothers. When Jasmine sought counseling for her marital problems and her husband's fourth open affair, her priest told her to be patient. He also told her that if she had affairs, she would encourage her daughters to do the same. Her mother offered similar advice.

Some women reported that their husbands suspected they had affairs and were possessive, jealous, and violent as a result. This contradictory way in which women and men are treated for extramarital affairs was articulated by some women with frustration. Eryna, a forty-eight-year-old woman from the Southern Nómwoneyas region of Chuuk, said her husband abused her early in their relationship over men calling on her. When men came around the house, he assumed she was having affairs and would leave, quiet and angry. He would return later that night, drunk, and physically harm her. She told me that when they made their marriage church-official several months later, he stopped drinking, and the abuse stopped as well.

Jasmine, frustrated with her mother's and priest's advice to never have an extramarital sexual relationship despite her husband's multiple partners, rejected the double standard. She asked what women the men were having affairs with if women did not engage in this practice, too. She never got a clear answer, but she thought that women have just as many affairs and are simply punished in much greater ways when caught. Kaylyn agreed, telling me she thought affairs were equally distributed, but "we won't really talk about the woman," whereas "the male, you know . . . we're very open to talk about it." Praise complained, "It's like they [men] are competing [in] how many girls they sleep with," and they gossip to each other afterward. All of these affairs, secretive or open, leave women vulnerable to STIs.

Surveilling Sexually Transmitted Infections

Nelly was the only woman I spoke with outside a clinic setting who openly shared her experience of being infected with an STI from her husband, but several women who sought prenatal care or family planning in Guam also discovered they had STIs when I was with them. Researchers and practitioners find STIs in Chuukese migrant communities to be disproportionately high when compared to host and other communities.[12] STI patterns in Chuuk and Guam are similar to those in the United States. Because migration to and from the States is much easier than it is with other countries, epidemiological profiles for communicable diseases reflect this migration access point.

When I asked women about their concerns regarding STIs, they expressed little knowledge or understanding of the effects on their bodies and had misconceptions about how they are spread. When Jessica and I were talking about her late husband's sexual partners, I asked her if she had been concerned about him bringing home STIs when he was still alive. Jessica said, "AIDS? Yeah, that's the one . . . scary, eh? . . . I don't want to sleep with him when he just came from another woman, you know?" Jessica proceeded to tell me that she argued with him and made him sleep elsewhere for a few nights to protect herself. I had a similar conversation with Siera. She told me she always scolded and lectured her now deceased husband that he needed to think about AIDS when he was with another person.

Women did not mention condoms and testing as strategies to protect themselves, although I ultimately asked about them during life history and family

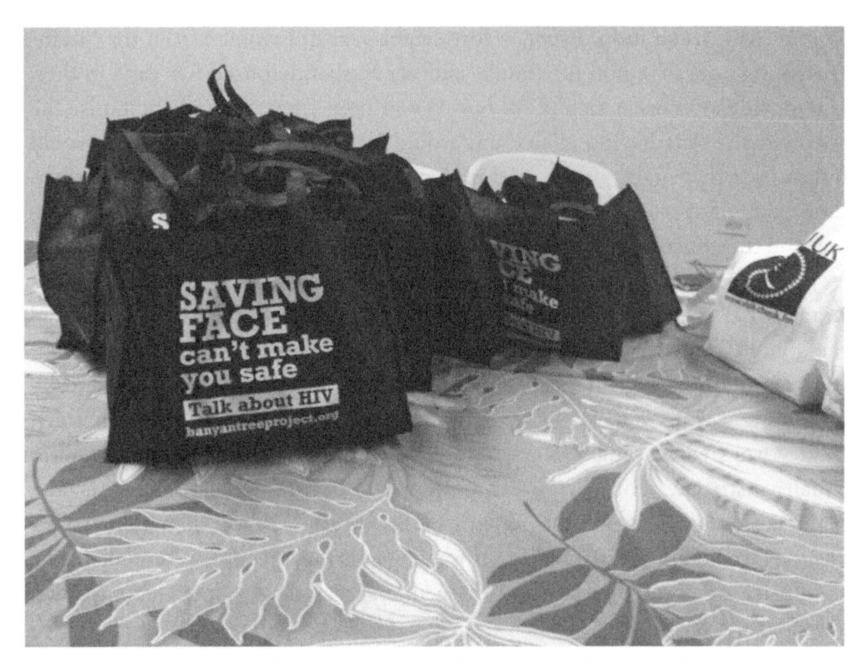
SAVING
FACE
can't make
you safe
Talk about HIV
banyantreeproject.org

FIGURE 16. Giveaway bags for pregnant women depicting HIV-stigma-reduction messages. Photo by Sarah Smith.

planning interviews.[13] A few survey-based studies indicate that condom use in Chuuk is minimal, with about half the people reporting ever using a condom.[14] This is likely due in part to the power women lack in heterosexual relationships to request condom use, and in part because of an association of condoms with unsanctioned sexual activity.

No women could name an STI besides AIDS. One research group studied HIV-risk behavior among Chuukese people aged thirteen to seventy-four after the first two locally transmitted cases were identified. They found that 72 percent of participants thought persons infected with HIV deserved it, and they were afraid of them; 58 percent of participants thought that persons with HIV should be imprisoned (Russell et al. 2007). As Jennifer Hirsch and colleagues (2009) report elsewhere, efforts to prevent HIV/AIDS in these communities are well funded by international donors, while STIs endemic to the community—but less globally visible—such as chlamydia, are not. HIV/AIDS prevention programming typically includes stigma reduction and testing; I witnessed well-funded projects in which the Chuuk Women's Council was tasked with these goals (see figure 16). In communities where there were few conversations about sexual risks and STIs, these stigma-reduction campaigns instead increased stigma. They alerted the community to the presence of HIV, confirmed the prevailing community view that immoral people contract this virus, and warned that men may bring it home when they have sex with other people.

Testing was rare, too. STIs embody two shameful events, both perceived to stem from moral transgressions: illness and unsanctioned sexual behavior (Mahony 1969). The stigma associated with STIs prevents women from voluntarily seeking care, increasing their vulnerability to poor outcomes. Women feared gossip and rumors spreading if they sought testing—especially in Chuuk, because the public health building is so small and visible. When you enter this building—the same one I described in chapter 4—there are very few reasons to be there: infant immunizations, prenatal care, family planning, and STI testing and treatment are at the top of the list. So even walking into the building may imply that a woman is pregnant or testing for STIs, both of which are indicators of sexual activity. Further, the women told me that when the nurse aides—all of whom were Chuukese—saw them walk into the actual STI testing room, they knew the news would spread. For many, it felt safer to avoid the clinic altogether.

In Guam, most women said that they did not know where to get tested when they suspected they had an STI or when their husband was having extramarital sex. Those who did, however, knew the specific room in the community health centers because of neighborhood gossip about others seen going there.[15] In each public health building, the STD/HIV office is marked by a sign outside its door, visible from hallways and waiting rooms; there is no possibility of sneaking in without being seen. One Chuukese woman who worked in an STD/HIV testing and treatment unit expressed the great shame she felt sneaking into her workplace every morning. This woman, full of energy and excitement over helping her community through public health, told me she had been given the job through an internship program at school. She told me she chose public health "because I thought public health is not STD and HIV yeah? I have totally no idea. First time [I go there] I was like 'what are these things?' Yeah, and really, I feel really uncomfortable talking about those things, especially when I go home. When I step out from that place? Like, going out to, outside the public health? I don't want people to see me!" She stuck it out and eventually started working there in a job full time (instead of as an intern), telling me about this initial fear with her always-infectious laughter. Years later, however, she continued to share discomfort talking to relatives about her job. Additionally, some women told me they felt shame seeking care not just because of the association with sexuality or the likelihood of being found out but also because they did not want to show their genitals to anyone (see also Wong and Kawamoto 2010).

While HIV instilled fear in women, chlamydia, human papilloma virus (HPV), and cervical cancer are of much greater concern to healthcare workers.[16] But in Chuuk, testing for STIs ebbs and flows depending on outside funding mechanisms. Typically, support for testing is through U.S. agencies (such as the

CDC) or international aid organizations. Funding is limited and inconsistent, a product of benign neglect, which means resources for testing are similarly limited and inconsistent. A consequence of these tight budgets through the COFA and international aid organizations is that the Department of Public Health in Chuuk does not typically have the resources for a fully functioning lab. All lab samples must be sent off to a private lab.[17] This lack of resources leads to higher costs for transporting samples, which ultimately reduces even further the ability to test. When I was last in Chuuk (in 2015), tests were not available, but data from the FSM government indicate that tests were available for 2019, and the positivity rate in Chuuk was 15 percent (Government of the FSM 2022a). The main prenatal health provider in Chuuk estimated that about 80 percent of her (prenatal) patients have cervicitis (infection of the cervix), mostly, she believed, caused by chlamydia. Chuuk public health workers presumptively provide antibiotics for chlamydia to all prenatal and occasional gynecological patients, pulling pink pills out of what looked like a candy jar. Pap smears had just been (re)introduced for pregnant women when I was last there, but abnormal results from the entire previous year had not been transmitted to women, and they had not been invited for follow-up. This is despite the finding in 2002 that cervical cancer was the leading cancer in the FSM (Government of the FSM 2004). The most recent data from 2020 indicate that 20 percent of women in Chuuk who get services in the Maternal and Child Health program received a Pap smear, but 2021 data indicate that only 1 percent did—more evidence of inconsistent services year by year. Regardless of Pap smear coverage, there are no providers in Chuuk to treat cervical cancer (Government of the FSM 2022a).

The workers in Guam's STD/HIV bureau expressed similar concerns about the disproportionately high rates of STIs in the Chuukese community, and they target the Chuukese population for much of their outreach work. Because Guam is officially a U.S. territory, it has more funding for regular testing, although it is still insufficient compared to that of the U.S. mainland. Because of these barriers, in concert with structural and clinical barriers, most STIs are identified during prenatal care.[18] One Guam prenatal provider estimated that 50 percent of his Chuukese patients have chlamydia. During my time in the Guam clinics, some women were diagnosed and treated for syphilis and HIV as well, presenting another threat to reproductive health outcomes.

Because most cases are diagnosed for pregnant women, data are unreliable and likely underestimate actual community prevalence. Further, not all pregnant women are tested, in part because not all women receive prenatal care. A 2014 study found that 26.8 percent of all births at GMH were not screened sufficiently early for syphilis to prevent adverse pregnancy outcomes, nor were they screened for HIV infection (31.1%), chlamydia (25.3%), or gonorrhea (25.7%) (Cha et al. 2017). While this study was not limited to Chuukese women, 26 percent of the sample was Chuukese. Prevalence data are therefore limited, but the data that are available yield concerning results. While the ethnic category of "other Micronesians" represented only 11.5 percent of Guam's population in 2016, it constituted 15.7 percent ($n = 147$) of all chlamydia cases in 2016, and 21.8 percent ($n = 214$) of all cases in 2015 (Government of Guam 2017). Micronesians suffer higher proportions of gonorrhea, HIV, and syphilis cases relative to their population in Guam as well (Government of Guam 2017). Knowing Chuukese migrants make up nearly three-quarters of FSM migrants in Guam, these data largely reflect their outcomes.

Hawai'i has seen similar trends. Researchers report disproportionately high rates of chlamydia, gonorrhea, syphilis, and cervical cancer.[19] Vanessa S. Wong and Crissy T. Kawamoto (2010) studied barriers to HPV (the virus that causes cervical cancer) and cervical cancer screening and prevention in Hawai'i (see also Yamada and Pobutsky 2009). When the interviewers asked women what they believed caused cervical cancer, women again spoke of shame as they posited that too much sex or poor hygiene caused it. They knew little about Pap tests, although many did know it was somehow associated with identifying cancer. A different study in Hawai'i found that breast and cervical cancer screening behaviors of women of several ethnic groups (including Chuukese women) were shaped by cultural beliefs, fear of bad news, lack of transportation, competing priorities (such as family obligations and work), and a lack of understanding of why they needed such screenings (Aitaoto et al. 2009). When data were disaggregated, Chuukese and Marshallese women were singled out as more likely than women from other communities to experience problems in English proficiency, economic vulnerabilities, and familial responsibilities.

Like Nelly, other women I followed in Guam asked very few questions when they received a positive STI diagnosis, most often chlamydia, and they received very little education from healthcare workers. I witnessed the delivering of positive test results all the time. A clinic nurse or provider would walk in with a chart and tell the patient she had an STI. The clinic worker would then typically either point to a chart on the wall explaining STIs (in English) or hand the patient a pamphlet about STIs (in English or Chuukese). The patient would remain silent, eyes averted. The healthcare worker would then begin to ask the patient about her male partner and their sexual exploits, telling her that she has an "infection from boyfriend or husband" (generally translated to the vague term rimpio if a Chuukese interpreter is present). Then they would ask if the male partner was present to be treated. When men were there, women would bring them into the room, and they would laugh awkwardly, uncomfortable about the diagnosis. A few times, I watched women look at their partners with great fury in their eyes, but they always remained silent.

Disproportionately high rates of STIs and limited testing and treatment enhance women's vulnerabilities to poor reproductive health outcomes, stratifying their reproduction. Providers indicate that they see babies born with eye problems (likely due to untreated chlamydia, gonorrhea, or syphilis) and that low birth weights and preterm births may be influenced by untreated STIs. The minimal data available are unreliable because of lack of adequate data collection funding or capacity in the region.[20] Epidemiological data highlighting the impact of STIs on birth outcomes—as well as the infertility caused by STIs such as chlamydia—are sorely needed to understand the depth and breadth of this problem.

Enduring Affairs and Violence, and Ending Marriages

Jasmine told me about her first marriage while we sat at her house in the village of Yigo, Guam. Though her house was usually full of her many teen or near-teen children, Jasmine insisted they go outside and play basketball at the nearby community park court so that we could be alone. Basketball is a popular sport among young Micronesian men, and any neighborhood will have a group of players at their community or school courts when the weather allows. I knew her family well; her boys respected her deeply and never questioned her, so they adhered to her directive to get out despite their desire to stay and hang out and play island tunes, as we usually did. We sat outside at her plastic table and chairs to escape the heat of her home—and the ears of her teenage daughter who stayed inside. While her children knew the circumstances of the divorce, she did not want them to hear her rehash the trauma they had all endured, thus wanting privacy. Jasmine prepared betel nut, pulling the leaf, tobacco, and lime powder out of a red and white striped plastic grocery bag (a typical betel nut kit), placed the preparation in her mouth, and settled in. As her three boonie dogs slept under our feet, she began to tell me the story of her first marriage.

Jasmine's marriage was tumultuous from the start. She and her husband, Danny, had a fast romance leading to marriage, and at her mother's insistence, they quickly began having children. Soon after her first birth, Danny had his first affair. He left for his home island and did not come back for months. When he returned, he bragged about his new girlfriend. This happened on a regular basis for years, as they continued to have more children each time they reconciled. But after several affairs and violent fights, Jasmine stopped letting him come back. Her mother told her she needed to accept him back; being a real woman included putting up with men's violence and their affairs: "Are you woman enough to have a family? . . . You have to be strong enough. You have to have that forgiving heart." Jasmine eventually allowed Danny back because of her mother's directive, but she refused to have sex with him. He raped her and blamed her for his use of force: "You hold yourself away from me like, it don't belong to me" (Smith 2019b, 157). Jasmine told me with fury that men like him simply thought their wives were objects to be owned and controlled. Jasmine divorced her husband after some ten more years of violence following that first incident. She explained that as much as she suffered, it took watching Danny hurt someone else and living in Guam (away from family) before she felt she had the right to divorce him.

Several women told me about physical violence they suffered from their husbands or former husbands. Rosie told me about her first husband: "He'd do things. He can even do things in front of my kids. The kids remember 'cause there are times that we, like, go to the motel or hotel in the middle of the night, two o'clock, three o'clock [to get away from him]. I was just lucky at the time that I work at the bank so I have a checkbook I can use . . . for us to, I mean like to check into a motel, hotel, just to sleep for the night." Kaylyn spoke of a brother who was physically violent toward his partner despite the many efforts of their father to intervene. She questioned how he had learned this behavior; she did not recall that her father was ever abusive. She never asked her brother, though, because the taboo between brothers and sisters made it unacceptable for her to talk to her brother about his relationship.

Findings from an FSM National Family Health and Safety Survey yielded similarly troubling results about physical and sexual violence in marriage. Forty-two percent of Chuukese women reported physical violence by their partner in their lifetime (Leon and Mori 2014). In addition, sexual assault and economic coercion were common, though women do not typically report these experiences to friends or family members. Thirty-four percent of Chuukese women reported that they experienced sexual violence by a partner (Leon and Mori 2014). The most common was a woman having sex against her will because she was afraid of how her partner would respond if she refused. For the women sharing their stories with me, this fear was warranted. Rosie would try to refuse sex if she knew her husband had another partner, and he would get angry and hit her. Several women tried to enforce pregnancy and postpartum sexual taboos they learned from their mothers, and an angry spouse would compel them to give in. Jessica never experienced violence but would succumb to sex if she refused the day before in order to keep the peace; she knew an argument would ensue if she said no. Jessica felt that since her husband did not hit her, she needed to respect his sexual desires. One avoidance strategy in Chuuk was to sleep in an all-women house, but this was not typically an option in Guam. For most women I spoke with, resisting or succumbing to unwanted sex was a relatively normal part of marriage, in which husbands are the head of the household.

The idea that husbands are the head of the household is relatively recent in Chuuk, supported by Christian nuclear family ideology. It contradicts Chuukese traditions, in which brothers are heads of extended families within one family compound. Women were taught as young girls that their brothers were the most important men in their lives, and that their kin—elders in particular—oversaw their well-being. Husbands, in contrast, were not very important. Jessica, for example, told me that women were not supposed to take husbands very seriously, since they do not belong to their clan. If a husband acts up, a woman supposedly drops him and gets another with her clan's permission.[21] Older literature also indicated that divorce was common, especially in early marriage, and that lineage oversaw decisions about divorce.[22] This reflects the general assumption of marriage as a contract between families; passionate love was fleeting, not expected to last (Caughey 1971).

When she was fighting with her husband early in her marriage, Jessica's mother told her "Oh nengin [girl], but we already go to church; that's why we cannot separate." Indeed, since missionaries arrived in the mid-nineteenth century, people were told that according to the church, husbands are the leaders of their (nuclear) families, and divorce is unacceptable. While men were previously unimportant in marriage, did not bring children into the clan, and did not inherit land, they gained such power through the imposition of German, Japanese, and then American patriarchal norms during colonization, in collusion with over a century of missionization. Indigenous scholar Myjolynne Kim (2020) argues that the colonial patriarchal system, along with militarization and environmental degradation, devalued many matrilineal practices.

Combining these two narratives, women were told that family elders and males remain the most important leaders in their lives, but listening to husbands is key in the eyes of the church. These opposing rules leave women confused and controlled by even more people, sometimes with contradictory directives. Rosie explained her frustration over this: "So yeah, that's very confusing, like, you respect your husband, but don't listen to him all the time. We [her family] come first." She continued: "[It's] very difficult. I think that's what causes more divorce in Chuuk. Some families break up because of that, 'cause the guy like 'ahh, I'm tired of this, I don't like this, that that family has to come in and ruin things.' . . . And to be honest with you, I'm still in that position until now." Rosie gushed over her kind and thoughtful second husband, but still struggled to negotiate the power dynamics between him and her parents.

Transnational movement resulting from the COFA also leaves women more vulnerable to intimate partner violence. Jan Shoultz and colleagues examined Chuukese women's perceptions of intimate partner violence in Hawai'i and found that women often blame their cultural role as a barrier to seeking help. Since their role in the family is to keep peace—which inevitably means keeping the family in good standing through silent obedience and quiet negotiations—speaking out or bringing attention to family violence is not acceptable (Magnussen et al. 2011; Shoultz et al. 2007). Marriages on family compounds in Chuuk can be mediated by family members when fights or violence occur or become more intense; now, families often live far away in various parts of the United States. Sometimes their family migrates to the same location, but they live in other apartments or houses due to limitations to the number of people allowed in households in U.S. jurisdictions.[23] Further, women are not supposed to discuss their marriages with male kin, yet brothers are expected to protect their sisters when they hear something; this is impossible if they are an ocean away.

Some have also argued that Chuukese women lose power when leaving Chuuk, where connection to their land is so important. This, combined with poverty, unemployment, and expanded access to alcohol, further increases the risks for intimate partner violence.[24] Yet since Chuukese men are already stereotyped as violent, women often do not call the police for help, as they fear contributing to the stigma associated with all Chuukese men in transnational spaces like Guam. Several women in these situations felt unable to leave Guam. Pamela endured an abusive marriage with no money or resources to leave her partner or return to Chuuk. Further, even if women like Pamela can return to Chuuk, they often feel obligated to stay in Guam for their children's education.

Several women, like Jasmine and Rosie, eventually separated or divorced their violent spouses. For some of the more economically advantaged women, mobility aids their efforts to get away. Of the fifteen women who shared their full life histories, nine were separated at some point, and each of these relationships ended with migration—either one spouse returning to Chuuk or the man (or increasingly, the woman) going to Hawai'i or the U.S. mainland, anticipating a family move but never sending for the partner. Pretta's husband left for the U.S. mainland and never sent for her and her kids; she could not afford to go there, so she continued to wait for him for years while listening to gossip about him and his new girlfriend. Some women are separated from their husbands for decades and have a live-in partner but are not officially divorced and remarried because of church doctrine. Transnational separation like this is what the community calls a Micronesian divorce.[25]

Despite these painful experiences, marriages are not all characterized by violence, jealousy, and extramarital affairs. Several women were still married to their first husbands or had found a loving husband the second or third time around; they genuinely enjoyed their relationships with kind, respectful Chuukese men. Many also indicated that the early years of their marriage were tumultuous, but extramarital affairs, possessive jealousy, and sexual violence are the actions of young men; as they aged, their husbands calmed down and respected them. Mary was advised by her relatives to be patient in the early years of her marriage. Others learned from that first experience. Rosie explained: "With my first husband I know that I [was] really very faithful to him, I really bowed down to him. [With my second husband] I can voice out what I want. And I learned from that so with him I stand up on my feet." Jasmine took a different approach, avoiding another marriage. When her cousins asked her why she did not want a man to take care of her, she said, "You know what? Men don't look for somebody to take care of. They look for somebody to control. . . . I have my freedom." Migration thus creates conditions for both increased vulnerability to poor reproductive and sexual health outcomes, and opportunities for resistance to the social conditions that foster it.

6 • CONTEMPT, CONFUSION, AND CARE IN GUAM'S IMPERIAL PUBLIC HEALTHCARE SYSTEM

When we met in the crowded waiting room, Marilynn was already thirty-five weeks pregnant. As I followed her through the prenatal clinic, telling her about my project, she explained that she gets treated better than others here. "I feel sorry for the ones who can't understand English. I know because I understand I get better treatment." Marilynn moved to Guam with her parents when she was in high school, and she was much more accustomed to Guam than were recent Chuukese migrants. She even had a friend who worked at the community health center, and she saw this as an advantage to getting good quality care. As we waited on metal bench seats in the large waiting room, and spoke over the constant sound of the intercom system calling patients to various consulting rooms, Marilynn told me her perspectives on health care. She thought Guam's health system was much better than Chuuk's, but even so, Chuukese people did not get fair treatment. She believed that this meant Chuukese people had to choose between Chuuk's deteriorating health system and Guam's discriminatory one. For Marilynn, it was not really a choice. She had moved to Guam in high school with her family and had not been back to Chuuk in over ten years. Guam was her home.

I saw Marilynn again in her thirty-seventh week; this time, I ran into her in a smaller waiting room a provider insisted be created specifically for the women's health section of the community health center.[1] This provider thought pregnant people might be treated better if they had a designated clerk, nurse aide, posting nurse,[2] and waiting room in a quiet spot near the clinic rooms used for consultations. The wait did not feel as long, and there was only one clerk, so there was no confusion over whom to ask if someone had questions. To me, the women appeared more comfortable once they had found this secluded space, although finding it was a challenge. The eight chairs were tightly packed in a small cold hallway behind several sets of double doors and larger hallways. Patients often wandered around the building trying to find this place, subject to being scolded by healthcare workers who walked by and noticed them unaccompanied. As a result, many patients waited in the larger waiting room (which felt like a holding pen) before being escorted back for intake with the medical records clerk.

Marilynn was late in her pregnancy and very familiar with exactly where to go, so she arrived on time and signed in, ready to be seen. She had already been there once that week, although I had missed her for that visit. She said, "The doctor is making me come twice a week now to make sure everything is OK. It is so annoying!" Hooked up to an older model heartbeat monitor for thirty minutes each time, her healthcare provider was making sure everything was still OK for Marilynn. He was concerned with her marginally high blood pressure readings and her body weight, so he insisted she come in regularly. On this day, as we sat and continued our conversation about life in Guam, the nurse came in and out, reading the output several times. "Something wrong?" Marilynn asked. "Your baby is not reactive," the nurse said and walked out of the room. Marilynn tensed, as did I, and we waited for her provider to return to the room. She spent another thirty minutes on the monitor before he arrived. During this long wait, I asked Marilynn about this pregnancy. She told me she was pregnant for the second time and was looking forward to her first girl baby. She repeated what many women said: girls in Chuuk are special because they inherit the land and belong to her clan. Her family was pampering her throughout this pregnancy. They were very excited about this addition to the family.

When the provider, Mike, came in, he read it himself but seemed to already know what to expect. "Your baby's heartbeat is not acting like I want it to. It might be nothing, but with your high blood pressure, I want you to be monitored tonight. I want you to go to GMH [Guam Memorial Hospital] tonight. I'm going to call them now and let them know you're coming." Mike left the room, and she asked me what that meant. I basically repeated Mike, saying, "I don't know; I think he said the baby's heartbeat isn't as reactive as he would like it, so he wants them to watch it at GMH." Marilynn grew frustrated: "Why won't he just say something's wrong? Why is he lying?" I said I was not sure he was lying. I told her he can only tell some things with the equipment he has, and that is probably why he wants her to go to the hospital.

After several more tense minutes, Mike came back with his prescription pad. "I'm writing exactly what I am concerned about and what I think they need to do, including admit you at GMH. I already called them, but in case they don't listen, give them this. They don't always listen to what I suggest." Mike was referring to the disconnect between the public hospital and the community health centers, which served mostly indigent and Medicaid populations in Guam. Most publicly insured women receive primary care at community health centers but then deliver with different hospital-employed providers at GMH. This means women seeking care at the community health centers do not have continuity of care from prenatal visits to birth.[3] Mike complained regularly that the hospital providers do not listen to community health center provider concerns or requests, and he thought some of his patients suffered unnecessarily as a result. Since Marilynn was told to go straight to the hospital, she called her partner. He left work early and came to pick her up. We said our good-byes, and I wished her good health.

Marilynn's friend who worked at the community health center pulled me aside the next week and told me what happened. According to her, GMH hooked Marilynn up to a fetal heart monitor, as they had at the clinic, and watched it for a few hours. They then gave her orange pills and sent her home. She reported that the providers told her to come back the next day if she was not feeling enough kicking. She did not want to leave because Mike had told her to stay there. Since it was the hospital doctor's orders, though, she did not feel she had a choice. At some point that evening, Marilynn realized that the baby had stopped kicking. She went back to the hospital as advised, but it was too late. She delivered a stillbirth.

Marilynn came in for a checkup the following week and told us herself what had happened. She was stoic in her storytelling, not displaying the pain from her loss. But she was also not her usual sassy self. She expressed a certain fatalism and said she would just try again for another girl when she healed. Her story of fetal loss highlights the vulnerability of migrants in a place with limited social or political power. Afraid to speak up at the hospital to reiterate what her clinic provider had told her, Marilynn went home and lost her pregnancy.

High blood pressure and gestational diabetes are endemic among Chuukese pregnant women. In Guam, the resources are better for managing these complications, but to do this, women must also manage their powerlessness throughout the public healthcare system. As Marilynn had described, she had an easier time than many other women in navigating the public health system, because of her English skills and insurance coverage. She was, however, still powerless in the face of contradictory medical advice given to her by clinic and hospital providers.

Kaylyn's overall experience of GMH was also negative, although without such a distressing conclusion. She had recently given birth in Guam, and her infant lay in her arms as we spoke in a quiet office at UOG. She described GMH as a dirty, dingy place in which she was completely ignored: "GMH—it's not what it used to be or maybe because when I was younger . . . or because I was used to the hospital back in Chuuk, I thought it was like the cleanest, most sanitary place ever! . . . And like now, you don't want to touch the walls, the nurses are angry, [laughs] and the doctors are tired" (Smith 2019a, 349). Glorida similarly said that GMH used to be "OK" in the 1990s, but now it was "crummy." Several other women told me they were ignored at the hospital and that they did not have an attendant when birthing. Other women said that they were attended to too closely and given emergency cesarean sections without being told why in a language they understood.

I did not have access to the hospital, so I only know the stories told to me by women who birthed there. Marilynn had a relatively easy time getting to the clinic, but this did not save her from the tragic loss of her pregnancy. Many women face barriers before they get to the hospital: they struggle with getting insurance, finding time and transportation, and getting an appointment at a clinic. Once they finally get in, they face challenging encounters with at times hostile and nearly always rushed healthcare workers, limiting the quality of care they receive. The structural and social barriers women face when seeking adequate reproductive health care inevitably contribute to the higher rate of cesarean deliveries and increased complications during pregnancy and birth for Chuukese women.[4] A lack of care can reduce the chances for early identification and prevention of many such outcomes. In addition to poor pregnancy-related outcomes, the rare women seeking other reproductive health services, such as Pap smears, often present too late and suffer significant morbidity and disproportionate death rates.[5] In this chapter, I elaborate on the structural and social factors inhibiting their access to adequate health care in Guam.

THE SETTING: PUBLIC HEALTH IN GUAM

Guam's first Department of Health was established in 1905 as the Department of Health and Charities. The then navy governor, George Dyer, oversaw this creation (Hattori 2004). Provision of health care, improved sanitation, and charity were all part of the imperial project of benevolent assimilation; the naval leaders saw themselves as philanthropists providing care to disease-ridden natives (Hattori 2004). The navy's unit for serving navy personnel was separate and did not have the name "charities," reflecting an early stratification of services in Guam. In the early years, this care took the form of dispensaries being opened throughout the island, which focused on hookworm eradication and other sanitation measures (Hattori 2004). They also segregated those who suffered from Hansen's disease (i.e., leprosy) and focused on birthing women.

Indigenous scholar Anne Hattori (2004) points to the ways in which American biomedicine was also a masculine effort to save (and control) Chamoru women, and thus all of (feminized) Guam, so attention to birthing became central to their benevolent savior cause. As a result and under the direction and fundraising efforts of a navy governor's wife, a hospital was built for birthing women in 1905 (Hattori 2004). Young women were trained to be nurse midwives in an attempt to push out patteras (indigenous, mostly elderly, midwives), but their work amounted to serving as maids to the U.S. nursing staff (Hattori 2004). These young women were trained to encourage pregnant women to use the hospital instead of home birthing with patteras. This pattern of training local women in the colonies to be some sort of medical aides who encourage hospital use was common throughout twentieth century colonial rule.[6] As I portray in this chapter, the stratification of roles in Guam's healthcare system continues to place female Chamoru employees overwhelmingly at the bottom.

Guam was not unique in receiving this type of colonial care. During the twentieth century, colonizers in the Pacific focused on keeping the "natives" or "workers" healthy through sanitation measures, often with a focus on reducing hookworm, isolating those with Hansen's disease, and managing cholera outbreaks (Anderson 2006; Manderson 1996; Hattori 2004, 2006). Strategies also included developing surveillance and statistical measures (Anderson 2006; Manderson 1996; Adams 2016a), many of which are now used in domestic health departments (Anderson 2006).

In Guam, these early dispensaries and hospital care eventually grew into the structure that exists today: the Department of Public Health and Social Services (DPHSS). The Guam DPHSS includes several arms of a traditional U.S. health department (e.g., surveillance, vital records, and preventive care) and the public hospital, GMH.[7] GMH was first built in 1946 as a military government hospital constructed with prefab buildings (Haddock 2010). It became civilian in 1950, and the navy moved its own hospital onto a permanent site in 1954. Much like the early twentieth-century health departments, the military in Guam continues to have a separate healthcare system. The Guam navy hospital services military personnel and dependents; it only assists with civilians in rare, large-scale, or complex emergency situations. This status reinforces the imperial circumstances by which the United States takes over one-third of the island's land but remains separate. It created a dual system whereby military personnel and their dependents receive different (better) health care, go to different (better) schools, and even have different (better, more affordable) grocery stores inaccessible to the local population.

GMH has been the only hospital open to civilians for most of its years serving Guam. A Catholic medical center (Medical Center of the Marianas) opened in 1976, but it closed shortly after (in 1978). The government of Guam bought the building, and GMH moved into this space (Haddock 2010). In 2015, another private hospital opened, but it sends nonemergency indigent patients back to GMH, and its acceptance of public insurance seems constantly in flux, so it is not a reliable option for underinsured (and uninsured) residents.

GMH experiences major funding problems, leading to supply and staff shortages and quality-of-care concerns. As I noted in the introduction, there is a severe nursing shortage at both GMH and the private hospital (Hattori-Uchima and Wood 2019; J. Taitano 2022b). In 2018, the hospital lost Joint Commission accreditation, which threatens its ability to be a Medicaid and Medicare-certified provider. As of this writing, the hospital has yet to be reaccredited. The isolation and small size of the island, and the limited spending by the United States on Guam's health care as compared to its mainland states, has left Guam's indigent residents with no other option, and all residents with very limited options for care.[8]

In efforts to get GMH reaccredited, the Department of the Interior ordered an assessment by the Army Corps of Engineers. Its report indicated unsafe buildings, outdated equipment, shared patient spaces that violate the Health Insurance Portability and Accountability Act (HIPAA), inadequate electric and fire safety systems, and more. The report estimated that more than $700 million would be needed to repair or simply build a new hospital, $21 million of which was needed immediately to fix the issues that caused the loss of accreditation (U.S. Army Corps of Engineers 2020). While capital improvements have begun, so has identification of a site to build a new hospital that is large enough to serve the island's needs. But the current proposed site in Mangilao is fraught with issues. The land was condemned by the U.S. Navy after World War II and taken from the original landowners (a common post–World War II practice in Guam); those former landowners have fought to get it back. Further, doctors are fighting against moving to a different village when their practices are set up near the old hospital (in the village of Tamuning) (Hernandez 2022). However, in Governor Lou Leon Guerrero's (2023) state of the island speech, she indicated she would be moving forward with signing a lease with the federal government to build on the Mangilao site.

GMH's financial woes and structural issues, a regular source of news,[9] are typically blamed on the average 26,000 uninsured/self-pay patients served by the hospital annually (Eugenio 2018). According to the Guam Memorial Hospital Authority, uninsured and underinsured patients cost the hospital $30 million per year (Limtiaco 2019a). News stories reporting such issues reflect what the communities assume: that all uninsured and underinsured residents are Micronesian, the vast majority Chuukese migrants. These circumstances have recently changed, as the final U.S. congressional spending bill of 2020 restored Medicaid to COFA migrants for 2021, increasing access (Diamond 2021).

The DPHSS also has three clinic facilities. The main facility, often referred to interchangeably as Central or Mangilao,[10] hosted one of the three clinics in which I undertook ethnographic work. Central primarily cares for uninsured people for prenatal care and family planning services, and conducts infectious disease surveillance, testing, and treatment (e.g., for HIV and tuberculosis). Central was in a Cold War–era nuclear fallout shelter with no windows, built in the mid-twentieth century, and it exuded an old sanitarium or prison-like ambiance. It was made of cinder blocks, was painted a hospital white, and always looked dingy while being quite cold, a sharp contrast to the sunny and hot tropical environment of Guam outdoors. This dark, dank, heavily air-conditioned building was characteristic of all public service buildings in Guam. The waiting room had a television, always broadcasting public health commercials, and the walls were covered with public health campaign materials—"How to get birth control" "Vaccinate your kids today!" "Caring for your baby." The building also hosted the central public health surveillance teams, an office for signing up for social services, and basic public health clinical services. When I followed patients in Central, they waited in a cold room on benches where there was one walk-up front desk, with plexiglass separating the patient from the attendant, and workers from other divisions running back and forth. A 2019 electrical fire at this site shut it down, resulting in various divisions being scattered throughout Guam in smaller office spaces. The DPHSS is seeking funds to rent one central office space again (J. Taitano 2022d). Until then, clinical services are limited to a small amount of space allotted at the Northern Community Health Center.

Guam also has two community health centers within the DPHSS structure, built originally in 1971 and 1984 (Haddock 2010). In 2003, Guam was awarded a grant to build out its Federally Qualified Health Centers, which provided significant support to these older clinical spaces, boosting their ability to provide a range of preventive and primary healthcare services. One is in the congested northern village of Dededo, and the second is in the quiet southern rural village of Inarajan. There are hundreds of Federally Qualified Health Centers throughout the country and in the U.S.-associated Micronesian islands (including Chuuk as of 2017). These centers support a holistic model of health care, whereby patients can come to one central processing facility to (1) sign up for services such as public insurance, Women, Infants and Children (WIC), and SNAP (i.e., food stamps); (2) receive a full range of primary medical care services; (3) complete lab work; (4) fill prescriptions; and (5) receive health education and social work services as needed.[11] The centers provide primary care, including but not limited to pediatrics, immunization, chronic disease management, STI testing and treatment, and women's health care in one single facility. The centers take insurance for primary care services, and chiefly serve those who are publicly insured. Most private clinics either do not accept public forms of insurance or have a very limited number of slots for publicly insured residents, who total 43,422 and make up over 30 percent of the island's population (U.S. Census Bureau 2022). These centers are a solution to the gaps in care throughout the United States (Arcangel 2019). Patients with Medicaid and those who qualify for the Medically Indigent Program (MIP) received much more comprehensive care at these centers than at Central's more traditional public health office. But to get in, they must first obtain that public insurance.[12]

GETTING INSURANCE: MEDICAID AND THE MEDICALLY INDIGENT PROGRAM

Guam has had a Medicaid program since 1975. It covers all U.S. citizens who meet income requirements set forth by the local government.[13] Although Medicaid is a national program, Guam's reimbursement is not like that of the states. While states get matching funding for all Medicaid recipients, territories like

Guam have a funding ceiling. This is one of the many ways in which the imperial status of Guam is reflected in U.S. policies that stratify funding and thus care in the colonies. This manifestation of benign neglect does not reduce the standards or expectations of U.S. healthcare institutions in Guam, however; it just reduces the funds available to meet them. Despite these funding obstacles, Guam also provides the MIP option, which covers non-US citizens who have been residents of Guam for at least six months. MIP was the primary mechanism through which low-income Chuukese migrant women were insured from shortly after the 1996 PRWORA (Personal Responsibility and Work Opportunity Reconciliation Act) decision (chapter 3), up to January 2021 when Medicaid access was restored.[14] Those who did not meet the requirements to be included in MIP and Medicaid (e.g., the six-month residency rule) are eligible for the Maternal and Child Health program. This short-term program covers pregnant people who have recently arrived in Guam, but only for clinic visits and a few lab tests, not delivery. MIP and Medicaid recipients are permitted to seek care only at the Northern and Southern Region Community Health Centers or at private clinics if they can get in (this is unlikely). Maternal and Child Health program recipients go to Central providers only (now housed at Northern since the electrical fire), but exceptions are made at the Northern Region Community Health Center for those who have high-risk pregnancies to see specialists. The rules about who can go where are in constant flux. Clerks told me they regularly enforce the rules, but they cannot keep up with who belongs at which clinic and what tests are covered based on insurance coverage.

Medicaid is the best public option. Very few services provided under Medicaid at the community health centers have co-pays.[15] MIP ultimately covers the same services as Medicaid except with many more co-pays. While they are often small (e.g., six or seven dollars for an immunization), I witnessed several patients who did not have sufficient funds to pay their portion of the cost under MIP.[16] Some patients did not show up for appointments when they did not have enough to pay for them, or if they did show up, providers would postpone tests, immunizations, and drugs until the patient could bring the money. This choice of the local government leadership to have two public insurance options in which Medicaid—for American citizens—allows more free services, while MIP—for noncitizen residents—requires patients to pay fees for visits, created a scenario that privileged certain groups (American citizens), stratifying who deserves free or reduced-cost care and who deserves to pay more.[17] I was told by more than one healthcare worker that co-pays for MIP recipients are a way to get back some of the "burdensome" costs of caring for migrants. Finding the money for the co-pays was a barrier only after women successfully completed their insurance application and received coverage, which was quite a challenge alone.

As I sat with Pamela, a thirty-nine-year-old woman from Chuuk's northwestern region, in her cramped apartment provided by Guam Housing and Urban

Renewal Authority (GHURA), she updated me on what was going on in her life. We sat at a small cluttered table in her galley kitchen, looking out the back window. Just beyond the dark, cramped space in which we sat, we could see a small courtyard filled with Guam's beautiful green foliage; more apartment buildings, with laundry hanging from every porch; and the endless bright blue sky. Pamela was rarely alone in her apartment, as her cousins and smaller children were always there with her. Even when they were gone, other cousins lived downstairs, and they treated each other's apartments as one big home. We cherished this brief respite from the crowd to talk about her recent separation from her husband, her pregnancy, and her clinical care. As we approached the subject of her pregnancy—she was then about three months along—I asked about her insurance coverage. Pamela told me she had lost her MIP coverage a few years prior because she did not follow through on a documentation requirement sent to her by mail. Her husband had always completed this type of paperwork, and in his absence, Pamela was intimidated by the process. I said I would be happy to help her fill it out. She excitedly accepted my offer, and we went through a very long and confusing application form together. As I started to read the thick collection of pages in the packet, I realized I did not understand what many of the questions meant. As a fully educated native English speaker, I wondered: How is someone with limited English skills supposed to fill this out if I do not understand it? We went through the questions I could help her with, and I suggested she ask for help at the application office for those I could not. Later that week, as I observed patients in Central's confined concrete facilities, I chatted with a medical social worker about the form and told her about my experience with Pamela. She told me I had given her the wrong advice; the Medicaid/MIP office would refuse to help her because of a conflict of interest. When I asked her what the conflict was, she was unable to give me a clear answer. She explained that the Medicaid/MIP application office would tell her to make an appointment with a medical social worker to receive help with the application. To me, these extra steps felt like just another delay for her in getting the insurance she needed.

When Pamela successfully applied for MIP with the help of a medical social worker, she began the first step in a very lengthy process. First, a person turns in an application and provides any proof required—immigration documents, proof of six months of residency from village mayors, and bank statements to show income requirements. Once this is submitted, the applicant is instructed to wait for a letter in the mail that either requests more documents or provides a time and date for the applicant interview.[18] After the interview is complete, applicants are expected to wait for a second letter in the mail, which will confirm eligibility or request more documents. Rebecca, a healthcare worker who often advocated for Chuukese women facing barriers to obtaining insurance, told me it was not uncommon for some Chuukese women to wait seven or eight months. My surprise encouraged her to continue. Rebecca told me that the public insurance workers "always reject them" and ask for more documents, delaying care. Fortunately, completing this complicated application form covers many social services, including the food stamp and supplemental income programs (for U.S. citizens in the household).[19] This is also the process for applying for Medicaid, so as COFA migrants have regained access, they are still subject to this bureaucratic process.

Jessica's MIP was unexpectedly cancelled mid-year as the result of a missing document. Jessica took time off from work to meet her caseworker at a scheduled time after reapplying but was told that the caseworker was out. She would need to come back a different day. This resulted in more lost workdays and wages. She said this was normal and that the caseworkers were always rude and short with her. She felt it was because she was Chuukese: "They don't like us. Whenever we go there, they really give us a hard time. They know that it's hard [to take off work], and they say, 'You come back tomorrow,' you know? I say, 'How come you said I come today but they, you know, they reschedule it?' . . . They make us go back and forth." Jessica also complained that there was always another document they needed to process coverage, making it take longer and longer. Her supervisor questioned why she had to take off so much to get coverage, which made her feel that her job was threatened just for trying to get insurance. Similarly, women who had housing through GHURA complained that they would get one day's notice to be at home for home visits, with no consideration of their work schedules.

When MIP recipients traveled back to Chuuk, they often lost coverage due to missing paperwork deadlines. Further, since they had then left the United States, if the MIP office learned they left, the original six-month residency clock to initiate coverage started all over again. Leena, an older Chuukese woman who had recently lost her son, told me how she went home to Chuuk for her son's last days and funeral. Upon returning, she found out that her MIP had been canceled. She explained why she had left, and they told her she needed to wait six months and then start a new application.

After learning of Jessica's and Leena's experiences, I offered to wait with another woman who had an appointment; we both agreed that my whiteness and primary English proficiency might help her get treated better in the process. It did not. The office was an add-on to a community health center and built much like a bank. There were four slots where caseworkers sat, walls dividing them to allow for some client privacy, and a long, single-file line to meet with them (despite this being an appointment-only office). We waited for over an hour, standing in the single-file line that stretched from the actual office to the patient waiting room. When we finally got to the front, we were told by a front-desk worker—with no apologies or attempts to help—that the caseworker assigned was at lunch and the client would have to reschedule.

Clients were not respected, were told to come back several times, and were told to show up for appointments that were then canceled; it thus became nearly impossible to get coverage. When services are withheld from women through concealment of vital information, providing misinformation, or continuously asking for extra documents, these women face what Leslie López (2005) describes as "de facto disentitlement" or what Shari Danz (2000) calls "bureaucratic disentitlement." These structural barriers to insurance render Chuukese women exceptionally vulnerable to accessing the already-limited reproductive health care available.

There is one major improvement to access in recent years, but not within the system. Since the Micronesian Resource Center One-Stop Shop (MRCOSS) opened (see chapter 3) and employed multi-lingual staff, one of their primary roles is to help COFA migrants complete applications for services and coverage like Medicaid. Not only are they helping with interpretation, but have assisted in streamlining the process by scanning and uploading all necessary client documents together to remove the common barrier of additional document requests. Additionally, they have fostered relationships with the Bureau of Economic Security (BES) office staff who process Medicaid applications to better address issues as they arise. Their efforts have been pivotal for improving COFA migrants' access to Medicaid.

GETTING INTO THE CLINICS

Pamela was given Maternal and Child Health coverage when she applied for insurance. This was supposed to be temporary while she waited for the more comprehensive MIP to process. That meant she had to go to Central public health in the meantime. Central is characterized by major funding issues and is known for constantly having supply shortages that affect patient care. The supply shortages in the lab change from week to week, and when there is a missing supply, patients are sent to a private lab to self-pay. So, if a pregnant patient is in the clinic on February 1, they may get five free lab tests in Central and be sent for a few tests to a private lab, but on February 8, they may get only three free tests. Uninsured people are expected to come up with anywhere from $40 to $140 to cover these private lab costs depending on current shortages. Pamela knew about possible lab fees at Central from her previous pregnancies. She did not have the money to cover them, so she waited for MIP to kick in to make an appointment at a community health center. By the time she was ready to call the community health center for a MIP-covered appointment, she had to wait another month to get in because of the center's full schedule. The center was constantly short-staffed and had insurmountable bureaucratic hurdles for hiring new staff, so its schedule was packed. Pamela's pregnancy was well into its second trimester at this point.

Pamela and several other women asked if I would meet them at the clinic for their next appointment, for support in this unwelcoming system, but then they would not show. Pamela did this during the application process. She apologized the next time I saw her. She did not have a bus fare or a load on her phone to call me.[20] I could have given her a ride. Pamela often did not have even one dollar with her, which is how much the bus costs each way. Like Pamela, transportation is by far the most prominent barrier to care for many Chuukese women in Guam. Often, a large family will have one car driven by the wage earner(s). If that person is at work, they must get a ride from someone else or take the bus. Guam is too big to simply walk or ride a bike to places. At 212 square miles, it is the size of a small spread-out suburban U.S. city. Like other small U.S. cities, the bus is notorious for being unreliable and slow. Women who are driven often wait for the wage earner to get off work to get a ride home. They are left to wait in the hot concrete parking lot when the clinic closes.

The second most prominent barrier is time. While some women work, those who do not often provide unpaid labor, taking care of several family members' children or elders. Chuukese women's family needs typically come first, and this often delays their care.[21] So, Chuukese women first must get insurance through an unfriendly and complex application system. If they do, often their busy lives supporting others inhibits early care-seeking, and transportation also proves to be a major barrier. If they get insurance, transportation, and time to seek care, they then must get through the phone system to make an appointment. Once they do that, they must navigate a rushed and often hostile system of care.

Waiting and Rushing through the Clinic

It took me months to enter the clinics. I called the main line dozens of times, and much to my dismay, it was rarely answered. I showed up a few times, but the director was always in meetings. And then, like magic, I got in. I was complaining to a colleague about my troubles when she told me she personally knew the director and would set up a meeting. This did the trick. I met with her, and all was clear after a few minutes of discussing my project and her confirming my ethical considerations and approvals. The barrier was really getting through to a person with connections to get a meeting with this very busy administrator. My initial experience led me to think it may be a formidable place for migrants seeking care.

Over the next several months, I learned that the phone is notorious for never being answered, likely a result of how overwhelmed the staff are in just processing patients. Providers complained that they cannot call into work when sick because of this. If a patient does get through on the phone, they are likely to be told to call back the following month, like Pamela. Further, a woman must confirm a pregnancy before getting a prenatal care appointment, which is the primary reason women seek care. Patients would come back several days in a row just to try to be seen to get a positive pregnancy confirmation and thus be allowed to make an appointment. The waiting was expected to take up to the full eight hours of the day, so work and family obligations could not be met on clinic days. This was only one of many hurdles to getting into the clinic for Chuukese

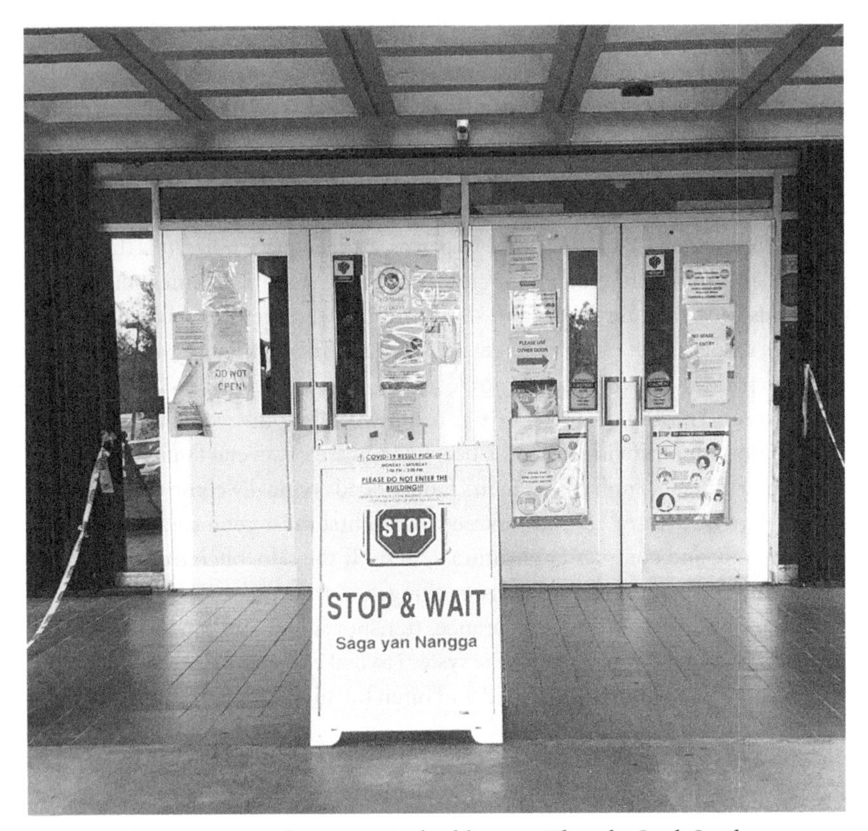

FIGURE 17. Front entrance of a community health center. Photo by Sarah Smith.

women. Since that time, COVID-19 protocols created even more barriers. Starting in 2020, the buildings had guards and a series of signs in the front that say Stop & Wait and indicated that only those with appointments were allowed in the building (see figure 17). That means women had to try to get through the impossible phone line to make an initial appointment and there is no online system to circumvent the phone line. During a visit in March 2023, I learned that people are allowed in the building again as pandemic restrictions loosen; and the line to make an appointment or get questions answered is typically very long.

On my first day in the clinic, the director cheerfully introduced me to everyone she could find, as I shifted left and right to let workers pass by during their clearly chaotic morning. After walking me through the clinic—a maze of concrete, clinic workers, and endless hallways—the director introduced me to Rebecca for further guidance. I was relieved; one tour of the clinic made me realize how big and overwhelming it was, and I did not want to be left alone. The director ran off to work on a grant, and Rebecca sat down with me to explain the clinic processes.

Like Central, women wait in a waiting room to be called, but unlike Central, instead of plexiglass, there was a (mostly unattended) front desk where they could ask questions while they wait. Through the first set of double doors near the waiting room are the medical clerks, who take patients at their cubicles to verify demographic and insurance information. Once patients get through this obstacle, they wait again in the main waiting room (or a side waiting room, depending on the purpose of their visit) until being called by a nurse aide to take vital signs and get medical history. Then they again wait until called into a clinic room to wait for their provider. If they successfully follow the many confusing signs pointing to multiple rooms labeled number one, for example, or find a worker to guide them, they can then get care.

As Rebecca explained the steps to get through the clinic, she also offered her own insights about my project topic: "They [clinic staff] check the sign-in sheet with the records. If they [patients] have records, they get in. If not treated well, women just go away because back in Chuuk [they will] just be pregnant until delivery. With the language barrier, sometimes they feel ignored and just go and leave and feel ashamed" (Smith 2016, 52). This was my first day, and I was already being told that Chuukese women are treated badly and often leave before receiving care as a result. This initial experience certainly colored my lens of the clinic. This first impression was not wrong though.

Healthcare workers often expect patients to wait for hours, chiding them for asking questions. Once in the clinic room, however, patients are rushed through the system. Ella, a healthcare worker who regularly assisted Chuukese patients, explained: "The doctors are not really, you know, answering their questions, they're just in a hurry to get them out from the room." Providers are just trying to get through their patients fast enough to see them all, but often this has a detrimental impact on their treatment of patients as they rush them through. Jevlyn, a Chuukese patient at one of the clinics for all eight of her births, was frustrated by how this rushed environment inhibited her from comfortably asking questions or getting more detailed explanations about her health. She shared her frustrations with me a few days after I accompanied her to a prenatal checkup. She complained that she was told she needed to rest due to concerns late in the pregnancy but with little explanation: "They just, need to be, really, explain what, what they give us, you know? Because sometimes when they go there they are just really fast because plenty patients. . . . They don't really . . . explain!" Jevlyn paused to catch her breath. "You know that time I went [and you were there]? The doctor so busy. . . . So that's why no, no time to explain because only one doctor. We just go in there just check, check, check OK go out, you know? Not really sit down and 'Oh, like this like this like this.' Didn't you see it, Sarah? It's really fast." I told her I did see it. The place always felt so rushed. I asked her, "Do you feel like you cannot ask questions because they are so busy?" She said,

"Yeah!" Jevlyn loved her doctor, but the rush was so overwhelming she felt it would mess up their flow to ask questions. Maria is a healthcare worker who felt the rushed environment affected nursing care as well: "I think yeah, because they've [nurses] been working here for too long, sometimes they feel like, because also the load of patients. . . . You want to get rid of the patient."

The social organization of waiting and rushing is not simply a logistical obstacle but an articulation of hierarchies of access to medical care. Elise Andaya (2019) studied clinical temporalities in publicly funded prenatal clinics in the United States. She perceived these notions of who waits and who is waited for as manifestations of neoliberal racism. Neoliberal racism occurs when divestment in public health—and particularly public prenatal care—means that pregnant minority and low-income women endure the most stressed systems, the longest wait times, and the most rushed care (Andaya 2019; Briggs 2017). Denise Spitzer (2004) explored the impact of strained, resource-poor publicly funded clinics on overworked nurses. She recognized that given their considerably limited energy surviving in these systems, nurses expended more energy on specific patients while ignoring and rushing others. This rationing of energy inevitably siphoned off the "easy" (white, Euro-American, English speaking) patients to whom they relegated more care from the more "difficult" (minority, non-English speaking) patients. Healthcare workers in the overburdened healthcare system try to care, Andaya (2019) argues, but they struggle to do anything but survive in such a dysfunctional setting. As the waiting and the subsequent rushed care fall on the most vulnerable, particularly in prenatal care settings, this is another example of what Dána-Ain Davis (2019) calls "obstetric racism." This term connects obstetric violence to medical racism—both the institutional or state-sanctioned practices (e.g., benign neglect) and professionals' perceptions and treatment decisions based on a patient's race. Andaya (2019) argues that the long wait times, rushed care visits, and overburdened healthcare providers in these public prenatal care settings are a manifestation of obstetric racism. This reflects the context for the community health centers in Guam.

While my feelings about the rushed environment did not dissipate with time, my understanding of how this rushed environment became a source of feeling disrespected and ignored among Chuukese women became increasingly complex. It was not simply that they felt pushed through by healthcare workers, although that was certainly part of it. They also experienced unfriendly care. Their care was often stratified by the roles of healthcare workers.

Getting Past the Front Desk

Women often told me they felt unwelcome at the clinics. I finally realized that it was not the entire clinic making women feel unwelcome but the reception area. This first impression of the clinic and the first step in the clinic process was often a very unfriendly and unwelcoming space. When we were talking about the community health center she had gone to and brought family members to sometimes, Kaylyn commented, "You know the [Location] clinic if you just, get past the receptionist and actually go into, into the women's clinic? You know, you know you start getting treated like a human being there like they are nice there, it's just like your initial, the initial thing" (Smith 2016, 52).

While scholars often focus on patient-provider interactions, patients do not simply interact with their providers. They see workers at the front desk, clerks updating patient records, medical assistants taking vital signs, and often nurses before or after being seen by advanced nurses and doctors. The front desk and medical records clerks are that first hurdle Kaylyn described. I witnessed patients walk up to the front desk several times and be told to wait for their name to be called before they even opened their mouths. Some women came in to ask how to make an appointment. These women were never going to hear their name called, since they did not have appointments that day. They had to keep approaching the clerks—eyes down and shooing them away—until one looked up and acknowledged them. Others were told that appointments were full. I observed this a few times when there were still walk-in triage appointments with a nurse. Front-desk workers chose when to acknowledge these facts and when to say there were no appointments to prospective patients who stood in front of them, deciding who deserved care (and who did not) that day. They had enormous power over patients (or would-be patients) venturing into the clinic.

Why these clerks would act as gatekeepers became more fascinating to me the longer I observed them: they had little power in the clinical structure but so much power over patients' access. It took months for clerks to feel comfortable with my white mainlander presence, but eventually they began to share their feelings about their work. They complained to me about how overworked they were, crowded into small spaces, with a great amount of pressure on their shoulders to get patients through the first step of their clinical visit in order to maintain the flow. This pressure inspired them to take shortcuts and ration care as they saw fit in the moment, making sure to get the scheduled patients through before providers or administrators got angry with them.

Front-desk workers felt pressure not just from above but from patients, whom they perceived as intentionally making their job more difficult. One clerk, Edith, revealed how misunderstandings were interpreted this way. She and others regularly accused patients of intentionally ignoring the signs posted—instead of just not seeing them—and told me how much this upset her. These clerks were the ones who had posted the signs, and they were vividly aware of them, as their intentions were to make them visible. However, to an outsider like me, there were posters and signs with rules and directions all over the place, and they blended in with the chaos. Further, the language barriers I witnessed were vast and complicated. When in doubt, however, these clerks believed there was something more fundamentally disrespectful in patients' behavior. They felt that the patients were ungrateful and impatient with the work they did, and they responded to these feelings with how they treated the patients.

My group conversations with the clerks also revealed larger discourses about Micronesians: that these people were ungrateful outsiders who used too much of Guam's resources. In these conversations, Katarina reflected on her frustration over Micronesian patient behavior: "I want to see how they, how they act in their clinic, compared to how they act when they come to our clinic? You know what I mean?" Dianna responded immediately, agreeing: "Like I said, because they are here, they think they have a right to be here and they have to be served and we have to be at their beck and call!" (Smith 2016, 53). Katarina and Diana alluded to sentiments heard throughout the community about Micronesian migrants.

While the poorest treatment of patients was consistently provided by the lowest-level providers, I also noticed that there was more respect shown to patients with each step up the hierarchy of the clinic. Nurse aides, for example, would lecture patients about their eating habits in derogatory ways and sometimes make fun of them (in ways largely not recognized or overheard by patients), but they were also playful and kind, and they often joked with patients, something also common among more senior posting nurses. The providers (nurse practitioners and physicians) were the friendliest group as a whole (with some racist exceptions). They were also the most accommodating to language, cultural, and access issues for Chuukese patients. One provider I followed frequently would introduce himself and shake the hand of patients, and help them up after an examination, small gestures that visibly released much of the tension patients were carrying from the first few stages of the clinic visit. Again, in this hierarchy, more power usually meant friendlier.

This division of roles and subsequent treatment reflected the hierarchy of Guam. Micronesians could not even get permanent jobs there.[22] The next most vulnerable group, Chamoru (women) of Guam, occupy the lowest permanent social position at the clinic with the lowest pay—medical clerks and frontline workers—mirroring the hierarchies from the first naval hospital in the early twentieth century. Their jobs are menial, repetitive, and, in their eyes, frustrating and unappreciated. Next in the hierarchy are the nurse aides and nurses—mostly Filipina—who stay connected to one another in the middle of the hierarchy. Then there are the advanced nurses and doctors, who are largely in charge. The providers were more diverse but were overrepresented by state-sider white males.

The indigenous Chamorus were forced to welcome many groups: the American military, Filipino/a workers, and now COFA migrants. Only the latter group was as poor or more poverty-stricken than the Chamorus themselves, and in the view of many—especially the clerks—these migrants self-righteously appropriated Chamoru resources. Their response was to view the Micronesians as suspect and ungrateful, which slowed down their frustrating daily work at the clinic. This frustration and suspicion manifested in harsh tones, cutting patients off before they could ask questions and, at times, purposely thwarting their access to care. The nurses and nurse aides were a bit more cheerful, although still at times short with the patients. Finally, providers provided care *nicely* (with some exceptions), though not always with enough explanations or time; still, they treated Chuukese patients, as Kaylyn said, "like humans," with dignity and respect.[23]

Researchers have acknowledged for decades the power that frontline workers within bureaucratic institutions have to implement public policies (Lipsky 1984). In these roles, many necessary exceptions to policies are made, providing a certain degree of discretion to their work. They must simplify their jobs to cope with the many demands of working in underfunded and overworked environments, and this simplification often takes the form of stereotyping individual clients to ease their workload. This is especially the case for the most powerless employees. Their sense of powerlessness and their suspicion that patients are often lying (Kingfisher 1996; Spitzer 2004; Bridges 2011) or stupid (Bridges 2011) helps them rationalize differential care.

Differential treatment is a complex form of agency within an under-resourced setting with poor working conditions. It may be how the most powerless health workers are asserting their power as gatekeepers over the only actors who have less power than them: the mostly migrant patient population (see also Andersen 2004). Anthropologist Khiara Bridges (2011) described a similar scenario in New York City public hospitals in which what she deemed the ancillary staff do not simply reflect the larger community but, as the most powerless employees, also try to distinguish their position from that of their patients. The local population also makes a great effort in Guam to distinguish themselves from their regional migrant neighbors who are backward and poor and not part of the United States, while grappling with their own ambiguous relationship with the United States and resulting second-class citizenship. The colonial environment of benign neglect and sanctioned migration by the United States has created this scenario of a largely impoverished indigenous group and an even poorer migrant group interacting and feeling as if they are competing for resources on this small island—one that is the richest in Micronesia and yet the poorest of the United States. The rushed environment of underfunded public clinics and clerks enacting power over patients through gatekeeping practices are important structural elements of obstetric racism but not the only way it manifests. Chuukese women also face issues with language access and cultural stereotypes inhibiting their care.

LANGUAGE, "CULTURE," AND CARE

Following mostly pregnant women in the clinics led to my witnessing many repetitive moments. For example, as women got closer to full term, healthcare workers would tell them the warning signs that should send them straight to the hospital. One day when I was with Anne, a healthcare worker with an inconsistent track record of respectful treatment of patients, she started an appointment with a Chuukese woman and her family interpreter with the long list of warning signs warranting an immediate hospital visit. She said, "If the baby stops moving, water bag breaks, bleeding, you need to go to the hospital. It is very, very important." The family interpreter, who did not have a very good understanding of English herself, said, "I'm sorry, when?" Anne, visibly annoyed at the language barrier, started laughing and sarcastically responded, "Well, I don't know." The family interpreter watched her silently for a moment, not really understanding what had happened. Then she responded, "I'm sorry, what did you say?" At the same speed as her original list, Anne repeated herself. The interpreter said "OK," and that was that. According to Anne, it was very important, and yet knowing there were interpretation issues, she sped through the list and laughed at a misunderstanding. While her sarcasm was a particularly hostile encounter and rare to witness, the speedy overview of important information that could save a woman or her pregnancy was a common tactic for overburdened healthcare workers, regardless of language proficiency.

Some Chuukese women speak English fluently. Others struggle with language skills. Those who struggle are more likely to be recent arrivals or women who do not work outside the home. Healthcare administrators recognize Chuukese as one of the primary languages spoken by patients and hired two Chuukese women just before I began visiting clinics. However, both Chuukese women were hired in other positions and had several duties in addition to translation. It was a creative way to hire them in the absence of a budget for interpreters but clearly not a permanent solution.

As I expected, women with whom I spoke both in the clinic and throughout the community expressed great appreciation for one clinic hiring Chuukese staff. They felt more respected, safer, and thought it would be easier for Chuukese patients to receive services. Jevlyn said, "It's good if Chuukese working here too. Before, no Chuukese, we treated like, you know, nobody wants to help us! [laughs]" (Smith 2018, 85). As we sat on her couch, with her newborn between us in a quiet house mid-morning, she told me her feelings about interpreters and their importance. Since the older children were at school, we could talk openly, and she told me a story of trying to help a family member give birth and not understanding the doctor's medical details to translate. Her cousin could not speak English and called for help because she was in labor, and so Jevlyn went to the hospital but, she told me, "We don't really understand those doctors, right?" I asked Jevlyn to explain what she meant because her English proficiency was excellent. She said, "How can we know what kind of sickness?" She proceeded to tell me that whether in Chuukese or English, she was not a medical expert, so she often did not understand what the doctor was trying to say to interpret for her cousin. She and others thus recognized the importance of having official interpreters instead of family. Women described the Chuukese interpreters as important advocates when they perceived women to be waiting too long for care.

At the same time, these same women often desired to change clinics or avoid care specifically because there were Chuukese women working there. It was not anything about the specific women hired but a consensus that Chuukese people do not respect confidentiality, and they do not want other Chuukese people becoming aware of their medical information. Women who had vastly different levels of education and English proficiency (ranging from stopping at fifth grade to finishing college, and from minimal English skills to fluency) told me they did not trust anyone who was Chuukese with their health information. Even Jevlyn, who was so happy to see them there, did not trust them with her information. Chuukese nurses in Chuuk similarly told me that Chuukese people do not understand the concept of confidentiality. Some women told me they left Chuuk to avoid Chuukese providers; they especially did not trust them in relation to sexual and reproductive health issues.

One recommended solution to improving clinical care in diverse communities is to increase the number of healthcare workers who "look like" (ethnically, culturally, linguistically) the patients being served, much like the one clinic's efforts to hire two Chuukese women. While efforts to ensure equal access to healthcare providers is a valuable one, the ideas underlying this strategy are problematic. When provider-patient matching is suggested as a solution, language, ethnicity, race, and cultural knowledge are conflated as all being the same (Shaw 2010). Moreover, underlying ideas about "sameness" and "difference" in hiring Chuukese providers could perpetuate the idea that Micronesians, and the Chuukese in particular, are a homogenous group, different from other Guam residents. But Chuuk has five distinct regional identities and many different dialects. While hiring Chuukese employees may be an important economic justice issue, it must not be assumed that these individuals can also serve as some sort of "cultural brokers," nor that all patients will want Chuukese nonrelatives providing care, even as interpreters. I discussed strategies with women to bring them much needed interpretation services while also ensuring their sense of privacy, but there was not a clear solution. Yet when patients do not share a common language with their healthcare workers, it can affect how much information is transmitted between healthcare workers and patients, whether patients understand the clinic processes, how well they can fill out forms or make appointments, and their comfort level in the clinic.

Knowing that most clinical interactions do not include official interpreters, I asked Mike, a healthcare worker in the women's health clinic, how he dealt with communicating with his patients. He told me that relatives are often helpful, but they do not translate everything; instead, they filter the information (I noticed this, too). I asked him how that worked for him. He paused for a moment, then reflected:

> If it's not working well, sometimes it's only 'cause I'm too lazy to go get the other translators. . . . I kinda like talk to the patient in a way that, I'll say the same thing in two or three different ways and find out if they're giving the right answer and really understanding me. So if I have a sense they're not understanding me, and I think it's important, then I'll go get the translator. Sometimes it's hard to figure out whether they don't understand you or they're just being really shy. You know because there's certain things, they're not gonna look you in the eye, and they don't talk to men who are strangers and different things like that. . . . There's [also] a certain amount that they're not gonna talk [about] with their relatives, or if their relatives are more senior to them, then they're letting their relative answer. They may know the language, but they're letting the relative answer.

As Mike described, women often come to the clinic with family members, who serve as the primary interlocutors for patient-provider interactions.[24] There is often an element of hierarchy and power in these relationships that leave women silent despite possible proficiency. Frequently I would watch the healthcare worker instruct the interpreter about contractions, when to go to the hospital, what signs are dangerous, and so forth, as if the patient were not there. When family members do not actually interpret but instead speak for the patient, it affects both patient care and women's levels of vulnerability within the family (see also Delafield et al. 2020; Delafield et al. 2021; Inada et al. 2019). Already in a vulnerable state as a generally younger (reproductive age) woman in a gender- and age-stratified community, translation by family members allows for increased control. Further, use of family interpreters can lead to reproductive coercion.

Mike also described more candidly than many others what I witnessed daily: often the interpreters were family members with limited English proficiency themselves, or the patient was alone, but the clinician would not opt to get an interpreter (if one was available) unless the topic was important to them (the clinician) and it was clear the patient did not understand anything. Each healthcare worker who did not claim to get interpreters every time had a personal system for figuring it out. Maria, for example, told me, "Well, when they smile a lot, that's when I think, 'Do they really (understand)?' That's like my cue: 'Do you really understand me or not?'" To which I responded, "So, what, the bigger the smile, the less likely they understand?" She emphatically answered "Yes!" Despite the smile, patients were often frustrated with not knowing what was going on with their own bodies.

Misunderstandings and Polite, Agreeable Patients

As healthcare workers often described, some Chuukese women are inclined to say yes or just smile to acknowledge something. This comes from a cultural environment in which people avoid conflict in public, or with family, and people are expected to keep their negative feelings "inside" so as not to negatively affect the group (Petersen 2009; Dernbach 2005). Similarly, hierarchies by birth order, generation, and gender are very important, and those with less familial power (such as young people and women) know they are to be seen but not heard, to listen but not speak. In the healthcare context, being a part of the clinic employee structure seems to automatically render healthcare workers as higher status than the patients; therefore, Chuukese patients often act with great deference. When women are brave enough to ask their questions, the interactions are often great, but when they do not ask, they leave without having their information needs fulfilled.

Such patient deference is not unique to Chuuk or Micronesia, however. Asian and Pacific Islander populations have been depicted as shy, deferent, and uncomfortable discussing concerns with providers (see, for example, Kim et al. 2000; Young and Klingle 1996), and Latinx patients are depicted as avoiding hostile confrontations (Flores 2000), worrying that asking questions may negatively affect the patient-provider relationship (American Medical Association 1994), and preferring to delegate healthcare decisions to their providers (Xu, Borders, and Ahmed 2004). In fact, in all underrepresented minority populations, this is a common argument used in "cultural competency" calls to providers. What these characterizations and subsequent arguments often do is perpetuate stereotypes about people and continue to blame the patient for not getting adequate care because of their deferent and polite culture, leaving them more vulnerable to poor health outcomes.

It is not just underrepresented minority patients. Studies have shown that regardless of background, patients rarely talk about all their concerns during visits (Korsch, Gozzi, and Francis 1968; Roter et al. 1997) and are often passive, asking for few further explanations (Kettunen, Poskiparta, and Gerlander 2002). Sociologists John Heritage and Douglas W. Maynard (2006) reviewed thirty years of patient-provider research, finding that studies consistently report patients not disclosing or self-censoring their needs. They, too, connected this finding to the power relations embedded in the clinical encounter. Just like the many ethnic groups who have previously been connected to patient politeness and deference, Chuukese women likely have a more pronounced version of something most patients share because of their vulnerability and powerlessness in the community and in the clinic.

Patient deference leads to some troubled interactions, wherein the healthcare worker does not trust the patient, or the patient does not trust the healthcare worker. Jonas, a provider, told me he struggled to trust his Chuukese patients: "They'll show [agreeability], they'll verbalize agreeability, and not do anything; they'll just do what they want." For healthcare workers, this concern is especially connected to taking medicine as prescribed and getting lab work completed, but it also leads to paranoia that everything their patients say is a lie.

The following example about food is revelatory of the resulting exchanges. I was baffled as I watched this conversation unfold. The nurse said, "What do you eat for lunch?" and the patient responded: "I eat local food." The nurse followed up, asking, "What is local for you?" "Breadfruit," the patient answered. "We boil, mash, and mix with coconut. And I eat chicken." The nurse said, "OK, so you eat chicken and breadfruit. Do you eat corned beef and Spam?" The patient said yes. The nurse's voice grew higher as she responded, scolding the patient, "No, you shouldn't eat that! Don't eat corned beef and Spam! It is not good for the baby. It gives you high blood [pressure] and your family has a history of high blood [pressure], so you don't want to do that, OK!" Then she followed up, asking, "How do you eat chicken if you eat corned beef and Spam?" The patient, as confused as I was by the question, asked, "I'm sorry, what do you mean?" The nurse clarified that she was suspicious of her answers: "You just said you eat chicken, and now you tell me you eat corned beef and Spam; how is that?" The patient said what I would have said: "Oh, each meal I eat different things." In reflecting on this encounter, I surmised that likely, at some point, it had been suggested to nurses that they provide nutrition education based on the U.S. model of nutritional foods, given the CDC posters all over the clinic's walls. But what this resulted in was an investigation of food habits, an accusation of lying, and a scolding. Given that many Chuukese community members do not have refrigeration, corned beef and Spam are important staples (as is rice) despite their high salt content. But the patient and nurse never got to the point of considering strategies and diet plans because the nurse accused the patient of not telling the truth and simply told her to stop eating bad food. This encounter demonstrated both the reach of the U.S. empire—influencing ideas about healthy foods—and the ways in which hierarchies of power are enacted in healthcare worker–patient interactions. I observed a similar interaction in which a healthcare worker accused a woman of not wanting prenatal vitamins because she never went to the pharmacy to get them (and thus she threatened to not refill the prescription) instead of what actually happened: the patient (with limited English skills) had not understood that they were free and did not have any money to purchase them. This type of interaction contributes to healthcare workers' suspicions over what they call "patient noncompliance," with little consideration for the structural, social, or individual barriers their patients face.

Patients are also suspicious at times that the clinic workers are purposely not helping them. Similarly, some patients believe that they are forced to wait longer because they are Chuukese, but often it is in a context in which all patients at the clinic are waiting a long time (see also Hattori-Uchima 2017). A unique element in the case of Chuukese patients is their not-infrequent concerns that healthcare workers are lying to them, purposely thwarting their care, as Marilynn experienced (described at the beginning of this chapter). If a woman does not trust her healthcare worker to be acting in her best interest, a deferent yes followed by the ignoring of directions (e.g., not filling prescriptions) is much more likely. Kaylyn agreed. She believed that Chuukese people often did not plan to do what they were told by providers: "They're just saying yes . . . so they can go on their way. . . . But they avoid confrontations at all costs."

Some of this mistrust of healthcare workers among patients is well founded. For example, Chuukese women's high fertility rates are a constant source of focus in these public health clinics. Derogatory comments are made regularly regarding their choices to have several children and not use birth control, reflecting fears that Chuukese bodies are invading Guam through (excessive) reproduction. Some clinic employees also indicated that they believed their patients' intentions in migrating are not to seek better health care but to get their child U.S. citizenship. Deteriorating healthcare conditions in Chuuk are rarely considered a reason for such migration.

Patient Competency

Some clinic employees recognized Chuukese patient shyness and deference and, instead of being suspicious, were genuinely concerned that this inhibited their ability to get all the information they needed. Maria explained: "Yeah, and that's the thing; they're just so, what's the word? . . . I mean, I honestly can't tell sometimes 'cause they're [Chuukese patients] some of my nicest patients. . . . I really want to make sure they understand. They always just say yes or nod or smile [emphasis] but I'm not really sure if they understand what I'm trying to say!" Some also worried that patients did not know their bodies well enough to understand, but their agreeable nods made it hard to tell, like Jonas: "I think sometimes there's a lack of deep understanding of what you are trying to tell them. I have taken hours literally to describe things to people and then they'll ask me a question at the end of it that lets me know that they didn't understand one twentieth of what I was talking to them about, you know?" Due to their often-rushed environment, seeing these patients as lacking biomedical understandings of their bodies, and knowing their patients would politely agree regardless of the information provided, some healthcare workers started to practice a "less is more" form of communication. Mike explained this when we were discussing early prenatal care tests, such as amniocentesis:

> Those are some of the things that are actually harder to get them to understand, 'cause that involves a huge education process to try to get them [to] understand why we wanna do this test. . . . You know, maybe I don't have the right words to explain what a Down syndrome baby is, you know what it looks like in their culture or something like that, so . . . So, I think, for me, I kinda gloss over . . . a lot of those kind of things, I—I just generally don't deal with them that much compared to what I might do if I was in another kind of clinic.

Mike's explanation was that he just does not discuss complicated issues like Down syndrome, glossing over biomedical details, although he would if he were in another kind of (presumably private) clinic. He found the education process to be "huge" and thus not worth the trouble. I appreciated Mike's candid discussion of his own faults in interacting with Chuukese women, but assuming one community may not need the same details or tests because of time constraints is problematic. And it directly inhibits Chuukese women's equal access to quality care.

Patient politeness compounded with lack of English language skills do not exist in a vacuum, however. How these presumed cultural characteristics influenced healthcare worker perceptions and treatment is also important to consider. Similarly, Linda Hunt and Katherine de Voogd (2005) studied physician perceptions of Latina patients, finding that when trying to be culturally sensitive, physicians provided less information to their Latina patients. They highlight an important phenomenon in these practices: physicians who have good intentions of being culturally sensitive and competent draw from their perceptions of Latinas as being in gender-unequal relationships and having ideas about reproduction that contradict reasons for amniocentesis, along with low education levels. Yet physician sensitivity to prescribed ideas about Latinas leads to these very particular stereotypes, removing the complexity with which pregnant people make decisions about their pregnancies. Thus, stereotypes fostered and perpetuated by efforts to be culturally competent with good intentions lead to differential or stratified care of ethnic "others" using the clinic.

Perceptions of Chuukese women held by healthcare workers even with the best intentions to be sensitive can and do similarly contribute to differential care in these clinics. Chuukese women may not be provided with all the necessary information as they would were they in a private clinic, as Mike indicated; they may be talked over as their culturally powerful male or elder interpreter discusses their care and makes decisions for them; or they may be perceived as traditional in a host of ways that could influence the ways in which various forms of healthcare options, such as birth control methods, are presented.

Anthropologists are critical of efforts to address cultural competency in general. Critiques include the concern that culture is turned into a static list of beliefs for "other" (nonwhite and/or immigrant) patients, which in turn perpetuates the idea of their difference, drawing attention to those who "have culture" while ignoring the culture of biomedicine and that of dominant groups.[25] This idea of having a list of traits is also problematic because it suggests a person's lifeworld can be reduced to a list to be memorized, resulting in the stereotyping of patients.[26]

Additionally, a focus solely on cultural competency takes attention away from issues like poverty, language, and insurance access, and the other structural and social elements that shape people's health (Taylor 2003b; Shaw 2010). Some have suggested that physicians need to be taught to recognize the complexity of cultural elements while also thinking of the structural factors shaping patients' health.[27] As I described in the introduction, the authors of the concept of structural vulnerability created a tool for clinicians to use. This tool addresses structural, symbolic, and individual factors shaping their patients' lives and is particularly fruitful for clinicians serving migrant communities (Carruth et al. 2021).

Treating Chuukese patients differently to accommodate presumed cultural characteristics may be problematic, but allowing space to learn their comfort level and time for follow up for questions, providing all patients equal high-quality care and information, and ensuring that all information is translated for all patients *is* possible. And some healthcare workers did this. Some would observe patients based on their current cultural knowledge and try to accommodate as they saw fit in the moment. For example, some of the more observant providers picked up on women's discomfort concerning vaginal examinations, leading these providers to allow women to keep their skirts on during exams. Some would ask family interpreters to step out, ask the patient whether they truly wanted and needed a family interpreter, and then proceed accordingly. While they did not use the structural vulnerability tool (as it did not exist yet), many would focus on the same important elements, asking patients about access to appointments, work schedules, family obligations, and financial concerns before making a care plan. Thus, despite these many obstacles and issues with care, there were administrators, community workers, and healthcare workers doing good critical work with Chuukese patients. Replication of these efforts could contribute to improved outcomes for Chuukese women.

7 • RESISTING IMPERIAL EFFECTS

On December 3, 2021, I opened my phone to a series of messages on WhatsApp about Kiki. The front screen told me that something was wrong, so I logged into my Facebook account to see what people were talking about and learned the heartbreaking news. Christina "Kiki" Poll Stinnett, president of the Chuuk Women's Council (CWC), had unexpectedly died. Along with hundreds of people across the globe, I was devastated. I still am. The outpouring of support and love at her passing is a testament to how much she did for Chuuk and Micronesia more broadly.

I met Kiki in Chuuk when I was there for the first time in 2012, and I instantly saw that her spark was contagious. She was managing the largest FSM Women's Conference ever, with numerous international visitors and hundreds of Micronesian women in attendance (see chapter 2). She ran around directing this person to take care of that one, and that person to cover this delegate, and so forth, losing track of nobody. In that short conference period of three days, she managed to give me tours of parts of Chuuk and the CWC, connect me to other researchers who had arrived for the conference, make sure I was fed, and, most importantly, tell me how I could work with the CWC in the future. She also made sure I was taken care of when I experienced food poisoning the last day of the conference, having someone check on me hourly with offers of crackers and Sprite before my flight back to Guam. I was twenty-nine at the time—a child by Chuukese standards. She mothered me even though I had only just met her.

When I returned that next summer to spend three months with Kiki, I got to see her in action daily. I realized that for her, the conference had not been a particularly busy time. Consultants regularly visited; programs constantly needed to be implemented, run, or evaluated; grants always needed writing; and various metaphorical fires consistently needed to be put out. When there were quiet moments, she would push everyone in the office to go into the conference room (the only room besides Kiki's that had a split-level air-conditioning unit, a very nice treat) and do some Zumba on an old DVD. After that summer, we remained close, although contact with people from Chuuk is always sporadic given the islands' limited Internet access. I visited her every time she came to Guam (where one of her children resided), and I went back to Chuuk for a few more months over the next several years.

Kiki and I got along great, but she had a special gift for connecting with people. I spent ample time with her, and we grew comfortable enough to playfully bicker sometimes, too. Kiki was insecure about her (fluent) English skills and insisted I read all her official-type emails, and I begrudgingly did so while insisting that my skills as a doctoral candidate with a master of public health degree went beyond being a primary English speaker. "Let me write grants, develop programs, train people in research skills!" I would insist. She eventually let me do all these tasks, but she never stopped asking me to read her emails. She requested this of every primary English speaker who volunteered at the CWC, whether they were consultants, Peace Corps or Jesuit volunteers, or researchers. We all laughed about it when we shared this requirement of our stay.

Kiki was a fierce leader of a council that brought together women's groups across all of Chuuk. She met with and managed the expectations of global development agencies, Micronesian political leaders, her own constituency—Chuukese families—and outsiders like me with power and grace. Her leadership led the CWC to grow from a vision her own mother had of a place for collective women's voices into a powerful NGO. In the years she was president, the CWC built a two-story center (dedicated to her late mother) with clinical space, education and conference rooms, a library, a childcare facility, and living quarters to host researchers and volunteers. She also led efforts (in partnership with other leaders, like the great Eleanor Setik, also an important mentor to me) to write grants that supported the funding of a Federally Qualified Health Center, a family violence prevention center, a community garden, exercise classes, environmental sustainability classes, advocacy efforts to change laws that hurt women and families, and much more. I intended to go back in 2020 to see the progress the organization had made over the last few years, but COVID-19 changed my plans, along with those of everyone else in the world.

Kiki was not just a leader of her extended family; she was like a powerful grandmother of the entire state of Chuuk. She ran the CWC in this way. She managed everyone and everything from a seat of power but also with a desire to use that force to improve the lives of the women and families of Chuuk. While she was particularly effective, Kiki's legacy will not end with her. She was surrounded by dozens of women who will continue to fight for women and families in Chuuk in every capacity they can imagine. I am deeply saddened by the loss of this mother figure and mentor, both personally and for Chuuk, but I know she will live on in others for generations to come. She is one of the reasons I wrote this book. One of the last times we spoke she asked me when I could share it with her. I never imagined she would not be around for me to give her my first copy.

When I heard of her passing, I was in the middle of writing this book. It led me to think about whether I had left space for the power of women like Kiki. Portraying structural vulnerabilities imprinted on their bodies does not always showcase Kiki or the other bossy grandmothers who run their families and any other younger people around them (like me) with very direct orders. Nor does it portray the playfulness of women when they start dancing in the middle of a meeting, encouraging everyone to join in while laughing and slapping their skirts. Everything I wrote is what I observed, but so are these moments in which I witnessed power and playfulness. Women's power and collective organizing are important forms of resistance to the structural, symbolic, and everyday violence Chuukese women have encountered at home and abroad. My goal in this chapter is to elucidate the forms of resistance in which women engage at each level of analysis.

RESISTING SYMBOLIC VIOLENCE

One form of resistance used by women is to joke about the imperfections of men. Myjolynne Kim (2020) notes that Chuukese women often quip that they should run every facet of government so that things will actually get done. Women like Jessica told me that men are expected to make mistakes. They are perceived as one big mistake; in saying this, women are joking with a play on words—mwáán means both "man" and "mistake" in the Chuukese language. Many made fun of their spouses, too. Mary told me her husband was like most (younger) men in that "he doesn't know how to be responsible. He always depends on somebody. He likes to enjoy. He cannot cope with hardship. When it comes to hard life, he is a crybaby." They describe women, on the other hand, as brave keepers of the culture, clan, and community. They call men unimportant while signaling their own importance as clan members and reproducers. These descriptions reverse the gender inequalities in their discourse, but the power of being important remains a mechanism to surveil and control women's bodies. It also justifies violence toward them when they step outside the modicum of acceptable behavior—and sometimes when they do nothing at all.

Some women resist narratives that women are not equal to men. Jasmine was by far the most vocal elder woman I met when it came to gender inequality. She told me stories of her mother's lessons on life, much of which had to do with how women should behave. While she missed her late mother dearly and revered her, she did not agree with her ideas about women. In Jasmine's older years—divorced and happily employed—she enjoys thinking through and critiquing these inequitable discourses of gender. When we were talking about the expectations of women to be pure and honorable, and men's freedom to explore and make mistakes, she complained: "They expect women to be as perfect as can be. But I don't know. The way my mom taught us is yes, men are allowed in our culture to do all the mistakes, but women are supposed to be very submissive and obedient and a perfect feature. A perfect figure in families. You know saying that [is one thing], but as you know life is not perfect." As Jasmine so clearly analyzed, the social expectations of women to be perfect seemed unreasonable to her. She resisted the idea that she was owned (her words) by men or her clan, and she enjoyed the freedom she had found in Guam. She resisted by speaking her opinions loudly, pursuing male partners openly, and standing up for women regularly.

Another way in which women challenge inequity and everyday inequalities is through the lens of age. Jessica explained not only how men are less important but that women gain value over time and with age: "Yeah because, women is more like, when they're older, that's, that's our custom we have to respect.... They're really important, yeah ... they are the ones, the leader of the clan.... And they have to run the community, so they were important, the women ... the woman is more important" (Smith 2019b, 159–160). Kaylyn similarly reflected on the stereotype that Chuukese women suffer gender inequities, laughing about the power of elder women: "You know, and it's kinda funny really, you know how, 'cause you look at the Chuukese culture you'd think women ... they get out of school early to have kids and you know, during meetings they are all the quiet ones. But it's kinda like behind the scenes they are the ones that kind of run the family" (Smith 2019b, 160). She pointed especially to the finniichi, the eldest woman in the family (see chapter 3). As Jessica also implied, older women have power in ways that younger women do not. Some women told me they were waiting their turn to be the powerful senior woman and so listened to their elders until that time came. These power structures are not new, but what women do with that power can be a form of resistance. Older Chuukese women have been called lobbyists, given their expertise on kinship and land histories and their ability to speak on behalf of others (Flinn 2010). They are the protectors and nurturers of the land and family (Kim 2020), and in recent years, they have used that power to improve the lives of younger women and children, often through women's groups (Smith and Katzman 2020).

RESISTING IMPERIAL VIOLENCE

When discussing gender roles, women I spoke with were not overly critical of the role of Christianity in stripping their power, although some complained that the church overemphasized that women listen to their husbands rather than their families. Christianity does play a role, however. Gender discourses in Chuuk are shaped by indigenous, Christian, and U.S. patriarchal ideologies (Dernbach 1998; Kim 2020). While women were already connected to the land prior to missionization, Christian ideologies reinforced their domestic roles and connections to home.[1]

Those domestic roles translated to mean that women did not belong in jobs in the U.S. political structure set up in Chuuk (see chapter 2). While women are not overly critical of Christianity, they are critical of U.S. imperialism. Women contend that the United States gave men power. Some argue that gender roles were complementary until the United States created a Micronesian government in its image. They recognize that new social ideas like gender roles are adopted and rejected in pragmatic ways by every colonized community. Unfortunately, women often feel that men adopted colonizer gender roles in ways that suited them, and women have been struggling to regain power while maintaining Chuukese customs of respect ever since. Members of women's groups complain that Chuukese women need to resist old customs and speak up; they protest that their education levels are equal to men's and therefore they should be electable.[2]

Organizing women's groups is one important way in which women collectively bring together elder power to effect community change. Acting as a collective is an older, historically important strategy among Chuukese communities, and specifically women's social organizations (Marshall and Marshall 1990; Dernbach 1998). Since missionization, however, the groups are largely centered around Christianity. While Christian missions in the Pacific reinforce Christian patriarchy in these groups, they also become spaces to mobilize (Maisonneuve 2006).

Women told me that their mothers or grandmothers first joined women's groups in the mid-twentieth century. This was during a time in which trust territory government support allowed easier access for missionaries to come to the region. The trust territory government itself also supported women's groups (Dernbach 1998). Empowering the community through improved education, nutrition, and health care, and through understanding their cultural histories, are all motivations for women to join groups. I learned that each group has different goals, such as teaching indigenous healing and birthing practices, resisting the dysfunctional biomedicine in Chuuk, encouraging improved biomedicine in Chuuk, bringing knowledge that they had prior to colonization back to the younger generation, and improving the lives of young girls who are often taken out of school too early or have unintended pregnancies. Some concentrate on growing indigenous crops and teaching people healthy eating through returning to indigenous diets. Some emphasize prayer and visiting the elderly and the sick. All of them, however, focus on collectively improving their communities. In doing so, they merge Christian ideologies with indigenous narratives to resist the structural and symbolic violence that affects their everyday lives.

Historically, Chuukese women formed groups along village, island, or career-specific lines. As a state created not by connections but by imperial forces, there are divisions among the islands in Chuuk (as described in chapter 3). Women did not automatically feel connected to women from different islands, but they resisted the narratives that they did not belong together and formed alliances. They increasingly recognized the importance of collectively working together as the state of Chuuk became more centralized.

As Wééné became a hub of commerce, education, and health care, women leaders began meeting to discuss community issues when they were there. One major issue affecting Chuuk in the 1970s and early 1980s was alcohol use among

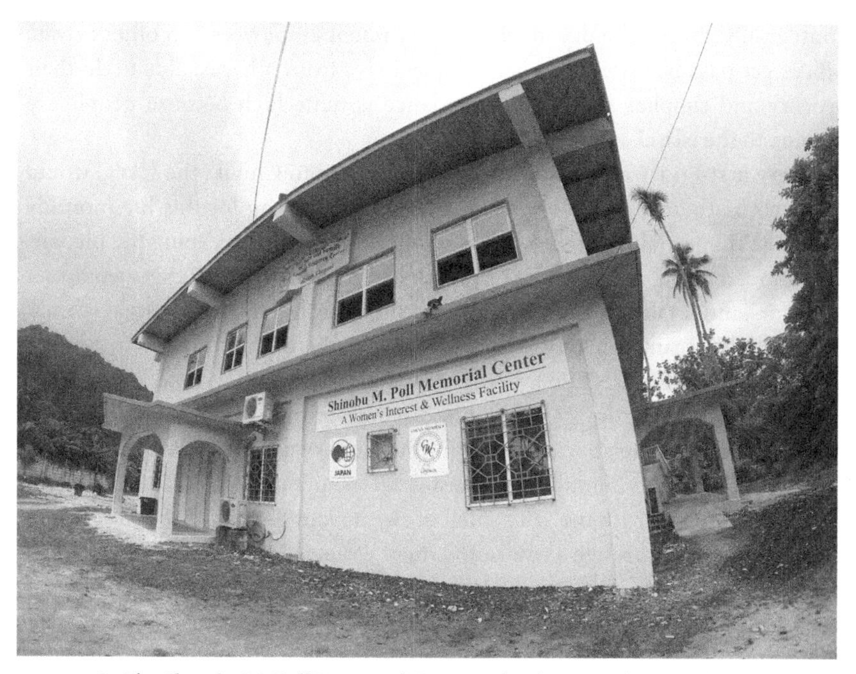

FIGURE 18. The Shinobu M. Poll Memorial Center, Chuuk Women's Council. Photo by Sarah Smith.

men. Women saw removing alcohol as key to reducing violence against women and violence between men (Marshall and Marshall 1990). They organized together and—contrary to their perceived silence—marched through the streets protesting alcohol sales. An alcohol ban was implemented after this march and much lobbying by elder women of their male relatives (Marshall and Marshall 1990). While the ban did not last long, women's understanding of what they could do together did. One of the march leaders, Shinobu M. Poll, saw the potential of state-level collective action. She and others began organizing a council to serve all Chuukese women. The Chuuk Women's Advisory Council, later renamed the Chuuk Women's Council, was born of this action and registered as an NGO in 1993.[3] Shinobu donated a parcel of her clan land to build a center that would house the council. This reflected her commitment and power to connect all Chuuk's women by using clan land she controlled. Kiki, the fearless leader I described at the beginning of this chapter, was her eldest daughter and took over this role. One of Kiki's first major accomplishments was to get funding to build the center named after her late mother. Through Shinobu and later Kiki, the CWC grew to become an umbrella organization that has registered over sixty-four groups in Chuuk (see figure 18).

The CWC mobilizes all the smaller women's groups through their strategic location in Wéénè. One Friday a month they hold a general meeting. They strategically choose the day in which government employees and other private offices get paid because it is when people arrive from other islands to do their grocery and supplies shopping. Attendance is quite high because people are coming to the island anyway.

Every first Friday of the month during my visits to Chuuk, the CWC would be abuzz as the regular volunteers ran around preparing for this big monthly meeting. They would all arrive early to help set up, some sweeping the big, air-conditioned room, enjoying the rare luxury of the cool space. Others would set up chairs and a table at the front, decorating it with floral island-style fabrics. Some would organize giveaway bags or other materials that came from outside agencies (UNICEF, UNFPA). When it was close to starting time, the women would start pouring in. Many donned mwárámwár (floral head coverings or necklaces) for the special occasion, but also sweat towels to manage the onslaught of sun and humidity, and dust from the unfinished roads. Thus, sweet floral smells mixed with the salty smell of sweat from the hot boat and car rides into town, wafting through as more and more women came in, talking, laughing, and catching up with one another. It was always in the morning, so most women came straight from the boat dock, making the CWC their first stop for the day. Kiki would spend time chatting with and greeting women as they entered before eventually taking a seat in the front and calling order. Then they would get down to business.

In these meetings, the CWC announces new funding opportunities, recruits for data collection for internal grants and external agencies seeking help, and provides updates on any ongoing projects (see figure 19). The women in turn hold meetings back on their home islands and villages to pass on the news they learn. Most of the islands do not have power, Internet, or reliable cell phone service, so this is how news gets spread.

It was at these meetings that I first witnessed elder women standing up to men, mostly outsider men (from the United States or other powerful nations), who came to speak to the CWC members. I watched thirty women sit and stare politely at leaders of church missions, such as those from the Church of Jesus Christ of Latter-day Saints, respectful but uninterested in the religion offered that day (most everyone was rather committed to their religious choices already). I also watched them grill members of initiatives who were trying to recruit workers from the CWC for labor, such as in coconut production or data collection. The elders spoke up in Chuukese (even if they spoke English); it was then interpreted by Kiki or some other English speaker (like adult daughters). The sweat poured down the temples of the outsider men as they tried to appease these women, explaining how people would be recruited, paid, or approached. As a group, the women snickered, napped, spoke to each other, and laughed through presentations of people who had garnered little respect. Only the elders, though. The younger women who sometimes accompanied the elders sat quietly and respectfully,

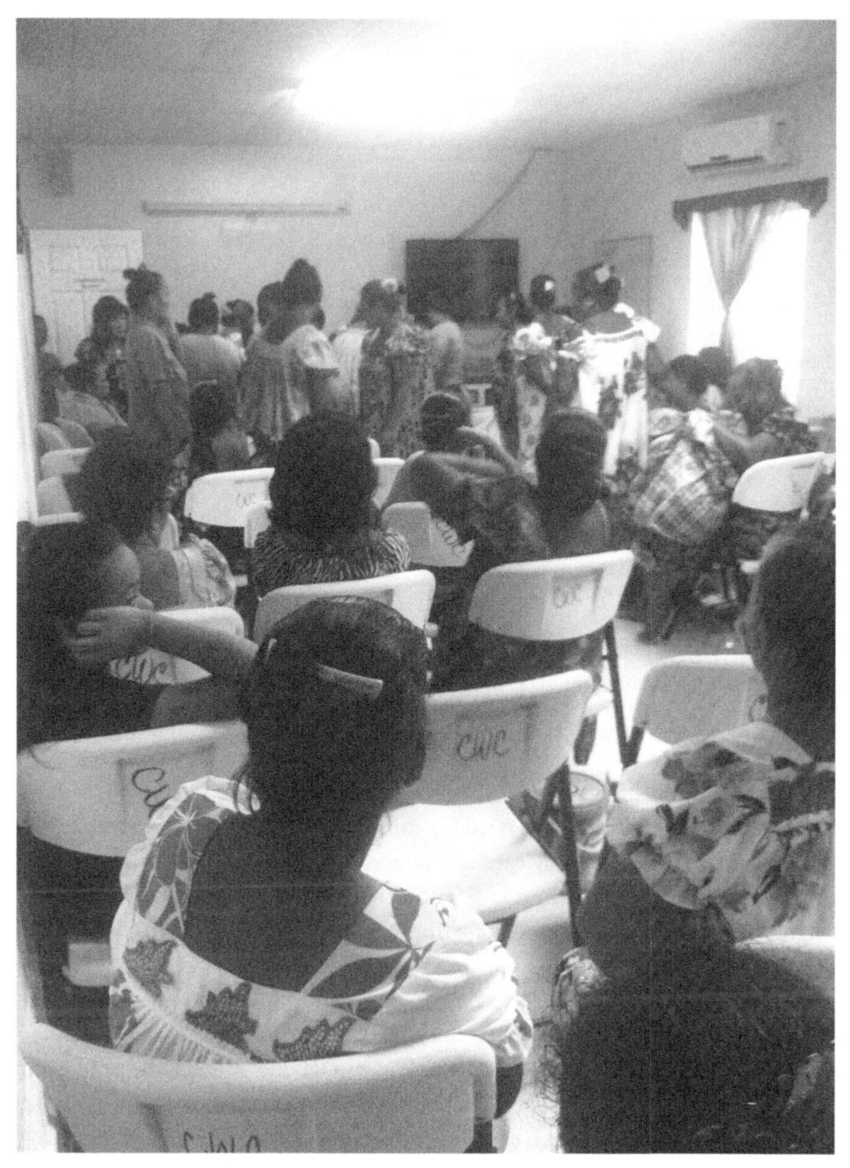

FIGURE 19. Women gathering for the Friday monthly meeting at the CWC. Photo by Sarah Smith.

their smirks revealing their amusement at their mothers' and grandmothers' words and actions.

Since its inception, the CWC has expanded its reach in every direction. As they witnessed the education system failing their children and grandchildren, CWC members organized tutoring and parent-teacher connections for school improvement projects. Recognizing that women were not getting sufficient

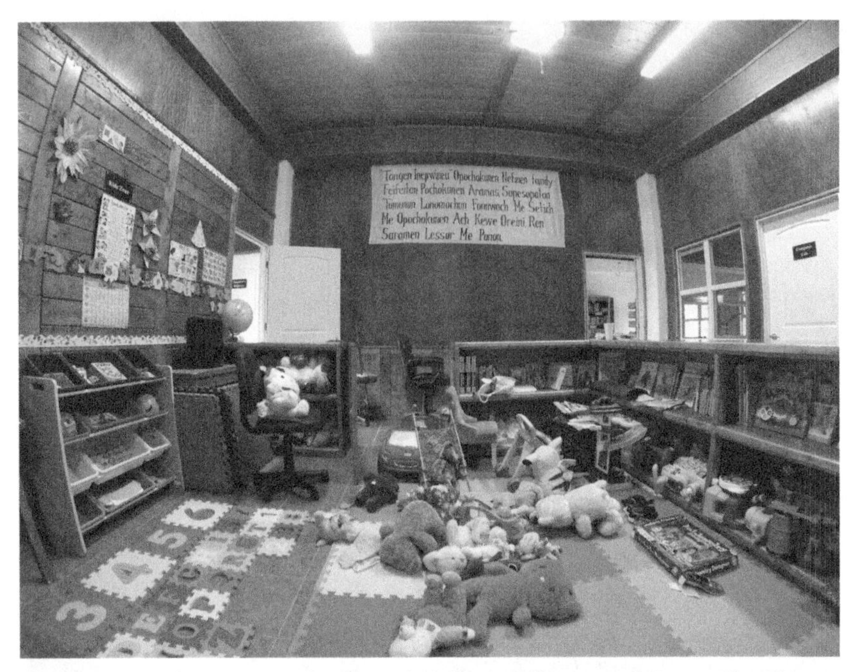
Tangen Inepwineu Opochokunen Nefinen famly
Feifeiten Pochokunen Aramas Sopesopaton
Tumunun Lanomochon Foumach Me Setich
Me Opochokunen Ach Kewe Oreini Ren
Saramen Lessor Me Panou

FIGURE 20. Childcare room in the CWC Shinobu M. Poll Memorial Center. Photo by Sarah Smith.

prenatal and family planning care, they created a clinical space and invited volunteer health providers. Seeing the need for childcare so that women could enter the workforce, they opened a day care and after-school play center (see figure 20). Recognizing the importance of indigenous healing, they organized workshops taught by local healers. For each issue they recognized, they acted to solve it.

One time when I was in Chuuk and working with the CWC, Kiki ran off to court to testify in a hearing. I knew it was a child molestation case, and the mother of the victim had come to the CWC for help. The CWC helped her report it to the authorities and made it public enough that it had to be processed (instead of being treated as a family affair, as the norm had been). I went about my day, chatting with women, editing grant reports, and planning events. Gossip, storytelling, and laughter always filled the air between moments of focus, and this day was no different as we all enjoyed one another's company. A few hours later Kiki returned, visibly frustrated and ready to vent: "What, are we social services now? We are not CPS!" By CPS, Kiki meant Child Protective Services. Child Protective Services is a well-known agency in Guam—because it is a U.S. territory—but it does not exist in Chuuk. In court that day, the judge's decision was to place the child with the CWC, as if it were a foster care or some other child services organization, and the CWC would be responsible for finding extended family members to take the child in. Despite her frustration over this unfunded mandate and the lack of an infrastructure in Chuuk to care for children like this victim, the CWC did just that, finding a foster placement for the child. Once again, Kiki transformed my understanding of the ways in which this umbrella group of women's organizations can and does have an impact in Chuuk, filling all the gaps despite limited—or often no—funding.

The CWC has memorandums of understanding with Chuuk state agencies and relationships with the international organizations working in Chuuk. They are replacing—rightfully so—the need for outside consultants, a role that anthropologists often played in colonization and then development. That is why when someone asks me how things get done in Chuuk—how to distribute a new vaccine, how to assess the needs of a particular region, how to do anything, really—I always say, "Contact the CWC."

The collective power of women's groups is not limited to Micronesia. These groups can be a powerful force across the globe, serving as mechanisms through which women share experiences and often start questioning gender inequities in their societies, challenging hegemony through collective processing. Further, like the CWC, they often work together to create the improved visions they have of their communities.[4] Women's groups have built up leadership roles in places where women in leadership was largely absent.[5]

Katherine Dernbach (1998) studied women's groups in Chuuk and saw not only the connections to Christianity and women's domestic roles reinforced through these groups but also the subversive ways in which women learned new leadership skills and were empowered in the very same light. She considered the ways in which women's groups globally are known to be feminist consciousness-raising spaces and argued that this was more complex. In Chuuk, she argued, they reinforced and resisted gender inequities in a multitude of ways. Twenty years later, I found the same to be true but also that women's groups grew on a grand scale, and feminist consciousness was far more pronounced as they did so. Religion is often the organizing force, but empowerment remains an explicit goal of these groups.

Pacific Islands women's groups are known to contribute to women entering politics, allowing their actions to become larger community change (Maisonneuve 2006; Scheyvens 2003). Their collective influence has been known to work in other ways even when women are not working from elected seats (Notwell 2014). The CWC does influence legislative decisions, such as when it lobbied successfully to get the age of consent increased from thirteen to eighteen. Given Chuuk's recent election of a woman, women are moving toward more successes in politics as well.

These grassroots organizations often transform into NGOs like the CWC, particularly in the era of global development. However, NGOs are critiqued for replacing, instead of improving, state functions in the neoliberal aid model, and the CWC is certainly one that replaces much needed state services.[6] Yet groups like this also provide spaces for people historically marginalized from the state (like women) to effect change (Bernal and Grewal 2014).

Unfortunately, NGOs like the CWC can be co-opted by powerful donors through their funding mechanisms with target- and metric- based requirements.[7] As I argued in chapters 2, 4, and 5, development metrics are often based on the priorities of former colonizers, which can perpetuate the imperial relationship but in a new form (Helms 2014; Adams 2016c; Richardson 2020). It also means, ironically, that the suffering must appeal to the perpetrators for money (Farmer 1999). In this case, Chuukese women are appealing to a host of U.S.-based aid or international aid organizations with considerable funding and influence.

Further, donor funding is usually short-term and limited to particular pieces that they (the donors) prioritize, so the NGOs are constantly searching for more funding to run their operations and keep their workers paid (Bernal and Grewal 2014). This structure can prevent grassroots organizations like the CWC from effecting real change as they chase funding and become service providers rather than activists (Alvarez 1999). Quickly putting together some sort of educational session becomes a norm (Hodžić 2014; Mukhopadhyay 2014). These quick one-off education sessions can also lead to a misunderstanding of real issues, such as when HIV education campaigns led to increased stigma (see chapter 5). They can also take away time devoted to structural change (Richardson 2020).

The CWC faces barriers of the development world as it grows in power and name, attracting large international donors. It became expected that the CWC could replace dysfunctional state systems with tiny fractions of the funding a state entity would have to perform such duties, such as providing prenatal care, STI testing, and violence prevention and treatment. The CWC is making important moves that the state is not making to improve Chuuk, but this only weakens the state's capacity to do what it is intended to do. However, this is the option women have because of their current inability to take over leadership positions in the state at any significant level. Long-term, and given the recent election of a woman, this may be changing.

Women also faced the unique challenge of having access to what might have been the shiniest, cleanest building in all of Chuuk. Some women told me they were intimidated to go into such a nice place: they felt unworthy. Indeed, this newly constructed cinder-block building was decorated with flowers and photos all over the walls, and the floors were regularly swept and mopped. There was a small computer lab donated by an international organization conducting a literacy project, a sewing room with brand-new donated machines, and newer office spaces. It did not resemble the deteriorating buildings throughout Chuuk, which had had little to no maintenance since the trust territory days, slowly rotting in the hot, wet tropical environment, evidence of benign neglect under the COFA. While members of the CWC welcomed all who walked through its doors, this shiny exterior and interior may have been a barrier to care for some of the more vulnerable women.

Regardless of its members' interest in the issues, the CWC is stuck looking for funding and applying for small projects because the larger donors are not always interested. The budget is then spread thin to try to cover what the CWC members find meaningful and important as well. But that means work for women is often short-term and underpaid, perpetuating the very gender inequities they seek to eliminate. However, while they do take on projects they are less interested in pursuing, they also push for projects they find important, learning from both. All these efforts lead to improved health, education, and economic outcomes for women and families in the state. They remain focused on their agenda of improving the lives of women and families in Chuuk in each project and program. Despite getting caught in the NGO world's limitations, they leverage the resources they obtain to improve their capacity to do more and more for Chuuk with time (see also Smith and Katzman 2020).

The CWC operates within the constraints it is dealt. Instead of giving up or doing nothing, it works with the limitations of development agencies, the structural violence of benign neglect, and the symbolic violence of gender inequities in their communities, and its members persevere. They make sweeping changes in some ways and mark small victories in others. While they do not use the term "pragmatic solidarity"—a phrase popularized by Paul Farmer to indicate the ways in which we should be helping people now even as we wait for structural change—that is exactly what CWC members are engaged in (Farmer 1999, 2003b).

All this work is recognized by members, who told me how the work leads to changes in policy (the body politic), conversations in the greater community about gender (the social body), and help for individuals seeking it (the individual body). As one group member told me, "CWC will help. We will step up, and we will help Chuuk. . . . We want to look out and see the importance and worth of women to our own [community]" (Smith and Katzman 2020, 1152–1153). But this collective action is happening largely in Chuuk. What about Guam?

RESISTING EVERYDAY VIOLENCE IN GUAM

In Guam, Chuukese women's transnational reproduction is stratified by poverty, gender inequities (see chapters 4 and 5), anti-immigrant sentiment (see chapter 3), and inaccessible clinical care (see chapter 6), but points of resistance are notable throughout, sometimes enabled by their migration to Guam. Jasmine told me how she felt like the pressure in Guam just changed; instead of challenging gender inequalities, she now must challenge the narratives that her people arrive only for food stamps, welfare, and other social safety net services. Women like Jasmine resist these narratives by getting jobs and supporting their families.

They show their power by pursuing college degrees, seeking careers, teaching their daughters to concentrate on education, and even removing men from their families when they are violent. But they do so while demonstrating clearly and symbolically who they are by wearing distinctive Chuukese skirts, dresses, and combs.

Vulnerabilities play out in the clinic, as does resistance to them. When flying to Guam, Chuukese women often navigate the hostile clinical spaces and insurance applications regardless of efforts to disentitle them from these services, as I have described (see chapters 3 and 6). That is why despite so many barriers to care, Chuukese women made up over half of all prenatal patients in Guam's community health clinics. Further, in the face of U.S.-inspired discourses about their reproductive bodies (being hyperfertile, driving up the debts of Guam), many continue to reproduce (see chapter 4). Reproduction is a source of power and pride for many women. And those who do not want to reproduce any longer start to ask for help with family planning. Some—hiding from their husbands and mothers—get these methods in secret. In these ways, some women practice agency over their reproductive bodies, resisting structural, social, and individual insults, enabling them to improve their lives and those of their children (see chapter 5). Yet despite these individual efforts to resist the vulnerabilities they face, Chuukese women still struggle with the worst sexual and reproductive health outcomes in Guam. Some of their grassroots efforts to collectively organize may, in fact, better contribute to long-term systemic change.

TRANSNATIONAL COLLECTIVE ACTION

Kiki always focused on Chuuk; she was from Kaylyn's parents' generation, and so she was taught to go abroad, learn what she could, and come home to improve Chuuk. She struggled to understand why so many people left for good. She wanted to make Chuuk more livable so that people did not have to make that choice. But while she wanted to remain focused on improving lives in Chuuk, she increasingly recognized that Chuukese communities abroad needed support and connection as well. When I last visited her, I learned that these connections were happening. Kiki told me how excited she was; she had about five women's groups in Guam and Hawai'i now registered with the CWC. Chuukese women's groups had become as transnational as women's lives.

When I interviewed women who had lived part or most of their lives in Guam, they all told me they participated in women's groups that had formed there. Most were church groups, primarily organized to host singing and dancing competitions and to raise money for their churches and community needs back in Chuuk (see figure 21). The first time I attended one of these competitions in Guam, I had no idea what to expect. I arrived at the community meeting space (usually a church or a school gymnasium) and saw hundreds of Chuukese

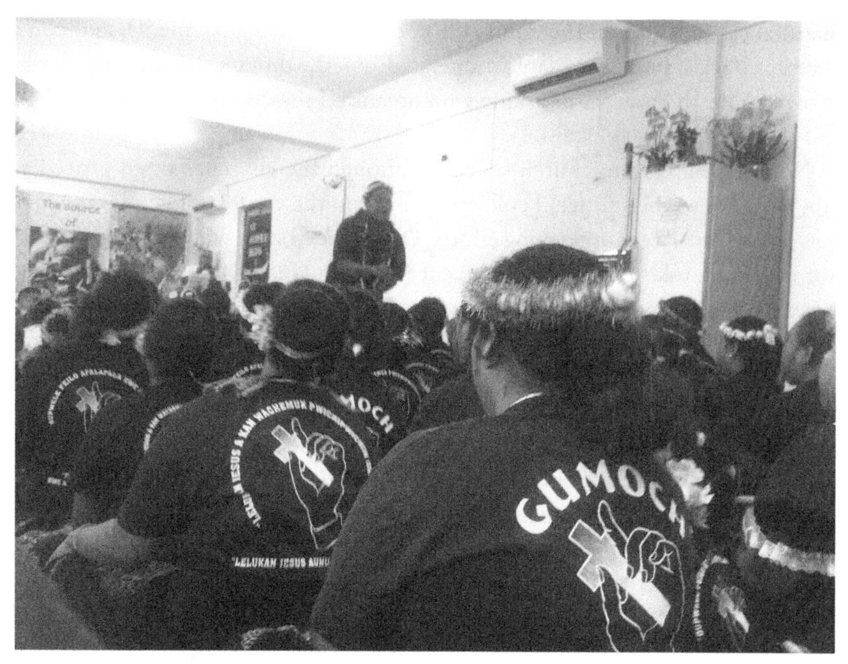

FIGURE 21. Chuukese groups host a singing competition in Guam. Photo by Sarah Smith.

women and children, all in matching team outfits. One group was adorned in yellow shirts that signified their island of origin; another wore pink shirts that signified a region; others wore green, blue, red, and orange. The groups on this occasion were from outer island communities, and the energy was abuzz as everyone waited for the competition to start. Most women wore mwárámwár, some with fresh flowers, but most were more permanent types with plastic flowers. The older children were all girls, dressed in the appropriate uniform for the competition and ready to sing. Younger children—mostly toddler aged—were girls and boys, watching the crowd grow while attached to their adult or older child caretaker. About an hour after the official start time, everyone sat on the floor in their respective groups, and the singing started. Each group sang a song while the others listened, all facing the stage of judges. Chuukese music is incredibly important and powerful, and it is typically sung in groups. The high notes women hit in these songs have a grating beauty to them, and the songs exude energy. This competition was followed by a party. Sometimes big feasts happened afterward, with everyone involved; sometimes the feasts happened in the homes of group members, each group going its own way. I always attended, leaving with Styrofoam containers full of ribs, rice, breadfruit, taro, and other Guam staples, such as noodles, BBQ chicken, and fish. These organizations and events were key to surviving in this hostile space, providing a social outlet, possibly financial support (when the competition prize included a payment), and connections back home. They largely operated quietly, though. I would not have known about them without asking who organized the competitions I attended and asking what else they did.

Not all groups were church specific, although the churches often proved a safe place for women to yield collective power in the context of gender inequities. Some were larger organizing efforts. One elder woman who had returned to live in Chuuk told me that in her twenty years in Guam, she had organized a larger COFA community group. Housed at UOG, she told me, the group would be called on to make handicrafts for big government of Guam events and were mobilized for any kind of community outreach. She was proud of the image this group promoted to greater Guam—one of a community that contributes meaningfully to Guam's social life. This was in the 1990s. She thought that organization was largely defunct now, but others have taken its place. There is a very active and engaged Chuukese Women's Association of Guam (Neechuumeres),[8] and a Catholic Chuukese Women's Association that I know of (and likely, several more). There is also an FSM Association of Guam,[9] which links all four states for expanded community connection. Neechuumeres and the FSM Association were both instrumental in mobilizing COFA communities around COVID-19 vaccination and testing. Both groups, along with MRCOSS, have been working closely with community partners to better reach COFA communities for a variety of projects. These groups demonstrate efforts to bridge differences across islands, regions, and even states to collectively work together to improve their circumstances on Guam. Wherever COFA communities settle, groups like this form,[10] and women are often at the center of such organizing.

While outside observers characterize transnational Chuukese women as quiet, submissive, and stuck in the domestic sphere in places like Guam, women are actively engaged in Guam and other places of residence culturally, politically, and economically. Chuukese women are working, going to school, caring for little ones and elders, maintaining extended family networks across transnational boundaries, and participating in their churches. Somehow, they also find time to organize and participate in various groups. These groups foster collective action and yield power in transnational spaces. While facing structural, social, and individual assaults on their bodies abroad, they organize to improve the lives of their people through such groups. Chuukese women provide a salient example of how gender is produced, stratified, and contested across transnational boundaries.

CONCLUSION

Formerly colonized communities disproportionately experience culture-blaming from both inside and outside communities for conditions and life experiences that actually reflect the structural and symbolic violence of benign neglect. In

Guam and Chuuk, culture is often blamed for Chuukese women's disproportionately poor reproductive health outcomes (as depicted in chapters 4 and 5). Historical processes shaping gender, relationships, and discourses about migration are largely ignored (chapters 1, 2, and 3). Culture is blamed for the lack of prenatal care, unintended pregnancies, intimate partner violence, and limited STI testing and treatment (chapters 4, 5, and 6). Rarely do former scholars, healthcare workers, or community leaders reference the violent history of colonization and the politics of benign neglect in analyzing stratified reproductive outcomes (see also Farmer 2003a). One of my objectives of this book has been to render visible the multilayered vulnerabilities at the structural (body politic), social (social body), and experiential (individual body) level instead of making the mistake of blaming culture for such inequities. Imperial domination, benign neglect, and resulting poverty and transnational migration, as well as the new forms of patriarchy that accompany such forces, contribute to women's stratified reproduction. The vulnerabilities resulting from this confluence of events contribute to the ways in which women's reproduction is stratified at individual, social, and structural levels, with powerful consequences for their sexual health and reproductive health.

I employed the concept of structural vulnerability (Quesada, Hart, and Bourgois 2011) and the politics of benign neglect to elucidate how Chuukese transnational women's reproductive bodies are stratified. I illustrated the vulnerabilities associated with the structural violence of imperialism and benign neglect, and how political, economic, and historical forces manage and surveil their bodies (the body politic). The gendered vulnerabilities I presented in this book (the social body) reflect the juxtaposition of pre-contact gender roles and masculine dominance associated with global capitalist expansion and Christian missionization (Dernbach 1998; Kim 2020). Considering how a study of stratified reproduction in the context of migration reveals public discourses over the economy, race, and immigration, I considered how women's bodies are represented (the social body)—as the oppressed gender in Chuuk and as the undesirable migrant in Guam—and how these symbolic articulations of their bodies perpetuate gender and racial inequities in their everyday lives. Finally, I illuminated these transnational bodies through women's personal stories of reproducing, forming relationships, seeking care, and seeking opportunities (individual body). Engaging with the politics of reproduction, these stories elicit how each layer of social life shapes and reflects women's experiences and, ultimately, their reproductive health. Behind every poor indicator of reproductive and sexual health is a structural, social, and individual set of circumstances that makes a community vulnerable to such outcomes. But there is also resistance to such violence, most notably through the power of collective action through women's groups.

As I argued in this book, decolonization is key to changing the circumstances stratifying women's reproduction. And yet calling for larger structural forces to change is not sufficient in this kind of work (Farmer 2003a). For human rights work more broadly, the late Paul Farmer (2003a) insisted on a new agenda two decades ago. He argued that we must do research and educate the public while also working to achieve independence from powerful governments and bureaucracies, many of whom are connected to or are the perpetrators of structural violence (Farmer 2003b). But this, too, is not sufficient. We must also make central the provision of services and the securing of more resources in the immediate future; that is, we must engage in pragmatic solidarity. Women running community organizations like the CWC already knew the principle of pragmatic solidarity: that to attempt to achieve only the biggest challenges may often result in achieving too little (Farmer 2003a). Instead, we must work on what we can while fighting for the larger changes that are necessary.

In consideration of pragmatic solidarity, I made suggestions for actions we can take now within clinical spaces and social service agencies throughout this book. I also provided my findings to the leadership and through training events at the Guam community health centers. But there are also important ways we can support community-level grassroots actions like those I have described in this chapter. These include involving more community leaders (i.e., religious leaders) in linking people to care, training more health outreach workers from COFA communities, and conducting community-driven research on the community's needs to better serve them.[11] Collective grassroots organizing and support from the larger community has been effective in reducing the vulnerabilities Chuukese communities face, and as this chapter portrays, women are often at the center of these efforts. The best work anthropologists and other supporters can do is assist these organizations in the ways they (the people in these organizations) see fit. Further, we can help with data collection, evaluation, and research, but the agenda needs to be born of collective community action (see also Inada et al. 2019; Rehuher et al. 2021). Finally, advocating for funding that is not siloed or metric based but that truly supports organizations like the CWC both in Chuuk and abroad is vital to supporting these communities in doing the work they need to do. In essence, Chuukese women are adept at organizing and working to improve their communities within the constraints they are dealt, and they are equipped to lead community efforts. Supporting these efforts is key.

ACKNOWLEDGMENTS

There are so many people who made this book possible. First, I am grateful to all the members of the Chuuk Women's Council—especially Kiki and Eleanor—who welcomed me into their hearts, homes, and activism as they led efforts to improve the lives of Chuukese women and their families. Any royalties from this book will be donated to the CWC to continue these efforts. I am also grateful to the entire Truk Stop family for taking me in each time I landed in Wééné, and Chuuk public health staff for supporting my presence in their clinics as I shadowed various providers and women seeking care.

This book would not have been possible without the support of so many people in Guam. My Guam family—the Weilbacher crew—were instrumental in supporting my move and taking me and my spouse into their world. Not only were Rosa, Walden, the girls, Meimei, and the rest of the family welcoming and supportive in everyday life in Guam, but they also helped me connect with various FSM leaders and community members. Other folks in Guam were important in this journey as well, especially colleagues at Guam's Department of Health and Social Services (DPHSS) and the University of Guam (UOG). Without the approval and patience of so many people at DPHSS for various projects over the last decade, there would be no book to write. I am also grateful to colleagues at UOG, Guam Behavioral Health, Healing Hearts Rape Crisis Center, and the Guam Coalition against Sexual Assault and Family Violence—colleagues in each of these organizations provided a listening ear as I processed my data in real time and offered important insights from their own work. Maira (Rios) Arriola was particularly helpful. I would also like to thank the many UOG students (now alumni!) and the Chuukese Student Organization for allowing me to spend time with you and learn your perspectives. Lulu, I am especially grateful to you for the language training and all your insights!

This book began when I embarked on my dissertation journey over a decade ago, and the training and support I received at the University of South Florida (USF) during the PhD and afterward was vital. First, I would like to acknowledge my dissertation committee members: Nancy Romero-Daza, Heide Castañeda, Keith "Mac" Marshall, Ellen M. Daley, and Elizabeth Bird. I am grateful to each of you for your consistent and continuous support, and your advice and expertise were invaluable. My major advisers Nancy Romero-Daza and Heide Castañeda provided exceptional support throughout the whole process, just as they did throughout my entire graduate career. You both are so amazing! Heide Castañeda continues to provide regular insights and support years later—even now, when I am a tenured associate professor; for this, I am truly grateful. Mac

Marshall also provided such important support and perspectives from afar. I am so indebted to Mac for his insights, connections, and constant cheerleading before we ever met in real life.

Since that time, my colleagues at my current institution, State University of New York (SUNY) Old Westbury, have also provided tremendous support for my research. I have had the privilege to present findings and have conversations that were integral to my analysis; I am so grateful for this environment. I am also eternally grateful to my colleagues Nathanial Dickey, Josealyn Eria, and Rahwa Haile, each of whom provided feedback on early versions of several chapters—thank you! And so many colleagues helped me in this process through conversations, presentation forums, and collaborations.

I would also like to acknowledge the financial support which made this possible: the University of South Florida through years of assistantship funding and the Fathauer Graduate Fieldwork Travel Grant; the University of Guam CLASS Faculty Travel Funding Grant, the UOG Cancer Center, and the U.S. Office of Minority Health Pacific Resource Center. I am also appreciative of the UOG Gender Studies Center for the office space and collegial support when I lived in Guam, especially through Seyda Turk-Smith. Since then, I have received significant support from my union, United University Professions (UUP), and SUNY Old Westbury through research grants that allowed me to travel back to Guam several times between 2015 and 2019, as well as the support of a sabbatical to begin planning this book in spring 2020 through the UUP Nuala McGann Drescher pre-tenure sabbatical program.

I am grateful to my *entire* family for all their support throughout this process. I am especially grateful to my parents for their love, patience, and pride, and to my father, Damon Smith, for his keen editing eye on early versions of these chapters. And the person I could not have done this without is my partner, Chris Comerford, who took on more of the emotional, domestic, and familial labor during each and every research project over the last decade. Thank you for always being patient and supportive when this book took over my time and my mind.

Most importantly, I am grateful for all the women, families, and healthcare workers who sat down to speak with me; let me follow them around in their workspaces, care settings, homes, churches, and group meetings; and shared honestly how their lives and work were shaped by the imperial circumstances of benign neglect. It was a great privilege to learn their stories and now share them in this book. Even when I could not be physically present in these recent pandemic years, social media allowed me to witness the continued collective actions of people working to improve their circumstances. But the precarity of their imperial circumstances remain. I hope that this book uncovers some of the hidden layers of the imperial strategy of benign neglect, revealing the deleterious consequences for health and well-being. In doing so, I aim to be complicit in decolonizing Micronesia.

NOTES

INTRODUCTION

1. For more on Panga design boats, see Heather Steinberger, "The History of the Panga," *Boating,* August 10, 2017, https://www.boatingmag.com/boats/history-panga/.
2. "Guamanian" is a term that originated specifically for the Chamoru of Guam. The term came into use during World War II, when the Japanese invaded Guam with the aid of Chamoru people from the Northern Mariana Islands; the term became a way to differentiate Chamorus from Guam from those of the Northern Mariana Islands. More recently, "Guamanian" has transformed into a catch-all term for all Guam residents, and "Chamoru" has been reappropriated specifically for indigenous Guam residents as part of the Chamoru rights movement.
3. "Micronesian" is a contested term. Technically, all people indigenous to the region of Micronesia are considered Micronesian, including the indigenous Chamoru from Guam and those from the Commonwealth of the Northern Mariana Islands. However, colloquial use of the term "Micronesian" in Guam specifically refers to people with indigenous ancestry in the FSM (including Pohnpei, Chuuk, Kosrae, and Yap), the Republic of the Marshall Islands, or the Republic of Palau. In this book, I use the term to evoke this colloquial meaning. In this region, "Micronesian" is used interchangeably with "COFA migrants," "FAS migrants," "COFA citizens," and "FAS citizens." "COFA" refers to the Compacts of Free Association between the United States and three island nations in Micronesia (which I describe later in this chapter), while "FAS" refers to the Freely Associated States, referencing the same three island nations and their compacts. All these terms refer to the same communities.
4. I use the spelling "Chamoru" instead of the standard spelling "Chamorro" to respect indigenous efforts to accurately reflect pronunciation and challenge the imposition of Spanish orthography (G. E. Taitano 2018). The Chamoru are indigenous to the entire Mariana Islands archipelago, of which Guam is the southernmost island. "CHamoru" (with a capital *H*) is another accepted indigenous spelling.
5. These data are very poorly tracked. The 2012 study by Hezel and Levin, combined with the 2020 U.S. census, provide the most updated estimates on COFA migration. These estimates are likely underreports, as COFA migrants are often part of hidden populations, and data collection is minimal at best even when they are accessible.
6. Some scholars have pointed out that people have always been mobile. This was not a new phenomenon in the 1990s; it was just the moment in which anthropologists found it theoretically convenient (Gupta and Ferguson 1997; Mintz 1998). Micronesian scholars have expressed similar sentiments (Puas 2021; Peter 2000).
7. See, for example, Basch, Glick-Schiller, and Blanc (1994); Glick-Schiller, Basch, and Blanc-Szanton (1992); Inda and Rosaldo (2008).
8. It was originally called Continental Micronesia or colloquially termed *Air Mike,* a subsidiary of Continental Airlines, and people still call it that despite the fact that United merged with Continental in 2010 (keeping the name United Airlines).
9. See Amundsen and Frain (2020); Mountz and Loyd (2014); Mountz (2011); Smith and Castañeda (2021).
10. There is a third hospital in Guam, the U.S. Naval Hospital. It is not open to civilians except in rare, severe, and emergency cases that are beyond the capacity of GMH until such persons can be transferred to Hawai'i, the Philippines or elsewhere for care (see chapter 6).

11. See, for example, Ardner (2006); Brown (1970); Ortner (1972); Weiner (1980).
12. On gender inequality, these anthropologists include Chodorow (1974); Ortner (1972); Rosaldo and Lamphere (1974). On the study of kinship, see, for example, Collier (1974); di Leonardo (1991); Rosaldo and Lamphere (1974).
13. See also Baer, Singer, and Susser (2003); Browner (2001); Browner and Sargent (2007); Greenhalgh (1995); Lock and Nguyen (2010); McElroy and Townsend (2015); Weiner (1995).
14. See Flinn (1987); Kawai (1987); Kim (2020); Moral (1996, 1998).
15. See Caughey (1971); Fischer (1963); Fitzgerald (2001); Flinn (1987); Moral (1996).
16. "Pregnant people" is a more appropriate term to reflect the variety of gender identities associated with who can become pregnant. This book, however, reflects only the experiences of cisgender women. For that reason, I use the term "pregnant women."
17. See Bautista (2010); Dernbach (2005); Marshall (2004).
18. This report, like many in the FSM due to its limited resources, does not differentiate fetal, neonatal, infant, and maternal deaths in this statement about the major causes of death. I elaborate on these data collection issues in chapter 4.
19. See, for example, Browner and Sargent (2011); Castañeda (2008); Ginsburg and Rapp (1995); Unnithan-Kumar and Khanna (2014).
20. I scheduled another monthlong trip for the spring of 2020, but the global COVID-19 pandemic did not allow that to happen. I rescheduled for early 2022, but a new variant again delayed travel. I was finally able to return for a short trip in March 2023.
21. See, for example, DeLisle (2015, 2016); Frain (2017); Kim (2020); Mack and Na'Puti (2019); Na'puti and Bevacqua (2015); Smith and Katzman (2020).

CHAPTER 1 IMPERIAL OCCUPATIONS

1. According to Puas, Chuukese people refer to their communities as remetaw *or* shon metaw (the people of the deep sea) (2021, 163).
2. The Gilbert Islands chain (encompassing the Republic of Kiribati) and Nauru are also in Micronesia, but differing colonial histories in the twentieth century kept these southernmost Micronesian islands separate from what is deemed "American Micronesia" (Kiste 1993).
3. See Diaz (2010); Kiste and Falgout (1999); Lutz (1984); Petersen (2004); Rogers (1995).
4. The Republic of Palau is also part of the Caroline Islands. They are located west of the islands depicted in figure 6 (see figure 5). Note that figure 6 has some misspelled names. The Marshall Islands have two ls in their name, and Phonpei (on the map) is actually spelled Pohnpei. Similarly, Truk was the name given to Chuuk by outsiders of this region. When these countries gained independence, they changed the spelling of several islands to reflect their own perspective on how their island states should be spelled and pronounced. It remains common to see a variety of ways of spelling island names throughout the region.
5. While historians have noted that the killing of a priest delayed colonization in the Caroline Islands, the killing of San Vitores did not delay anything in the case of Guam. Instead, it led to the Spanish-Chamoru Wars. I believe this was because Guam was such an important strategic location, as it remains today under U.S. control.
6. Puas (2021), citing Mac Marshall (1979) and Francis X. Hezel (1983), differentiated between lagoon Chuukese people (perceived as violent) and Mortlockese people, who were perceived as friendly by outsiders such as Dumont D'Urville, Captain Alonso de Arellano, and Andrew Cheyne. These stereotypes remain today.
7. Chuuk lagoon is an atoll lagoon, which forms when a larger island completely subsides under water, leaving a ring of coral that continues to grow upward. It is about 64 kilometers in diameter and formed by a barrier reef that encloses an area of 2,125 square kilometers.

8. This was also the year (1901) in which the U.S. Supreme Court heard a series of cases dubbed "the insular cases" after acquiring new territories during the Spanish-American War. In reviewing these cases, the court determined that the U.S. Constitution does not automatically apply to U.S. territories, and that unincorporated territories and their residents specifically do not fall under full protection, even if they are U.S. citizens (Rogers 1995).
9. The difference between congressional and constitutional citizenship is that the U.S. Congress can repeal Guam's citizenship at any time with a simple majority. The citizenship of state-based American citizens is protected by the U.S. Constitution, changes of which are rare, as it requires a higher threshold of congressional support and ratification by state legislatures.
10. Bonilla (2015) calls this paradox in which small island states in the Caribbean are neither fully sovereign nor independent "non-sovereignty." She argues that there is not yet a word to describe these iterations outside the organizing political framework of sovereignty.
11. While the navy no longer controls immigration in Micronesia, several of these islands are still denied access to people from any country that cannot travel through Guam (U.S. territory), since all flights go through Guam.
12. There is debate over the context in which he made this statement. Some have indicated that he made this remark in regard to debates over whether the United States should use eminent domain to take the land of Micronesians during the trust territory period. Others have indicated that this was in reference to discussions of whether or not to conduct nuclear testing in the Marshall Islands. Regardless of which context, the sentiment remains the same: Micronesians were a small, forgettable body politic.
13. Robert Kiste (1994b) noted that despite the United States not seeing itself as a colonizer, the U.S. Departments of War, State, and the Interior all fought over control of this region. The Department of the Interior won the battle, signaling that the region is part of the United States.
14. The Northern Mariana Islands were under Japan's control from 1914 to 1944.
15. The people of Palau took longer primarily because they wanted the agreement to be antinuclear. The years leading up to the agreement were tumultuous, as Palauans—led by powerful women—refused to stand down to their antinuclear requirement. Despite CIA attempts to intervene and change the power dynamics and decision-makers in Palau, they persevered. Palau's is the only COFA that explicitly does not allow nuclear devices on its land (Dé Ishtar 1994).
16. Some have argued that this denial clause indicates that the FSM does not have sovereignty, but others argue that the denial clause "does not and cannot usurp the FSM's Constitution" (Puas 2021).
17. See, for example, Kiste (1994b); Hanlon (1998); Lutz (1986); Barker (2004).
18. Since these changes, the Joint Economic Management Committee Office (JEMCO) has become a sort of "fourth branch" of government to control compact funds; three of the five members of the committee are American, providing a clear control of JEMCO decisions. Leaders of the FSM have challenged this committee and the management of their funds; so far, they have been ignored (Puas 2021, 112–113).
19. On May 20, 2022, the China First Policy was publicly rejected by the president of the FSM, David Panuelo, who perceived this as more of a colonizing agreement than an establishment of international relations. In March 2023, right after FSM national elections, outgoing FSM President Panuelo wrote another letter about China that was leaked to the press. In this letter he accused China of "political warfare," detailing, in fourteen pages, several attempts made by China to interfere in FSM governance (Perry 2023).
20. During my last visit, the decades-long paving project for the main roads was nearly complete.
21. For this summary, I included those who designated one "race" or ethnic identity. These numbers are a bit higher when including those who identify as having multiple ethnicities or

"race" identities on the island. Chamoru alone and in combination increases to 41 percent, and Filipino alone or in any combination increases to 35.3 percent.

22. See also Mountz (2011).

CHAPTER 2 IMPERIAL OBSERVATIONS

1. Flying the same day after a dive can trigger decompression sickness, so divers typically do another activity on their last day of a trip requiring a flight.

2. Many tourists I spoke with were given the impression that going outside the hotel was unsafe for them. Chuuk is stereotyped as the most dangerous place in Micronesia (see chapter 3).

3. During my last trip to the FSM in 2017, WorldTeach (https://www.worldteach.org/) was also filling a large portion of high school teacher positions.

4. These observations are from prior to the COVID-19 pandemic, when the FSM shut down its borders to both citizens and noncitizens. They were not completely open again until late 2022. See https://fm.usembassy.gov/covid-19-information/.

5. I have been a longtime member of this organization, and I am a graduate of an applied program. I believe we must address our historical application of advancing imperialism.

6. Chilean academics were informed of this study and promptly told Chilean government officials, who sent notice to the U.S. Department of State of their opposition to this project and went public. The U.S. Department of State was unaware of the project, which was funded by the U.S. Department of Defense.

7. See, for example, Asad (1973); Dirks (1992); Gough (1967); Pels (1997); Pels and Salemink (1994); Price (2016).

8. Many observations and suggested changes to decolonize the discipline were made in this era. See, for example, Agar (1996); Behar and Gordon (1995); Clifford (1986); Coffey (1999).

9. See, for example, Rosaldo (1989); Trouillot (1991); Harrison ([1991] 1997); Pels and Salemink (1994).

10. This does not mean that all anthropologists simply began to resist imperial regimes. A minority of anthropologists continued to serve colonial and military interests, the most recent example being the Human Terrain System (HTS) of the U.S. Department of Defense. The HTS was meant to serve the military and help them to better understand local populations in order to reduce violence (Forte 2011). The AAA meetings again marked contentious debates over this program, and the executive board outright condemned the project (Forte 2011; American Anthropological Association Executive Board 2007). Pressure from members responding to this work led to an overhaul of the AAA's ethics code in 2009 (and updated again in 2012). This new code expresses the importance of research independent of government intervention and of recognizing the possible ways in which findings could be used by imperial or military organizations prior to publishing (Price 2016; American Anthropological Association 2012).

11. For some, however, working in development is an avenue to resist recolonization and better advocate for more nuanced, in-depth understandings of communities (see, for example, McPherson 2016; Adams 2016b).

12. See, for example, Alcalay (1992); Heine (1974); Kiste and Falgout (1999); Kiste and Marshall (1999); Kroll (2003).

13. There is a deeper ethnographic history with human "zoos." Early researchers in colonized zones often brought human body parts or living people back from the colonies and put them on display as subjects (or rather objects) of scientific study (Manderson 2018). These displays further perpetuated racial hierarchies developed by colonial administrations with a scientific bent added to them (Manderson 2018). Micronesia was not immune to these racialized zoos; the World's Fair in St. Louis had people from Guam on display. Heine's reference, however, was internal. Instead of being brought for display to imperial centers, Micronesians under the USTTPI were kept in the confines of Micronesia, not allowed to leave because of U.S. naval control of immigration while being observed by scientists from CIMA and SIM.

14. See, for example, F. B. Caughey (1971); J. L. Caughey (1977); A. Fischer (1963); J. L. Fischer (1951); Fischer and Swartz (1960); Gladwin and Sarason (1953); Goodenough (1949, 1978); Swartz (1958).

15. See, for example, Manderson and Jolly (1997); Manderson (1996); Anderson (2006); Wendland (2016).

16. This analysis of studies of gender, sexuality, and reproduction focuses on heterosexuality and cisgender women. Very little literature exists that discusses the lives of people who identify as LGBTQIA+ in Micronesia. HIV healthcare workers in Chuuk told me that there are men who secretly have sex with men outside their heterosexual marriages but very few openly queer men. In terms of gender identity, some scholars argue that prior to colonization (and early in colonization), when Christian patriarchal norms were not infused throughout the islands, transgender people were ceremonially accepted into Micronesian communities (Ward 1989). More recently, openly queer individuals from greater Micronesia often migrate and participate in the LGBTQIA+ community in Guam and other U.S. jurisdictions. Some shared with me that to be openly queer and feel safe, they feel they must leave their home islands.

17. See J. L. Caughey (1977); Gladwin and Sarason (1953); Goodenough (2002); Mahony (1969).

18. European missionary accounts from the early twentieth century also participated in the colonial gaze of sexuality. Laurentius Bollig (1927), for example, discussed moonlight dances and parties celebrating the goddess Inemes, which openly celebrated love and sex (Bollig 1927, as cited in Dernbach 2005).

19. See Ashby (1993); Dernbach (1998, 2005); Dobbin and Hezel (1995); Hezel (1995, 2001, 2004); Marshall (1976); Marshall and Marshall (1979, 1980, 1982); Rauchholz (2008, 2009).

20. Stooping is when people bend over or get on their knees to be physically lower as they walk (or scoot) by people they perceive as more powerful than them. Children are taught to do this regularly, and women often do it in the presence of men. People do this in front of high-ranking clan members as well. It is a physical and symbolic gesture of respect and acknowledgment of hierarchies of power.

21. At the time, some islands had adopted patriarchal ideas about land ownership from missionaries and former colonizers; others still respected matrilineal land ownership.

22. See Anne Hattori (2006) for a history of the U.S. agenda to "save" women through biomedicine in Guam.

CHAPTER 3 IMPERIAL MIGRATIONS

Themes from portions of this chapter were previously published in other forms in *PoLAR: Political and Legal Anthropology Review* (Smith and Castañeda 2021).

1. A woman named Mary, who is also a finniichi, said it is not all about being spoiled. "There is advantage and disadvantage to be an eldest," she told me, "'cause like you got all the respect and all that, but then, the responsibilities."

2. This was before the COVID-19 pandemic. The FSM shut down its borders for nearly two years to even its own citizens, followed by an opening with a strict return and quarantine policy in late 2021. In late 2022, the FSM removed the quarantine policy, although vaccination requirements remain in effect. See https://fm.usembassy.gov/covid-19-information/.

3. See Hezel and McGrath (1989); Hezel (2001); Rubinstein and Levin (1992); Marshall (2004); Bautista (2010).

4. See also Bautista (2010); Gladwin and Sarason (1953); Marshall (2004); Petersen (2009); Puas (2021).
5. See also Flinn (1987); Kawai (1987); Moral (1996, 1998).
6. See, for example, Alkire (1989); Bautista (2010); Dernbach (2005); Flinn (1987); Marshall and Marshall (1990); Moral (1996).
7. Xenophobia is also a major issue in Hawai'i. However, women perceived Guam as "the worst" option regarding anti-Micronesian sentiment.
8. Of the elderly who are convinced to or desire to live abroad (often for medical care), many still want to be buried in Chuuk. Flights to Chuuk are almost always carrying those who die abroad, with funeral processions from the plane nearly every week. During the COVID-19 pandemic, several bodies were sent back on planes without family members to accompany them due to the border closing. Family members who were in Chuuk would receive the body and proceed with the funeral. Once the borders opened, family members who missed these momentous events began planning visits to see their relatives' graves in Chuuk.
9. Outsiders experience xenophobia in Saipan as well. However, to Rosie, the community was much friendlier toward Chuukese people than it was in Guam.
10. For example, Supplemental Security Income, Temporary Assistance for Needy Families, the Supplemental Nutrition Assistance Program, and Medicaid coverage.
11. See also Hezel (2001); Hezel and McGrath (1989).
12. See, for example, Daleno (2013); Daleno (2015); Gilbert (2019); Limtiaco (2019b).
13. See, for example, Sablan (2014); Stole (2016). Similar reactions occurred in Hawai'i, including a change of insurance that drastically reduced coverage.
14. Shortly after this began, U.S. Immigration and Customs Enforcement began working with the governor to officially deport these people (Tomas 2016).
15. See Bautista (2010); Hezel (2012, 2013); Hezel and McGrath (1989); Marshall (2004); Rubinstein and Levin (1992).
16. See, for example, Castañeda (2010); Castañeda et al. (2015); Chavez (2001, 2004).
17. My colleague Heide Castañeda and I also provide a brief portrayal of Kaylyn's migration story in Smith and Castañeda (2021).
18. The University of Guam Chuukese Student Organization formed a writing group in 2014 to help process experiences with discrimination through creative writing. I was the group's faculty sponsor at the time.
19. There is now a Department of the Interior–funded Micronesian Resource Center One-Stop Shop located in Guam (see https://www.manelu.org/micronesian-resource-center-one-stop-shop-1), which should help in navigating Guam's systems. COFA community groups and leaders in Guam's government advocated for such a center for more than a decade, and it finally happened. Largely staffed by people with COFA ancestry, it provides multilingual support, including interpretation services, case management, and outreach in the community. This was a very important win, as the center and its staff help migrants fill out forms for social services and navigate Guam's bureaucracies for housing and employment, and simply provide a friendly space to seek help. Staff members also hold regular Virtual Village Meetings on Facebook to keep the community connected to their efforts and the larger Guam community (see https://www.facebook.com/MRCOSSGuam/).
20. The name Zero Down is a nickname assigned to this community by its residents for the lack of a down payment needed to buy plots, an important incentive for Micronesian families with limited incomes and a desire to own their own spaces.
21. Sociologist and film director Lola Quan Bautista wrote and directed a film about the Gil Baza settlement. The film told the story of when the Guam Environmental Protection Agency required residents to get plumbing or vacate, and the residents came together to sue the origi-

nal developer to get what should have been installed before purchase. It also highlights the comfort and familiarity of these homes for COFA migrants, and the sense of community they built in Gil Baza (Bautista 2013).

22. While these dynamics make community-building more of a challenge, it can still happen. See Bautista (2013) for a good example of a diverse COFA community successfully working together to assert their needs and rights. The COVID-19 pandemic also brought communities together to care for each other; see chapter 7 for more on collective action.

23. See, for example, Basch, Glick-Schiller, and Blanc (1994); Kearney (1995); Ong et al. (1996); Tsing (2008); Appadurai (2008).

CHAPTER 4 REPRODUCING IMPERIALISM IN THE BODY

Themes from portions of this chapter were previously published in another form in the journal *Medical Anthropology* (Smith 2019a).

1. Throughout this book I use the term "local" when referring to indigenous Chuukese healing and medicine. I chose to use this term because the Chuukese people I interviewed preferred it when speaking English and comparing it to biomedicine. Safei is the Chuukese term for medicine and healing. Biomedicine in Chuukese is typically called sefein piiuiing, translated literally as "hospital medicine."

2. See also Fischer (1963); Fitzgerald (2001); Mahony (1969); Swartz (1958).

3. A few women were taught menstrual taboos, such as not handling food, sharing cups with male relatives, or going into the ocean when menstruating. Others told me they heard about menstrual huts from their grandmothers. These practices are reflected in the literature as well (see Fischer 1963; Fitzgerald 2001; Gladwin and Sarason 1953; Goodenough 1978). While the women told me most were no longer practiced, Dernbach (2005) found that some elder Kuttu women blamed sea-level rise on their discontinuation of menstrual taboos.

4. Older accounts exoticizing Chuukese sexuality do report whispers of elders "teaching" youth about sex in this way (see chapter 2), and Rauchholz (2016) pointed to this as still occurring. Families I spoke with were quick to discount any truth to these stories. Missionaries made clear how unacceptable any kind of sex within the family would be, so if it did happen that openly and acceptably in the past, it did not by the time I asked about it. The Chuuk Women's Council successfully lobbied to change a law that allowed sexual consent at age thirteen to age eighteen, another indicator that sex with youth is not acceptable.

5. Tupu ngeni aat means to easily fall for whatever boys say or do or to be compelled to have sex with boys. Tupu is short for tuputa—"to easily believe," "gullible," or "being naïve." When you say "kosapw/kesapw tupu ngeni aat," it can mean "do not fall for their sweet words (and have sex)." It can also mean "don't let boys have sex with you" (A. Lodge, personal email to the author, 2012).

6. Love magic was less frequently used for romantic love and more often for sexual coercion, which I depict in chapter 5 (see also Dernbach 2005; Mahony 1969).

7. This is not uncommon; Micronesia has some of the highest suicide rates in the world and was the leading cause of death for adolescent males in Chuuk (Rubinstein 1995). Further, those from the FSM account for a disproportionate amount of suicides on Guam (Workman and Rubinstein 2019).

8. While this practice is generally discussed as a form of dating for young people, the women I interviewed often pointed to the fact that given the proximity in which entire families sleep at night in Chuuk, married couples also "night crawl" just to get some alone time, as do those people seeking sex outside their marriage. Privacy is in short supply in family compounds in

Chuuk and in crowded apartments in Guam, so night is the time to find privacy with a lover, whether sanctioned or secret (see also Dernbach 2005; Gladwin and Sarason 1953).

9. See also Flinn (1987); Kawai (1987); Moral (1996, 1998a, 1998b).

10. Josealyn Eria, personal email to the author, March 1, 2022.

11. See also Flinn (2010); F. B. Caughey (1971); Kim (2020).

12. Historically, some were arranged by families. Some women said their grandparents' era experienced arranged marriages, but they were uncommon by the time these women reached adolescence. Arranged marriages often included exchange of familial land or maintenance of land by marrying an acceptably distant relative (Goodenough 1949; Gladwin and Sarason 1953).

13. Two women told me this form of elopement could also be a form of kidnapping, in which the man tricks the woman to go to a different island and keeps her there with his family long enough for everyone to notice. Her time in the man's compound would then solidify the need for her family to agree to marriage. One woman reported that she was tricked into her elopement, but others indicated that it was more of a romantic decision shared between the couple.

14. See also Fischer (1970).

15. Julianna Flinn (1987) argued that female Chuukese (specifically Pulapese) college students in the United States may use pregnancy as a coping mechanism in handling the pressure and stress of going abroad to college. In an environment where these women are experiencing the normal stress of entering college, the culture shock of the United States, and the discrimination and discomfort associated with being a migrant, pregnancy can be a way to feel empowered (Flinn 1987). Additionally, she explained how this was a way to be sent home without "giving up"—by taking on a new status as mother. Flinn also analyzed the potential conflict felt between this notion of empowerment and U.S. messages of unintended and illegitimate pregnancy, noting how stressful the experience can become for a young Chuukese woman to give birth outside marriage in a U.S. hospital without her female kin.

16. Josealyn Eria, personal email to the author, March 1, 2022.

17. "Boonie dog" is a term used in Guam for the mixed-breed dogs that live all over the island—some wild, some adopted by families and living in the family yard.

18. See, for example, Dernbach (2005); Fischer (1963); F. B. Caughey (1971).

19. See, for example, Anderson (2006); Browner and Sargent (2011); Jolly (1998, 2002); Lock and Nguyen (2010); Manderson (1996); Ram (1998).

20. The Japanese chose a different nearby island (Tonoas) for the central island of Chuuk. Remnants of the Japanese hospital remain there today.

21. During the trust territory period, Chuukese people began to be trained in biomedical care; some were chosen because they were already local practitioners, while others were not, creating a divide between "local" and the biomedically trained "health officer" or "midwife." Since that time, this inconsistent trend continues, as many island-specific practitioners are trained in local and biomedical methods, while on other islands, these separate roles mean that there are two or more distinct practitioners.

22. For a historical overview of how biomedicine operated globally, see Lock and Nguyen (2010). For Pacific examples, see Anderson (2006); Hattori (2006); Manderson (1996); Jolly and Macintyre (1989). Anne Hattori (2004, 2006) provides the best comparison in her historical account of colonial medicine in nearby Guam.

23. For example, Hattori (2006); Jolly (1998); Smith (2019a).

24. This is a global phenomenon. See, for example, Baer (2003); Broom, Doron, and Tovey (2009); Lambert (2012).

25. UNICEF also reports data, but it is suspicious given all the stories I heard. The organization reports that 100 percent of women in Chuuk give birth with skilled attendants (UNICEF 2016).

26. See the following for more analysis of data concerns in Micronesia specifically: Hoy et al. (2017); Aitaoto and Ichiho (2013); Cash et al. (2021); FSM (2012a, 2022b); UNICEF (2017).
27. With the exception of Praise, who revered home births.
28. See also Ashby (1993); F. B. Caughey (1971); Fischer (1963); Fitzgerald (2001).
29. The cited study focused on FSM citizen-women, but it is important to note that data collected on this population in the United States is typically based on ethnic identity. This means that the reproductive outcomes often include FSM or U.S. citizens who identify as ethnically Micronesian.
30. Chang and colleagues compared these outcomes because physicians anecdotally note that women from these communities had more cesarean sections because of poorly managed gestational diabetes and pre-eclampsia. There are many other indicators for a cesarean that were not measured for this study.
31. What is deemed objective versus subjective in this study is based on the U.S.-biomedical model of birth. The authors (in concert with U.S.-trained obstetricians) coded subjective indicators to include: (1) non-reassuring fetal heart tracing (NRFHT) and (2) arrest of labor (e.g., arrest of dilation and arrest of descent). All other indicators were coded as objective (e.g., malpresentation).
32. For example, Alur et al. (2002); Fox, Parker, and Palmer (2005); Haddock et al. (2008); Hattori-Uchima (2017).
33. Although some researchers did; see, for example, Delafield et al. (2020); Delafield et al. (2021); Yamada (2011).

CHAPTER 5 DISCOURSES OF IMPERIAL SEXUALITY

Themes from portions of this chapter were previously published in another form in the *Journal of Aggression, Maltreatment & Trauma* (Smith 2019b).
1. Many women began supplementing with powdered milk and later formula during the trust territory period (Marshall and Marshall 1979). This was likely influenced by the popularity of bottle-feeding among the U.S. biomedical establishment at the time, and the new availability of such products with the U.S. occupation (Marshall and Marshall 1979, 1980). Older research shows a steady decline in exclusive breastfeeding (Marshall and Marshall 1979, 1980). More recent data reported that only 35 percent of infants were still being exclusively breastfed at six months in Chuuk (Government of the FSM 2022b). Guam researchers have also seen a decline in exclusive breastfeeding among Chuukese women (Wood and Qureshi 2017). Despite these contradictory findings, women talk about breastfeeding positively and indicate how important it is for mothers and babies (Wood and Qureshi 2017). I witnessed many women in the clinics feeding babies formula during infant checkups while also stating that they breastfed. I believe the data available are not completely clear because a distinction between exclusive and some breastfeeding is not always made when interpreting between languages.
2. Chuuk's total fertility rate in the FSM 2010 census was 3.57, and the average family size was 4.8. Each census in recent decades has demonstrated a declining fertility rate (Government of the FSM 2012b).
3. Researchers found similar attention to Chuukese women's fertility among providers in Hawai'i (Inada et al. 2019).
4. Delafield et al. (2020) reported similar concerns among obstetricians in Hawai'i. They observed family members involved in or making the decisions for women.
5. The only exception for Fischer was the occasional fetus or infant deemed to be a "ghost" (and thus not a child), who was aborted or killed at birth; she said this happened when children were born with some sort of "deformity."

6. Roe v. Wade, 10 U.S. 113 (1973) is a landmark U.S. Supreme Court case that argued for a woman's right to abortion without government intervention. It invoked the Fourteenth Amendment's right to privacy and struck down laws criminalizing abortion throughout the United States. In a shocking and uncommon reversal of a long-standing decision, it was overturned by a largely conservative court on June 24, 2022, in the *Dobbs v. Jackson Women's Health Organization* decision. For a depiction of how *Roe v. Wade* was interpreted, debated, and resisted in Guam in the decades before the 2022 Supreme Court decision, see Rubinstein (1992); Dames (2003); Raidoo, Kaneshiro, and Stowers (2021).
7. When the last abortion provider left the island, telehealth appointments were not legal, but in September 2021, an injunction was issued by a district court judge, which temporarily allowed people to have telehealth appointments for abortions.
8. Since the *Dobbs* decision, Guam's attorney general also fought to restrict abortion, specifically by filing to lift the injunction to stop telehealth access to abortion for pregnant people in Guam (J. Taitano 2022a). As of March 24, 2023, the federal district court in Guam denied the attorney general's request (American Civil Liberties Union 2023).
9. See also Caughey (1971); Caughey (1977); Fischer (1963); Gladwin and Sarason (1953); Rauchholz (2016). Another older practice was that if a spouse died, the widow would marry one of the late spouse's siblings to keep the marriage in the family (Goodenough 1978). One woman shared that she was asked to do this by her family; she agreed, but the marriage ended poorly. She indicated that some families still do this, while others have discontinued the practice.
10. The women were being accused of being lamelam tekiya: arrogant, loud, boastful, brash, disrespectful (Dernbach 2005).
11. Mahony (1969) also discussed love magic and concluded that various forms of safei (local medicine) and magic are used to control women: "All the spirit powers of Group I, some of which we have already discussed, emphasize contingent behavior. It is rather interesting to note how many of these are concerned with restraining, controlling, and channeling the behavior and activities of women, either by threats to their own health, or to the health of their children. The spirits seem to be supporting the established social authority which, of course, has been in the hands of men" (Mahony 1969, 246).
12. See Katz et al. (2009); Wong and Kawamoto (2010); Yamada and Pobutsky (2009).
13. After interviews, I always discussed and explained the efficacy of condoms and testing, and ultimately helped some women navigate the STD/HIV testing and treatment program in Guam.
14. See CWC (2011); Government of the FSM (2012a).
15. The Chuukese community is not unique in Guam for avoiding STD/HIV testing and counseling services. This is an issue in the entire Guam island community and in the rest of the United States as well.
16. Chlamydia was also noted as a likely cause of infertility in Micronesia during the trust territory days (Brewis 1993, 1992); no data on Chuukese infertility are presently available.
17. In 2017, the CDC awarded Chuuk public health funding for a Federally Qualified Health Center, which I describe in chapter 6. This (temporarily) resolved some of the inconsistent lab funding issues.
18. Prenatal population STI testing is voluntary, but women are rarely told they have a choice; instead, it is conducted as the standard of care in both Chuuk and Guam; thus, it serves more as a mandatory test measure. The only other common way in which people are tested, specifically in Chuuk, is through work permits that require STI testing. The type of testing depends on the availability of tests at the time.
19. See Pobutsky et al. (2005); Pobutsky, Krupitsky, and Yamada (2009); Wong and Kawamoto (2010).

20. See Aitaoto and Ichiho (2013); Cash et al. (2021); Hoy et al. (2017).
21. There are contradictory stories, however. Older accounts describe men beating their wives as an act of love, and some men told me, unsolicited, that if a man beats his wife, it shows that he really loves her (see also Dernbach 2005; Rauchholz 2016). Others told me this type of violence is new and was imported by colonizers. Love magic, also occasionally used by women to make men love them, is sometimes blamed for men's violence toward their wives (Dernbach 2005).
22. See Caughey (1971); Caughey (1977); Fischer (1963); Gladwin and Sarason (1953); Goodenough (1978); Swartz (1958).
23. This is particularly a concern when migrants have housing support through the GHURA, which imposes restrictions on how many people can reside in one household.
24. See, for example, Magnussen et al. (2011); Shoultz et al. (2007); Smith (2019b).
25. See also Dernbach (2005); Marshall (2004).

CHAPTER 6 CONTEMPT, CONFUSION, AND CARE IN GUAM'S IMPERIAL PUBLIC HEALTHCARE SYSTEM

Themes from portions of this chapter were previously published in other forms in *Social Science & Medicine* (Smith 2016) and *Hawaii Journal of Medicine & Public Health* (Smith 2018).
1. Guam is very small and has very few people serving in each role in which I shadowed. I purposely use vague language so as not to reveal the identity of the nurse aide, nurse, nurse midwife, or physician to which I am referring and protect their confidentiality.
2. Posting nurses carry out the provider's orders at the end of the visit. They are registered nurses and licensed practical nurses.
3. At the time, one hospital obstetrician did about ten hours per week of contract work for community health centers. If he were a provider for a woman and on-call when she went into labor, it is possible someone could have that continuity of care.
4. See also Alur et al. (2002); Delafield et al. (2020, 2021); Fox and Parker (2005).
5. See Hagiwara et al. (2016); Pobutsky, Krupitsky, and Yamada (2009); Wong and Kawamoto (2010).
6. For example, Anderson (2006); Jolly (1998); Manderson (1996, 1998). The introduction of reproductive biomedicine in Chuuk by the U.S. Navy and trust territory government is discussed in chapter 4.
7. GMH is officially Guam Memorial Hospital Authority (GMHA), but Guam residents colloquially refer to it as GMH.
8. As of this March 2023, there is no other place for people to birth on Guam. There is a birthing center that accepts a small number of publicly insured patients after they complete a minimum of four prenatal visits at the community health centers, but during the COVID-19 pandemic, they stopped providing birth services. The private hospital also does not accept birthing patients.
9. See, for example, Akimoto (2019); Eugenio (2019); Hernandez (2022); Limtiaco (2019a); J. Taitano (2022b).
10. Mangilao is the name of the village in which Central was housed (see figure 3).
11. At the time of this study, only one community health center had offices for MIP/Medicaid and other social services (social workers, WIC, and so on).
12. They also have the option to self-pay on a sliding scale, but even the lowest fees are far beyond what some Chuukese patients can afford.
13. The income limits are different depending on the size of the family. For example, since January 2021, a family of four must have a monthly gross income under $2,373, with approximately $406 added per household member after that.

14. The processes for applying for MIP and Medicaid are the same, so these hurdles remain.
15. Co-pays, or co-payments, are standard payments made by patients at the time of service required by most U.S. health insurance providers, usually ranging from $5 to $30 for primary care.
16. I inquired several times with the Division of Public Welfare office about its decision-making in terms of coverage and co-pays and requested a coverage and co-pay schedule for each. I never received a response. Since that time, some details about Medicaid coverage have been posted on their website: http://dphss.guam.gov/resources-bhcfa/.
17. While I am critical of this decision of the local government, it is more generous than the U.S. federal government, which simply removed coverage for noncitizens.
18. This is further complicated as extended families in Guam often share one post office mailbox, delaying women's access to any requests they receive by mail.
19. Supplemental Food and Nutrition Assistance (food stamps) and Supplemental Security Income (welfare) are still not available for COFA-nation citizens, but often there are children in the household who are U.S. citizens and therefore eligible.
20. A "load" is a term that refers to minutes that can be loaded on a SIM card for a cellular phone. Residents of Guam can buy small (five- or ten-dollar) prepaid cards at gas stations to load their phone with minutes when they have the money. As the phone will not ring when there is no load, this was also a barrier to getting in touch with women.
21. See also Aitaoto et al. (2009); Hattori-Uchima (2017); Wong and Kawamoto (2010).
22. There were two Micronesians working in low-level temporary positions. They were both were gone by the time I returned in 2016.
23. Not all providers were created equal. The low wages, lack of overall providers in Guam, and difficulty in hiring people through the government of Guam system create a severe shortage of providers. So regardless of how *well* or how *badly* a provider treats patients, the providers are very unlikely to be fired or even reprimanded. Thus, the structural constraints in Guam allow for bad providers, too. Some people perceive Guam as a haven for physicians (and particularly surgeons) who have lost their licensing in U.S. states.
24. Delafield et al. (2020) reported this common practice in Hawai'i as well.
25. See Kleinman and Benson (2006); Taylor (2003a, 2003b); Shaw (2010).
26. See, for example, Kleinman and Benson (2006); Taylor (2003b); Willen (2013).
27. See Kirmayer (2012a, 2012b); Willen and Carpenter-Song (2013).

CHAPTER 7 RESISTING IMPERIAL EFFECTS

Some themes from portions of this chapter were previously published in another form in *Global Public Health* (Smith and Katzman 2020).
1. See, for example, Dernbach (1998); Flinn (2010); Kim (2020); Marshall and Marshall (1990).
2. Some women at the CWC and other smaller women's groups had little to no education; others had completed high school; and some had college degrees at the associate, bachelor, and master levels. This is quite variable and does not reflect hierarchies as much as clan status, birth order, and age do. The woman I was speaking with who explicitly compared degrees in thinking about access to government leadership had a bachelor of arts from UOG.
3. See Chuuk Women's Council (n.d.).
4. For example, Atteraya, Gnawali, and Palley (2016); Molesworth et al. (2017); Notwell (2014); Scheyvens (2003).
5. For example, Maisonneuve (2006); Molesworth et al. (2017); Notwell (2014); Scheyvens (2003).

6. See, for example, Aksartova (2009); Alvarez (1999); Helms (2014); Schuller (2009); Silliman (1999).
7. See, for example, Adams (2016b); Aksartova (2009); Helms (2014); Schuller (2009); Silliman (1999).
8. See Neechuumeres (2021).
9. See FSM Association of Guam (2019).
10. Additionally, every college and university hosting FSM students has at least an FSM club and often state-specific clubs. The Chuukese Student Organization at UOG did all kinds of outreach when I was its faculty sponsor. Students in this group worked with the DPHSS and other organizations to interpret for community events (mass immunization campaigns, TB testing), assisted UOG researchers to provide betel nut prevention education to communities, collected donations of food and clothing for more vulnerable or recently arrived residents, and much more. There are also groups doing great work in Hawai'i, such as We Are Oceania (https://www.weareoceania.org/) and Micronesians United—Big Island (https://www.mu-bi.org/). The COFA Alliance National Network is a well-known group based in Oregon (https://cann.us/), which now has chapters in Washington, Texas, East Oregon, and Arizona. There is also the COFA Community Leadership & Advocacy Network (CLAN) (https://www.facebook.com/groups/COFACLAN/about/).
11. See Hagiwara et al. (2016); Inada et al. (2019); Rehuher et al. (2021); Shek et al. (2021).

REFERENCES

Adams, Vincanne. 2016a. Introduction to *Metrics: What Counts in Global Health*, edited by Vincanne Adams, 1–18. Durham, NC: Duke University Press.

———. 2016b. "Metrics of the Global Sovereign: Numbers and Stories in Global Health." In *Metrics: What Counts in Global Health*, edited by Vincanne Adams, 19–54. Durham, NC: Duke University Press.

———, ed. 2016c. *Metrics: What Counts in Global Health*. Durham, NC: Duke University Press.

Agar, Michael H. 1996. *The Professional Stranger: An Informal Introduction to Ethnography*. 2nd ed. San Diego: Academic Press.

Aguon, Julian. 2022. *No Country for Eight-Spot Butterflies*. New York: Astra House.

Aguon, Mindy. 2013. "Victim Was 16 When Working at Blue House." *Kuam News*, August 23, 2013. https://www.kuam.com/story/23236215/2013/08/Friday/victim-was-16-when-working-at-blue-house.

———. 2017. "Blue House Defendants Spared Prison Time, Plead to Not Be Deported." *Guam Daily Post*, April 2, 2017. https://www.postguam.com/news/local/blue-house-defendants-spared-prison-time/article_96484b7e-15f4-11e7-9f48-0b2e3b404e80.html.

Aitaoto, Nia, and Henry M. Ichiho. 2013. "Assessing the Health Care System of Services for Non-communicable Diseases in the US-Affiliated Pacific Islands: A Pacific Regional Perspective." *Hawaii Journal of Medicine and Public Health* 72 (5 suppl. 1): 106–114. https://www.ncbi.nlm.nih.gov/pmc/articles/PMC3689460/.

Aitaoto, Nia, JoAnn Tsark, Danette W. Tomiyasu, Barbara A. Yamashita, and Kathryn L. Braun. 2009. "Strategies to Increase Breast and Cervical Cancer Screening among Hawaiian, Pacific Islander, and Filipina Women in Hawai'i." *Hawaii Medical Journal* 68 (9): 215–222. https://www.ncbi.nlm.nih.gov/pmc/articles/PMC4850232/.

Akimoto, Vincent Taijeron. 2019. "Solutions to GMH's Life Threatening Problems." *Guam Pacific Daily News*, September 7, 2019. https://www.guampdn.com/story/opinion/readers/2019/09/07/solutions-gmhs-life-threatening-problems/2239259001/.

Aksartova, Sada. 2009. "Promoting Civil Society or Diffusing NGOs." In *Globalization, Philanthropy, and Civil Society: Projecting Institutional Logics Abroad*, edited by David C. Hammack and Steven Heydemann, 160–191. Bloomington: Indiana University Press.

Alcalay, Glenn. 1992. "The United States Anthropologist in Micronesia: Toward a Counter-Hegemonic Study of Sapiens." In *Confronting the Margaret Mead Legacy: Scholarship, Empire, and the South Pacific*, edited by Lenora Foerstel and Angela Gilliam, 173–201. Philadelphia: Temple University Press.

Alkire, William H. 1989. "Land, Sea, Gender, and Ghosts on Woleai-Lamotrek." In *Culture, Kin, and Cognition in Oceania: Essays in Honor of Ward H. Goodenough*, edited by Mac Marshall and John L. Caughey, 79–96. Washington, DC: American Anthropological Association.

Alur, Pradeep, Priya Kodiyanplakkal, Amanda Del Rosario, Sanjay Khubchandani, Radha Alur, and John J. Moore. 2002. "Epidemiology of Infants of Diabetic Mothers in Indigent Micronesian Population-Guam Experience." *Pacific Health Dialog* 9 (2): 219–221.

Alvarez, Sonia E. 1999. "Advocating Feminism: The Latin American Feminist NGO 'Boom.'" *International Feminist Journal of Politics* 1 (2): 181–209. https://doi.org/10.1080/146167499359880.

American Anthropological Association. n.d. "Statement on Ethics." Accessed November 25, 2021. https://www.americananthro.org/LearnAndTeach/Content.aspx?ItemNumber=22869.

American Anthropological Association Executive Board. 2007. "Statement on the Human Terrain System Project." October 31, 2007. https://www.americananthro.org/ConnectWithAAA/Content.aspx?ItemNumber=1952.

American Civil Liberties Union. 2023. "Federal Court Preserves Abortion Access in Guam." March 24, 2023. https://www.aclu.org/press-releases/federal-court-preserves-abortion-access-in-guam.

American Medical Association. 1994. *Culturally Competent Healthcare for Adolescents: A Guide for Primary Care Providers.* Chicago: American Medical Association.

Amundsen, Fiona, and Sylvia C. Frain. 2020. "The Politics of Invisibility: Visualizing Legacies of Nuclear Imperialisms." *Journal of Transnational American Studies* 11 (2). https://doi.org/10.5070/T8112049588.

Andaya, Elise. 2019. "Race-ing Time: Clinical Temporalities and Inequality in Public Prenatal Care." *Medical Anthropology* 38 (8): 651–663. https://doi.org/10.1080/01459740.2019.1590826.

Andersen, Helle Max. 2004. ""Villagers": Differential Treatment in a Ghanaian hospital." *Social Science & Medicine* 59 (10): 2003–2012. https://doi.org/10.1016/j.socscimed.2004.03.005.

Anderson, Warwick. 2006. *Colonial Pathologies: American Tropical Medicine, Race, and Hygiene in the Philippines.* Durham, NC: Duke University Press.

Appadurai, Arjun. 2008. "Disjuncture and Difference in the Global Cultural Economy." In *The Anthropology of Globalization,* edited by Jonathan Xavier Inda and Renato Rosaldo, 47–65. Malden, MA: Blackwell.

Arcangel, Maria Theresa L. 2019. *Division of Public Welfare FY 2018 Expenditure and Demographic Report.* Mangilao: Guam Department of Public Health and Social Services.

Ardner, Edwin. (1975) 2006. "Belief and the Problem of Women." In *Feminist Anthropology: A Reader,* edited by Ellen Lewin, 47–65. Malden, MA: Blackwell.

Asad, Talal, ed. 1973. *Anthropology and the Colonial Experience.* London: Ithaca and Humanities Press.

Ashby, Gene, ed. 1993. *Micronesian Customs and Beliefs.* Eugene: Rainy Day Press.

Atteraya, Madhu Sudhan, Shreejana Gnawali, and Elizabeth Palley. 2016. "Women's Participation in Self-Help Groups as a Pathway to Women's Empowerment: A Case of Nepal." *International Journal of Social Welfare* 25 (4): 321–330. https://doi.org/10.1111/ijsw.12212.

Baer, Hans A. 2003. "Contributions to a Critical Analysis of Medical Pluralism: An Examination of the Work of Libbet Crandon-Malamud." In *Medical Pluralism in the Andes,* edited by Joan Koss-Chioino, Thomas L. Leatherman, and Christine Greenway, 42–60. New York: Psychology Press.

Baer, Hans A., Merrill Singer, and Ida Susser. 2003. *Medical Anthropology and the World System.* 2nd ed. Westport, CT: Praeger.

Baldacchino, Godfrey. 2010. "'Upside Down Decolonization' in Subnational Island Jurisdictions: Questioning the 'Post' in Postcolonialism." *Space and Culture* 13 (2): 188–202. https://doi.org/10.1177/1206331209360865.

Barker, Holly M. 2004. *Bravo for the Marshallese: Regaining Control in a Post-Nuclear, Post-Colonial World.* Edited by John A. Young. *Case Studies in Contemporary Social Issues.* Belmont, CA: Wadsworth Cengage Learning.

Basch, Linda G., Nina Glick-Schiller, and Christina Szanton Blanc. 1994. *Nations Unbound: Transnational Projects, Postcolonial Predicaments, and Deterritorialized Nation-States.* Langhorne, PA: Gordon and Breach.

Bautista, Lola Quan. 2010. *Steadfast Movement around Micronesia: Satowan Enlargements beyond Migration*. Lanham, MD: Lexington Books.
———. 2011. "Building Sense Out of Households: Migrants from Chuuk (Re)create Local Settlements in Guam." *City and Society* 23 (1): 66–90. https://doi.org/10.1111/j.1548-744X.2011.01049.x.
———. 2013. *Breadfruit and Open Spaces*. DVD. Breadfruit Educational Productions. https://breadfruiteducational.com/filmsandvideos/breadfruit-and-open-spaces.
Baxi, Pratiksha. 2014. "Sexual Violence and Its Discontents." *Annual Review of Anthropology* 43:139–154. https://doi.org/10.1146/annurev-anthro-102313–030247.
Behar, Ruth, and Deborah A. Gordon. 1995. *Women Writing Culture*. Berkeley: University of California Press.
Benjamin, Jefferson B. 2000. "Community Perceptions of the Quality of Health Care Services in the Federated States of Micronesia." PhD diss., University of Hawaii.
Berg, M. L. 1992. "Yapese Politics, Yapese Money and the Sawei Tribute Network before World War I." *Journal of Pacific History* 27 (2): 150–164. https://doi.org/10.1080/00223349208572704.
Bernal, Victoria, and Inderpal Grewal. 2014. "Introduction: The NGO Form: Feminist Struggles, States, and Neoliberalism." In *Theorizing NGOs: States, Feminisms, and Neoliberalism*, edited by Victoria Bernal and Inderpal Grewal, 1–18. Next Wave: New Directions in Women's Studies. Durham, NC: Duke University Press.
Bevacqua, Michael Lujan. 2012. "The (Un)exceptional Life of a Non-voting Delegate: Guam and the Production of American Sovereignty." *Pacific Asia Inquiry* 3 (1): 58–75.
———. 2019. "Guam's Liberation Didn't Set Us Free." *Pacific Daily News*, July 4, 2019. https://www.guampdn.com/opinion/bevacqua-guams-liberation-didnt-set-us-free/article_34f6b5a5-9cbf-56dc-b80c-d8471adbcba6.html.
Bollig, P. Laurentius. 1927. *The Inhabitants of the Truk Islands: Religion, Life and a Short Grammar of a Micronesian People*. Translated from the German in 1942 for the Yale Cross-Cultural Survey in connection with the Navy Pacific Islands Handbook Project. Human Relations Area Files.
Bonilla, Yarimar. 2013. "Ordinary Sovereignty." *Small Axe. A Caribbean Journal of Criticism* 17 (3): 152–165. https://doi.org/10.1215/07990537-2378973.
———. 2015. "Non-sovereign Futures." In *Non-sovereign Futures*. Chicago: University of Chicago Press.
Bourdieu, Pierre. 1977. *Outline of a Theory of Practice*. Cambridge: Cambridge University Press.
———. 2001. *Masculine Domination*. Palo Alto, CA: Stanford University Press.
Bourgois, Philippe, Seth M. Holmes, Kim Sue, and James Quesada. 2017. "Structural Vulnerability: Operationalizing the Concept to Address Health Disparities in Clinical Care." *Academic Medicine: Journal of the Association of American Medical Colleges* 92 (3): 299–307. https://doi.org/10.1097/ACM.0000000000001294.
Brewis, Alexandra A. 1992. "Sexually-Transmitted Disease Risk in a Micronesian Atoll Population." *Health Transition Review: The Cultural, Social, and Behavioural Determinants of Health* 2 (2): 195–213. https://www.jstor.org/stable/40651984.
———. 1993. "Age and Infertility in a Micronesian Atoll Population." *Human Biology* 65 (4): 593–609. https://www.jstor.org/stable/41465126.
Bridges, Khiara M. 2011. *Reproducing Race: An Ethnography of Pregnancy as a Site of Racialization*. Berkeley: University of California Press.
Briggs, Laura. 2003. *Reproducing Empire: Race, Sex, Science, and US imperialism in Puerto Rico*. Berkeley: University of California Press.

———. 2017. *Reproductive Justice: A New Vision for the 21st Century.* Vol. 2, *How All Politics Became Reproductive Politics: From Welfare Reform to Foreclosure to Trump.* Berkeley: University of California Press.

Broom, Alex, Assa Doron, and Philip Tovey. 2009. "The Inequalities of Medical Pluralism: Hierarchies of Health, the Politics of Tradition and the Economies of Care in Indian Oncology." *Social Science & Medicine* 69 (5): 698–706. https://doi.org/10.1016/j.socscimed.2009.07.002.

Brown, Judith K. 1970. "A Note on the Division of Labor by Sex." *American Anthropologist* 72 (5): 1073–1078. https://doi.org/10.1525/aa.1970.72.5.02a00070.

Browner, Carole H. 2001. "Situating Women's Reproductive Activities." *American Anthropologist* 102 (4): 773–788. https://doi.org/10.1525/aa.2000.102.4.773.

Browner, Carole H., and Carolyn F. Sargent. 2007. "Gender: Engendering Medical Anthropology." In *Medical Anthropology: Regional Perspectives and Shared Concerns,* edited by Francine Saillant and Serge Genest, 233–251. Malden, MA: Blackwell.

———. 2011. "Toward Global Anthropological Studies of Reproduction: Concepts, Methods, and Theoretical Approaches." In *Reproduction, Globalization, and the State: New Theoretical and Ethnographic Perspectives,* edited by Carole H. Browner and Carolyn F. Sargent, 1–18. Durham, NC: Duke University Press.

Bryce, Bindi. 2017. "First Woman to Enter Chuuk State Senate Promises to Bring Big Changes." *Pacific Beat.* March 16, 2017. ABC Radio Australia.

Calvo, Eddie Baza. 2014. "State of the Island Address." Office of the Governor. February 25, 2014. https://governor.guam.gov/press_release/state-island-watch-read-governor-calvos-address/.

Camacho, Keith L. 2011. *Cultures of Commemoration: The Politics of War, Memory, and History in the Mariana Islands.* Honolulu: University of Hawai'i Press.

Carruth, Lauren, Carlos Martinez, Lahra Smith, Katharine Donato, Carlos Piñones-Rivera, and James Quesada. 2021. "Structural Vulnerability: Migration and Health in Social Context." *BMJ Global Health* 6 (suppl. 1): e005109.

Carucci, Laurence Marshall. 2012. "You'll Always Be Family: Formulating Marshallese Identities in Kona, Hawai'i." *Pacific Studies* 35 (1): 203–231.

Carucci, Laurence M., and Lin Poyer. 2002. "The West Central Pacific." In *Oceania: An Introduction to the Cultures and Identities of Pacific Islanders,* edited by Andrew Strathern, Pamela J. Steward, Laurence M. Carucci, Lin Poyer, Richard Feinberg, and Cluny Macpherson, 183–249. Durham, NC: Carolina Academic Press.

Cash, Haley L., Stacy De Jesus, A. Mark Durand, Si Thu Win Tin, Dana Shelton, Rebecca Robles, Amber R. Mendiola, Suzette Brikul, Maybelline Ipil, and Molly Murphy. 2021. "'Hybrid Survey' Approach to Non-Communicable Disease Surveillance in the US-Affiliated Pacific Islands." *BMJ Global Health* 6 (10): e006971. https://gh.bmj.com/content/6/10/e006971.abstract.

Castañeda, Heide. 2008. "Paternity for Sale: Anxieties over 'Demographic Theft' and Undocumented Migrant Reproduction in Germany." *Medical Anthropology Quarterly* 22 (4): 340–359. https://doi.org/10.1111/j.1548–1387.2008.00039.x.

———. 2010. "Im/Migration and Health: Conceptual, Methodological, and Theoretical Propositions for Applied Anthropology." *NAPA Bulletin* 34:6–27. https://doi.org/10.1111/j.1556-4797.2010.01049.x.

Castañeda, Heide, Seth M. Holmes, Daniel S. Madrigal, Maria-Elena DeTrinidad Young, Naomi Beyeler, and James Quesada. 2015. "Immigration as a Social Determinant of Health." *Annual Review of Public Health* 36:375–392. https://doi.org/10.1146/annurev-publhealth-032013-182419.

Caughey, Frances Blossom. 1971. "The Social Context of Pregnancy and Childbirth on Uman, Truk." Master's thesis, University of Pennsylvania.

Caughey, John L. 1977. *Fa'a'nakkar: Cultural Values in a Micronesian Society.* Philadelphia: Department of Anthropology, University of Pennsylvania.

Cha, Susan, Tasneem Malik, Winston E. Abara, Mia S. DeSimone, Bernadette Schumann, Esther Mallada, Michael Klemme, Vince Aguon, Anne Marie Santos, and Thomas A. Peterman. 2017. "Screening for Syphilis and Other Sexually Transmitted Infections in Pregnant Women—Guam, 2014." *MMWR: Morbidity and Mortality Weekly Report* 66 (24): 644. https://doi.org/10.15585/mmwr.mm6624a4.

Chang, Ann Lee, Eric Hurwitz, Jill Miyamura, Bliss Kaneshiro, and Tetine Sentell. 2015. "Maternal Risk Factors and Perinatal Outcomes Among Pacific Islander Groups in Hawai'i: A Retrospective Cohort Study Using Statewide Hospital Data." *BMC Pregnancy and Childbirth* 15 (1): 239–246. https://doi.org/10.1186/s12884-015-0671-4.

Chavez, Leo R. 2001. *Covering Immigration: Popular Images and the Politics of the Nation.* Berkeley: University of California Press.

———. 2004. "A Glass Half Empty: Latina Reproduction and Public Discourse." *Human Organization* 63 (2): 173–188. https://doi.org/10.17730/humo.63.2.hmk4momfey1on51k.

Cheyney, Melissa. 2015. "Of Missing Voices and the Obstetric Imaginary: Commentary on Jankowski and Burcher." *Journal of Clinical Ethics* 26 (1): 36–39.

Chodorow, Nancy. 1974. "Family Structure and Feminine Personality." In *Woman Culture and Society,* edited by Michelle Zimbalist Rosaldo and Louise Lamphere, 43–66. Stanford, CA: Stanford University Press.

Chuuk Women's Council. n.d. "Our History." Accessed January 20, 2022. http://www.cwcfiinchuuk.org/index.php/about/history.

Clifford, James. 1986. "Introduction: Partial Truths." In *Writing Culture: The Poetics and Politics of Ethnography,* edited by James Clifford and George E. Marcus, 1–26. Berkeley: University of California Press.

Coddington, Kate, R. Tina Catania, Jenna Loyd, Emily Mitchell-Eaton, and Alison Mountz. 2012. "Embodied Possibilities, Sovereign Geographies, and Island Detention: Negotiating the 'Right to Have Rights' on Guam, Lampedusa, and Christmas Island." *Shima: The International Journal of Research into Island Cultures.* 6 (2): 27–48.

COFA. 2003. Compact of Free Association Amendments Act of 2003. Pub. L. No. 108–188, 117 Stat. 2720 (2003).

Coffey, Amanda. 1999. *The Ethnographic Self: Fieldwork and the Representation of Identity.* London: Sage.

Colen, Shellee. 1986. "'With Respect and Feelings': Voices of West Indian Child Care and Domestic Workers in New York City." In *All American Women: Lines That Divide, Ties That Bind,* edited by Johnetta B. Cole, 46–70. New York: Free Press.

———. 1995. "'Like a Mother to Them': Stratified Reproduction and West Indian Childcare Workers and Employers in New York." In *Conceiving the New World Order: The Global Politics of Reproduction,* edited by Faye Ginsburg and Rayna Rapp, 78–102. Berkeley: University of California Press.

Collier, Jane Fishburne. 1974. "Women in Politics." In *Woman, Culture and Society,* edited by Michelle Zimbalist Rosaldo and Louise Lamphere, 89–96. Stanford, CA: Stanford University Press.

Congress of the Federated States of Micronesia. 2021. "Dr. Konman Seated as First Woman in the FSM Congress." December 13, 2021. https://www.cfsm.gov.fm/index.php/public-info/this-week-in-congress/514-dr-konman-seated-as-first-woman-in-the-fsm-congress.

Council of the American Anthropological Association. 1967. "Statement on Problems of Anthropological Research and Ethics." March 1967. https://www.americananthro.org/ParticipateAndAdvocate/Content.aspx?ItemNumber=1656.

CWC (Chuuk Women's Council). 2011. *Chuuk HIV and STI Behavioral Survey with Women Who Exchange Sex for Money or Goods.* July 2011. https://www.aidsdatahub.org/sites/default/files/resource/chuuk-hiv-sti-behavioral-survey-fsw-fsm-2011.pdf.

Daleno, Gaynor Dumat-ol. 2013. "Compact-Impact Cost $125M in Fiscal '12." *Pacific Daily News,* April 1, 2013.

———. 2015. "More Compact Migration Expected: Calvo: GovGuam Agencies Already at 'Breaking Point.'" *Pacific Daily News,* February 25, 2015.

———. 2020. "Governor Wants to Curb Regional Migrants' Entry." *Guam Daily Post,* April 25, 2020. https://www.postguam.com/news/local/governor-wants-to-curb-regional-migrants-entry/article_e447480c-861c-11ea-977d-ef5665dedca6.html.

Dames, Vivian Loyola. 2003. "Chamorro Women, Self-Determination, and the Politics of Abortion in Guam." In *Asian/Pacific Islander American Women: A Historical Anthology,* edited by Shirley Hune and Gail M. Nomura, 365–375. New York: New York University Press.

Danz, Shari M. 2000. "A Nonpublic Forum or a Brutal Bureaucracy? Advocates' Claims of Access to Welfare Center Waiting Rooms." *New York University Law Review* 75 (4): 1004–1044. https://heinonline.org/HOL/LandingPage?handle=hein.journals/nylr75&div=34&id=&page=.

David, Annette M., on behalf of the Guam SEOW. 2018. *Guam State Epidemiological Profile: 2016 Update.* Hagatna, Guam: Prevention and Training Branch, Guam Behavioral Health and Wellness Center. https://gbhwc.guam.gov/sites/default/files/REV_FINAL_Guam%20State%20Epidemiological%20Profile%202016_August%202018.pdf.

Davis, Dána-Ain. 2019. "Obstetric Racism: The Racial Politics of Pregnancy, Labor, and Birthing." *Medical Anthropology* 38 (7): 560–573. https://doi.org/10.1080/01459740.2018.1549389.

Dé Ishtar, Zohl. 1994. *Daughters of the Pacific.* North Melbourne, Australia: Spinifex Press.

Delafield, Rebecca, Jennifer Elia, Ann Chang, Bliss Kaneshiro, Tetine Sentell, and Catherine M. Pirkle. 2020. "Perspectives and Experiences of Obstetricians Who Provide Labor and Delivery Care for Micronesian Women in Hawai'i: What Is Driving Cesarean Delivery Rates?" *Qualitative Health Research* 30 (14): 2291–2302. https://doi.org/10.1177/1049732320942484.

———. 2021. "A Cross-Sectional Study Examining Differences in Indication for Cesarean Delivery by Race/Ethnicity." *Healthcare* 9 (2): 159–170. https://doi.org/10.3390/healthcare9020159.

DeLisle, Christine Taitano. 2015. "A History of Chamorro Nurse-Midwives in Guam and a 'Placental Politics' for Indigenous Feminism." *Intersections: Gender and Sexuality in Asia and the Pacific* 37. http://intersections.anu.edu.au/issue37/delisle.pdf.

———. 2016. "Destination Chamorro Culture: Notes on Realignment, Rebranding, and Post-9/11 Militourism in Guam." *American Quarterly* 68 (3): 563–572. https://doi.org/10.1353/aq.2016.0052.

Dernbach, Katherine Boris. 1998. "Enacting Motherhood: Strategies of Grass-Roots Community-Building by Catholic Women in Chuuk, Micronesia." Master's thesis, University of Iowa.

———. 2005. "Popular Religion: A Cultural and Historical Study of Catholicism and Spirit Possession in Chuuk, Micronesia." PhD diss., University of Iowa.

Diamond, Dan. 2021. "How 100,000 Pacific Islanders Got Their Health Care Back." *Politico,* January 1, 2021. https://www.politico.com/news/2021/01/01/marshall-islands-health-care-453215.

Diaz, Vicente M. 1994. "Simply Chamorro: Telling Tales of Demise and Survival in Guam." *Contemporary Pacific* 6 (1): 29–58. https://www.jstor.org/stable/23701589.

———. 1995. "Bye Ms. American Pie: The Historical Relations between Chamorros and Filipinos and the American Dream." *ISLA: A Journal of Micronesian Studies* 3 (1): 147–160.

———. 2010. *Repositioning the Missionary: Rewriting the Histories of Colonialism, Native Catholicism and Indigeneity in Guam. Pacific Islands Monograph Series 24.* Honolulu: University of Hawai'i Press.

di Leonardo, Micaela. 1991. "Introduction: Gender, Culture, and Political Economy: Feminist Anthropology in Historical Perspective." In *Gender at the Crossroads of Knowledge: Anthropology in the Postmodern Era,* edited by Micaela di Leonardo, 1–48. Berkeley: University of California Press.

Dirks, Nicholas B. 1992. *Colonialism and Culture.* Ann Arbor: University of Michigan Press.

Dobbin, Jay D., and Francis X. Hezel. 1995. "Possession and Trance in Chuuk." *ISLA: A Journal of Micronesian Studies* 3 (1): 73–104.

DOJ, Office of Public Affairs. 2012. "Guam Bar Owner Sentenced to Life in Prison for Sex Trafficking and Related Crimes." September 20, 2012. https://www.justice.gov/opa/pr/guam-bar-owner-sentenced-life-prison-sex-trafficking-and-related-crimes.

Douglas, Mary. 1966. *Purity and Danger: An Analysis of the Concepts of Pollution and Taboo.* London: Routledge.

———. 1970. *Natural Symbols.* New York: Vintage.

———. 1973. *Natural Symbols: Explorations in Cosmology.* New York: Random House.

Ekeroma, Alec, Rachel Dyer, Neal Palafox, Kiki Maoate, Jane Skeen, Sunia Foliaki, Andrew J. Vallely, James Fong, Merilyn Hibma, Glen Mola, Martina Reichhardt, Livinston Taulung, George Aho, Toakase Fakakovikaetau, David Watters, Pamela J. Toliman, Lee Buenconsejo-Lum, and Diana Sarfati. 2019. "Cancer Management in the Pacific Region: A Report on Innovation and Good Practice." *Lancet Oncology* 20 (9): e493–e502. https://doi.org/10.1016/S1470-2045(19)30414-0.

Eria, Josealyn, Rebecca Hofmann, and Sarah A. Smith. 2022. "Micronesian Conceptions of Home and Gender in Chuuk and the US: Between the Presence of Absent Islanders and Island Imaginaries Abroad." *Pacific Geographies* 58 (July/August): 11–18. https://doi.org/10.23791/581118.

Escobar, Arturo. 2011. *Encountering Development: The Making and Unmaking of the Third World.* Princeton, NJ: Princeton University Press.

Eugenio, Haidee V. 2018. "Chamber Business Panel Suggests Property Tax Increase, Federal Help for Migrants in GMH Funding Woes." *Guam Pacific Daily News,* February 1, 2018. https://www.guampdn.com/story/news/2018/02/01/chamber-business-panel-suggests-property-tax-increase-federal-help-migrants-gmh-funding-woes/1081089001/.

———. 2019. "Diverted Patients, Broken Elevators, Costly Fixes: Senators Hear GMH's Pile of Woes." *Pacific Daily News,* October 16, 2019. https://www.guampdn.com/story/news/2019/10/16/diverted-patients-broken-elevators-costly-fixes-gmh-woes-pile-up/3982671002/.

Falgout, Suzanne. 2012. "Pohnpeians in Hawai'i: Refashioning Identity in Diaspora." *Pacific Studies* 35 (1): 184–202.

Falgout, Suzanne, Lin Poyer, and Laurence Marshall Carucci. 2016. *Memories of War: Micronesians in the Pacific War.* Honolulu: University of Hawai'i Press.

Farmer, Paul. 1999. "Pathologies of Power: Rethinking Health and Human Rights." *American Journal of Public Health* 89 (10): 1486–1496.

———. 2003a. Introduction to *Pathologies of Power: Health, Human Rights, and the New War on the Poor,* 1–22. Berkeley: University of California Press.

———. 2003b. "Rethinking Health and Human Rights: Time for a Paradigm Shift." In *Pathologies of Power: Health, Human Rights, and the New War on the Poor*, 224–246. Berkeley: University of California Press.

Fischer, Ann. 1956. "The Role of the Trukese Mother and Its Effect on Child Training." PhD diss., Radcliffe College.

———. 1963. "Reproduction in Truk." *Ethnology* 2 (4): 526–540. https://doi.org/10.2307/3772961.

Fischer, John L. 1951. "Applied Anthropology and the Administration." *American Anthropologist* 53 (1): 133–134. https://doi.org/10.1525/aa.1951.53.1.02a00320.

———. (1957) 1970. *The Eastern Carolines*. 3rd ed. New Haven, CT: Human Relations Area Files Press.

Fischer, John L., and Marc Swartz. 1960. "Socio-Psychological Aspects of Some Trukese and Ponape Love Songs." *Journal of American Folklore* 73 (289): 218–224. https://doi.org/10.2307/537974.

Fitzgerald, Maureen H. 2001. *Whisper of the Mother: From Menarche to Menopause among Women in Pohnpei*. Westport, CT: Bergin and Garvey.

Flinn, Juliana. 1987. "Pregnancy and Motherhood among Micronesian Students in the United States." In *Encounters with Biomedicine: Case Studies in Medical Anthropology*, edited by Hans A. Baer, 119–146. New York: Gordon and Breach Science.

———. 1990. "We Still Have Our Customs: Being Pulapese in Truk." In *Cultural Identity and Ethnicity in the Pacific*, edited by Jocelyn Linnekin and Lin Poyer, 103–126. Honolulu: University of Hawai'i Press.

———. 2010. *Mary, the Devil, and Taro: Catholicism and Women's Work in a Micronesian Society*. Honolulu: University of Hawai'i Press.

Flores, Glenn. 2000. "Culture and the Patient-Physician Relationship: Achieving Cultural Competency in Health Care." *Journal of Pediatrics* 136 (1): 14–23. https://doi.org/10.1016/S0022-3476(00)90043-X.

Flores, Jayne. 2019. "Wanted: a culture where rape is NOT acceptable." *Pacific Island Times*, November 5. https://www.pacificislandtimes.com/post/2019/11/06/wanted-a-culture-where-rape-is-not-acceptable.

Forte, Maximilian C. 2011. "The Human Terrain System and Anthropology: A Review of Ongoing Public Debates." *American Anthropologist* 113 (1): 149–153. https://doi.org/10.1111/j.1548–1433.2010.01315.x.

Foucault, Michel. 1978. *The History of Sexuality*. Vol. 1, *An Introduction*. Translated by Robert Hurley. New York: Pantheon.

Fox, Andrew M., and Theodore Parker. 2005. "Stillbirths in the Commonwealth of the Northern Mariana Islands." *Pacific Health Dialog* 12 (1): 75–80.

Fox, Andrew M., Theodore Parker, and Karen S. Palmer. 2005. "Prenatal Care in the Commonwealth of the Northern Mariana Islands." *Pacific Health Dialog* 12 (1): 67–74.

Fox, Chloe. 2014. "11 Reasons Guam Is the Most Exotic Destination in America." *Huffington Post*, March 18, 2014. https://www.huffpost.com/entry/guam-travel-destination_n_4953530.

Frain, Sylvia C. 2017. "Women's Resistance in the Marianas Archipelago: A US Colonial Homefront and Militarized Frontline." *Feminist Formations* 29 (1): 97–135.

FSM Association of Guam. 2019. Facebook: Created July 5, 2019. https://www.facebook.com/FSMCommunityCorp.

Gavey, Nicola. 2013. *Just Sex? The Cultural Scaffolding of Rape*. London: Routledge.

Gelardi, Chris. 2021. "Guam: Resisting Empire at the 'Tip of the Spear.'" *Nation*, 2021. https://www.thenation.com/article/world/guam-resistance-empire/.

Gilbert, Haidee Eugenio. 2019. "'Unacceptable': Census Error in Hawaii to Result in $12M Compact Funding Loss for Guam." *Pacific Daily News*, December 6, 2019. https://www.guampdn.com/story/news/2019/12/06/12-m-mistake-census-error-hawaii-means-guams-compact-funding-loss/2625680001/.

Ginsburg, Faye, and Rayna Rapp. 1991. "The Politics of Reproduction." *Annual Review of Anthropology* 20:311–343. https://doi.org/10.1146/annurev.an.20.100191.001523.

———. 1995. "Introduction: Conceiving the New World Order." In *Conceiving the New World Order: The Global Politics of Reproduction*, edited by Faye D. Ginsburg and Rayna Rapp, 1–17. Berkeley: University of California Press.

Gladwin, Thomas, and Seymour B. Sarason. 1953. *Truk: Man in Paradise*. Edited by A. Irving Hallowell. Viking Fund Publications in Anthropology 20. New York: Wenner-Gren Foundation for Anthropological Research.

Glick-Schiller, Nina. 1995. "From Immigrant to Transmigrant: Theorizing Transnational Migration." *Anthropological Quarterly* 68 (1): 48–63.

———. 2003. "The Centrality of Ethnography in the Study of Transnational Migration: Seeing the Wetlands Instead of the Swamp." In *American Arrivals: Anthropology Engages the New Immigration*, edited by Nancy Foner, 99–128. Santa Fe: School of American Research Press.

Glick-Schiller, Nina, Linda Basch, and Cristina Blanc-Szanton, eds. 1992. "Towards a Transnational Perspective on Migration: Race, Class, Ethnicity, and Nationalism Reconsidered. Edited by Bill Boland." Special issue, *Annals of the New York Academy of Sciences* 645 (1).

Gomberg-Muñoz, Ruth. 2018. "The Complicit Anthropologist." *Journal for the Anthropology of North America* 21 (1): 36–37.

Good, Mary-Jo DelVecchio. 2001. "The Biotechnical Embrace." *Culture, Medicine and Psychiatry* 25 (4): 395–410. https://doi.org/10.1023/a:1013097002487.

Goodenough, Ward H. 1949. "Premarital Freedom on Truk: Theory and Practice." *American Anthropologist* 51 (4): 615–620. https://doi.org/10.1525/aa.1949.51.4.02a00070.

———. 1978. *Property, Kin and Community on Truk*. 2nd ed. Hamden, CT: Archon Books. 1951.

———. 2002. *Under Heaven's Brow: Pre-Christian Religious Tradition in Chuuk*. Philadelphia: American Philosophical Society.

Gough, Kathleen. 1967. "Anthropology and Imperialism." *Monthly Review* 19:12–27.

Government of Guam. 2017. *2016 Guam Statistical Yearbook*. Prepared by the Bureau of Statistics and Plans, Office of the Governor. Hagatna, Guam. http://bsp.guam.gov/wp-bsp-content/uploads/2018/01/GuamStatistcalYearbook_2016.pdf.

———. 2020. *Title V MCH Block Grant FY 2020 Need Assessment*. Prepared by the Bureau of Family Health and Nursing Services, Department of Public Health and Social Services. Mangilao, Guam.

———. 2021. *2020 Guam Statistical Yearbook*. Prepared by the Bureau of Statistics and Plans, Office of the Governor. Hagatna, Guam. https://bsp.guam.gov/wp-bsp-content/uploads/2021/12/2020-GSY_Final.pdf

———. 2022. *Title V MCH Block Grant Program FY 2022 Application and FY 2020 Annual Report*. Prepared by the Bureau of Family Health and Nursing Services, Department of Public Health and Social Services. Mangilao, Guam. https://mchb.tvisdata.hrsa.gov/Admin/FileUpload/DownloadStateUploadedPdf?filetype=PrintVersion&state=GU&year=2022.

Government of the FSM (Federated States of Micronesia). 2004. *FSM Strategic Development Plan, 2004–2023: The Next 20 Years; Achieving Economic Growth and Self-Reliance*. Prepared by the Department of Transportation, Communications and Infrastructure. Palikir, Pohnpei.

———. 2012a. *Health Progress Report: 2008–2011*. Prepared by the Department of Health and Social Affairs. Palikir, Pohnpei.

———. 2012b. *Summary Analysis of Key Indicators from the FSM 2010 Census of Population and Housing*. Prepared by the Division of Statistics, FSM Office of Statistics, Budget, Overseas Development Assistance and Compact Management (SBOC). Palikir, Pohnpei.

———. 2022a. *STD Detection Rate 2019*. Prepared by the Bureau of Communicable Diseases, Department of Health and Social Affairs. Palikir, Pohnpei. https://hsa.gov.fm/sexually-transmitted-diseases. Accessed January 4, 2023.

———. 2022b. *Title V MCH Block Grant Program FY 2023 Application and FY 2021 Annual Report*. Prepared by the Department of Health and Social Affairs. Palikir, Pohnpei. https://mchb.tvisdata.hrsa.gov/Admin/FileUpload/DownloadStateUploadedPdf?filetype=PrintVersion&state=FM&year=2023.

Green, Caitlin, Charity Ntansah, Meghan T. Frey, Jamie W. Krashin, Eva Lathrop, and Lisa Romero. 2020. "Assessment of Contraceptive Needs and Improving Access in the US-Affiliated Pacific Islands in the Context of Zika." *Journal of Women's Health* 29 (2): 139–147. https://doi.org/10.1089/jwh.2020.8302.

Greenhalgh, Susan. 1995. "Anthropology Theorizes Reproduction: Integrating Practice, Political Economic, and Feminist Perspectives." In *Situating Fertility: Anthropology and Demographic Inquiry*, edited by Susan Greenhalgh, 3–28. Cambridge: Cambridge University Press.

Grieco, Elizabeth M. 2003. *The Remittance Behavior of Immigrant Households: Micronesians in Hawaii and Guam*. New York: LFB.

Grimshaw, Patricia. 1989. "New England Missionary Wives: Hawaiian Women and the Cult of True Womanhood." In *Family and Gender in the Pacific: Domestic Contradictions and the Colonial Impact*, edited by Margaret Jolly and Martha Macintyre, 19–44. Cambridge: Cambridge University Press.

Guam Police Department. 2023. *Crime in Guam 2021: Uniform Crime Report*. January 23, 2023. https://gpd.guam.gov/wp-gpd-content/uploads/2023/01/UCR-2021.pdf.

Guerrero, Wilfred Leon, and John C. Salas. 1995. "Issues for the United States Pacific Insular Areas: The Case of Guam." *ISLA: A Journal of Micronesian Studies* 3 (1): 139–145.

Gupta, Akhil, and James Ferguson. 1997. "Beyond "Culture": Space, Identity, and the Politics of Difference." In *Culture, Power, Place: Explorations in Critical Anthropology*, edited by Akhil Gupta and James Ferguson, 33–51. Durham, NC: Duke University Press.

Haddock, Robert L. 2010. *A History of Health on Guam*. Hagatna, Guam: Crushers Football (Soccer) Club.

Haddock, Robert L., Margaret Murphy-Bell, Cynthia L. Naval, and Carolyn Garrido. 2008. "Lack of Prenatal Care—a Re-emerging Health Problem on Guam." *Hawai'i Journal of Public Health* 1 (1): 40–44.

Hagiwara, Megan Kiyomi Inada, Jill Miyamura, Seiji Yamada, and Tetine Sentell. 2016. "Younger and Sicker: Comparing Micronesians to Other Ethnicities in Hawai'i." *American Journal of Public Health* 106 (3): 485–491. https://doi.org/10.2105/AJPH.2015.302921.

Hanlon, David. 1994. "Patterns of Colonial Rule in Micronesia." In *Tides of History: The Pacific Islands in the Twentieth Century*, edited by K. R. Howe, Robert C. Kiste, and Brij V. Lal, 93–118. Honolulu: University of Hawai'i Press.

———. 1998. *Remaking Micronesia: Discourses Over Development in a Pacific Territory; 1944–1982*. Honolulu: University of Hawai'i Press.

———. 2009. "The 'Sea of Little Lands': Examining Micronesia's Place in 'Our Sea of Islands.'" *Contemporary Pacific* 21 (1): 91–110. https://doi.org/10.1353/cp.0.0042.

Harrison, Faye V. (1991) 1997. *Decolonizing Anthropology: Moving Further towards an Anthropology for Liberation*. 2nd ed. Washington, DC: American Anthropological Association.

Hattori, Anne Perez. 2004. *Colonial Dis-Ease: US Navy Health Policies and the Chamorros of Guam, 1898–1941.* Honolulu: University of Hawai'i Press.

———. 2006. "'The Cry of the Little people of Guam': American Colonialism, Medical Philanthropy, and the Susana Hospital for Chamorro Women, 1898–1941." *Health and History* 8 (1): 4–26. https://doi.org/10.2307/40111527.

Hattori-Uchima, Margaret. 2017. "Chuukese Migrant Women in Guam: Perceptions of Barriers to Health Care." *Asian/Pacific Island Nursing Journal* 2 (1): 19–28. https://doi.org/10.9741/23736658.1049.

Hattori-Uchima, Margaret, and Kathryn Wood. 2019. "Nursing Leadership in Guam." *Nursing Administration Quarterly* 43 (1): 19–25. https://doi.org/10.1097/NAQ.0000000000000332.

Health Resources and Services Administration. 2021. "III.B. Overview of the State - Guam—2021." Accessed March 28, 2023. https://mchb.tvisdata.hrsa.gov/Narratives/Overview/08312f4f-d1b8-4988-a861-b6aa9678a13e#:~:text=Guam%20has%20ten%20specialty%20and,pharmacies%20for%20prescription%20drug%20needs.

Heine, Carl. 1974. *Micronesia at the Crossroads: A Reappraisal of the Micronesian Political Dilemma.* Canberra, Australia: Australian National University Press.

Helms, Elissa. 2014. "The Movementization of NGOs? Women's Organizing in Postwar Bosnia-Herzegovina." In *Theorizing NGOs: States, Feminisms, and Neoliberalism,* edited by Victoria Bernal and Inderpal Grewal, 21–49. Durham, NC: Duke University Press.

Heritage, John, and Douglas W. Maynard. 2006. "Problems and Prospects in the Study of Physician-Patient Interaction: 30 Years of Research." *Annual Review of Sociology* 32:351–374. https://doi.org/10.1146/annurev.soc.32.082905.093959.

Hernandez, Julianne. 2022. "GMHA CEO: Some Doctors Object to New Hospital Site." *Pacific Daily News,* July 13, 2022. https://www.guampdn.com/news/gmha-ceo-some-doctors-object-to-new-hospital-site/article_851a5992-0279-11ed-a316-93c4ce1ceb79.html.

Hezel, Francis X. 1970. "Catholic Missions in the Caroline and Marshall Islands: A Survey of Historical Materials." *Journal of Pacific History* 5 (1): 213–227.

———. 1983. The First Taint of Civilization: A History of the Caroline and Marshall Islands in Pre-colonial Days, 1521–1885. Honolulu: University of Hawai'i Press.

. 1995. *Strangers in their Own Land: A Century of Colonial Rule in the Caroline and Marshall Islands. Pacific Islands Monograph Series 13.* Honolulu: University of Hawai'i Press.

———. 2001. *The New Shape of Old Island Cultures: A Half Century of Social Change in Micronesia.* Honolulu: University of Hawai'i Press.

———. 2004. "Chuuk: A Caricature of an Island." In *Pacific Places, Pacific Histories: Essays in Honor of Robert Kiste,* edited by Brij V. Lal, 102–119. Honolulu: University of Hawai'i Press.

———. 2012. *Pacific Island Nations: How Viable Are Their Economies?* East-West Center (Honolulu). https://www.eastwestcenter.org/publications/pacific-island-nations-how-viable-are-their-economies.

———. 2013. *Micronesians on the Move: Eastward and Upward Bound.* East-West Center (Honolulu). http://hl-128-171-57–22.library.manoa.hawaii.edu/bitstream/10125/30616/1/pip009.pdf.

Hezel, Francis X., and Michael J. Levin. September 2012. *Survey of Federated States of Micronesia Migrants in the United States including Guam and the Commonwealth of the Northern Mariana Islands (CNMI).* FSM Office of Statistics, Budget & Economic Management, Overseas Development Assistance and Compact Management (Palikir, Pohnpei). https://prd.psc.isr.umich.edu/files/Resources_Report%20on%20PI%20Jurisdictions.pdf.

Hezel, Francis X., and Thomas B. McGrath. 1989. "The Great Flight Northward: FSM Migration to Guam and the Northern Mariana Islands." *Pacific Studies* 13 (1): 47–64.

Hirsch, Jennifer S., Holly Wardlow, Daniel Jordan Smith, Harriet Phinney, Shanti Parikh, and Constance A. Nathanson. 2009. *The Secret: Love, Marriage, and HIV.* Nashville: Vanderbilt University Press.

Hodžić, Saida. 2014. "Feminist Bastards: Toward a Posthumanist Critique of NGOization." In *Theorizing NGOs: States, Feminisms, and Neoliberalism,* edited by Victoria Bernal and Inderpal Grewal, 221–247. Durham, NC: Duke University Press.

Hofmann, Rebecca. 2018. "Localizing Global Climate Change in the Pacific: Knowledge and Response in Chuuk, Federated States of Micronesia (FSM)." *Sociologus* 68 (1): 43–62.

Hofschneider, Anita. 2022. "The Fight over Abortion Access in Guam Has Broad Implications for Women in the Pacific." *Honolulu Civil Beat,* December 22, 2022. https://www.civilbeat.org/2022/12/the-fight-over-abortion-access-in-guam-has-broad-implications-for-women-in-the-pacific/.

Horowitz, Irving Louis. 1966. "The Life and Death of Project Camelot." *American Psychologist* 21 (5): 445–454.

Hoy, Damian, A. Mark Durand, Thane Hancock, Haley L. Cash, Kate Hardie, Beverley Paterson, Yvette Paulino, Paul White, Tony Merritt, and Dawn Fitzgibbons. 2017. "Lessons Learnt from a Three-Year Pilot Field Epidemiology Training Programme." *WPSAR: Western Pacific Surveillance and Response Journal* 8 (3): 21–26. https://doi.org/10.5365/wpsar.2016.7.4.005.

Hunt, Linda M., and Katherine B. de Voogd. 2005. "Clinical Myths of the Cultural 'Other': Implications for Latino Patient Care." *Academic Medicine* 80 (10): 918–924. https://journals.lww.com/academicmedicine/Fulltext/2005/10000/Clinical_Myths_of_the_Cultural__Other__.11.aspx.

Inada, Megan Kiyomi, Kathryn L. Braun, Parkey Mwarike, Kevin Cassel, Randy Compton, Seiji Yamada, and Tetine Sentell. 2019. "Chuukese Community Experiences of Racial Discrimination and Other Barriers to Healthcare: Perspectives from Community Members and Providers." *Social Medicine* 12 (1): 3–13. https://www.ncbi.nlm.nih.gov/pmc/articles/PMC6853624/.

Inda, Jonathan Xavier, and Renato Rosaldo. 2008. "Tracking Global Flows." In *The Anthropology of Globalization,* edited by Jonathan Xavier Inda and Renato Rosaldo, 3–46. Malden, MA: Blackwell.

Jolly, Margaret. 1998. "Introduction: Colonial and Postcolonial Plots in Histories of Maternities and Modernities." In *Maternities and Modernities: Colonial and Postcolonial Experiences in Asia and the Pacific,* edited by Kalpana Ram and Margaret Jolly, 1–25. Cambridge: Cambridge University Press.

———. 2002. "Introduction: Birthing beyond the Confinements of Tradition and Modernity?" In *Birthing in the Pacific: Beyond Tradition and Modernity?,* edited by Vicki Lukere and Margaret Jolly, 1–30. Honolulu: University of Hawaiʻi Press.

Jolly, Margaret, and Martha Macintyre. 1989. *Family and Gender in the Pacific: Domestic Contradictions and the Colonial Impact.* Cambridge: Cambridge University Press.

Katz, Alan R., Adrianne M. Cadorna, Maria Veneranda C. Lee, Alan Komeya, Mandy Kiaha, and Roy G. Ohye. 2009. "Investigation of a Cluster of Syphilis, Gonorrhea, and Chlamydia Cases among Heterosexual Micronesians Living on Oahu." *Journal of Community Health* 34:357–360. https://doi.org/10.1007/s10900-009-9170-8.

Kawai, Toshimitsu. 1987. "Females Bear Men, Land and Eterecke s: Paternal Nurture and Symbolic Female Roles on Truk." *Senri Ethnological Studies* (21): 107–125.

Kearney, Michael. 1995. "The Local and the Global: The Anthropology of Globalization and Transnationalism." *Annual Review of Anthropology* 24:547–565. https://doi.org/10.1146/annurev.an.24.100195.002555.

Kettunen, Tarja, Marita Poskiparta, and Maija Gerlander. 2002. "Nurse–Patient Power Relationship: Preliminary Evidence of Patients' Power Messages." *Patient Education and Counseling* 47 (2): 101–113. https://doi.org/10.1016/S0738-3991(01)00179-3.

Kihleng, Emelihter S. 2015. "Menginpehn Lien Pohnpei: A Poetic Ethnography of Urohs (Pohnpeian skirts)." PhD diss., Victoria University of Wellington.

Kim, Min-Sun, Renee Storm Klingle, William F Sharkey, Hee Sun Park, David H. Smith, and Deborah Cai. 2000. "A Test of a Cultural Model of Patients' Motivation for Verbal Communication in Patient-Doctor Interactions." *Communications Monographs* 67 (3): 262–283. https://doi.org/10.1080/03637750009376510.

Kim, Myjolynne Marie. 2007. "Combatting 'Dreaded Hogoleu': Re-centering Local Histories and Stories of Chuukese Warfare." Master's thesis, University of Hawai'i at Manoa.

———. 2020. "Nesor Annim, Niteikapar (Good Morning, Cardinal Honeyeater): Indigenous Reflections on Micronesian Women and the Environment." *Contemporary Pacific* 32 (1): 147–163. https://doi.org/10.1353/cp.2020.0007.

Kingfisher, Catherine P. 1996. *Women in the American Welfare Trap.* Philadelphia: University of Pennsylvania Press.

Kirmayer, Laurence J. 2012a. "Cultural Competence and Evidence-Based Practice in Mental Health: Epistemic Communities and the Politics of Pluralism." *Social Science & Medicine* 75 (2): 249–256. https://doi.org/10.1016/j.socscimed.2012.03.018.

———. 2012b. "Rethinking Cultural Competence." *Transcultural Psychiatry* 49 (2): 149–164. https://doi.org/10.1177/1363461512444673.

Kiste, Robert C. 1993. "New Political Statuses in American Micronesia." In *Contemporary Pacific Societies: Studies in Development and Change,* edited by Victoria S. Lockwood, Thomas G. Harding, and Ben J. Wallace, 67–80. Englewood Cliffs, NJ: Prentice Hall.

———. 1994a. "Pre-colonial Times." In *Tides of History: The Pacific Islands in the Twentieth Century,* edited by Kerry Ross Howe, Robert C. Kiste, and Brij V. Lal, 3–28. Honolulu: University of Hawai'i Press.

———. 1994b. "Towards Decolonization: United States." In *Tides of History: The Pacific Islands in the Twentieth Century,* edited by Kerry Ross Howe, Robert C. Kiste, and Brij V. Lal, 227–257. Honolulu: University of Hawai'i Press.

———. 1999. "A Half Century in Retrospect." In *American Anthropology in Micronesia: An Assessment,* edited by Robert C. Kiste and Mac Marshall, 433–467. Honolulu: University of Hawai'i Press.

Kiste, Robert C., and Suzanne Falgout. 1999. "Anthropology and Micronesia: The Context." In *American Anthropology in Micronesia: An Assessment,* edited by Robert C. Kiste and Mac Marshall, 11–51. Honolulu: University of Hawai'i Press.

Kiste, Robert C., and Mac Marshall, eds. 1999. *American Anthropology in Micronesia: An Assessment.* Honolulu: University of Hawai'i Press.

Kleinman, Arthur, and Peter Benson. 2006. "Anthropology in the Clinic: The Problem of Cultural Competency and How to Fix It." *PLoS Medicine* 3 (10): e294. https://doi.org/10.1371/journal.pmed.0030294.

Korsch, Barbara M., Ethel K. Gozzi, and Vida Francis. 1968. "Gaps in Doctor-Patient Communication: Doctor-Patient Interaction and Patient Satisfaction." *Pediatrics* 42 (5): 855–871.

Kroll, Gary. 2003. "The Pacific Science Board in Micronesia: Science, Government, and Conservation on the Post-War Pacific Frontier." *Minerva* 41:25–46. https://doi.org/10.1023/A:1022205821483.

Lambert, Helen. 2012. "Medical Pluralism and Medical Marginality: Bone Doctors and the Selective Legitimation of Therapeutic Expertise in India." *Social Science & Medicine* 74 (7): 1029–1036.

Leon, Carlued, and Eleanor S. Mori. 2014. *Federated States of Micronesia Family Health and Safety Study.* Palakir, Pohnpei: FSM Department of Health and Social Affairs.

Leon Guerrero, Lourdes (Lou) A. 2019. "State of the Island Address 2019." Office of the Governor. April 11, 2019. https://governor.guam.gov/wp-content/uploads/2021/05/STATE-OF-THE-ISLAND-ADDRESS-2019.pdf.

———.2020. "State of the Island Address 2020." Office of the Governor. February 24, 2020. https://governor.guam.gov/wp-content/uploads/2021/05/STATE-OF-THE-ISLAND-ADDRESS-2020.pdf.

———.2023. "State of the Island Address 2023." Office of the Governor. March 15, 2023. https://governor.guam.gov/wp-content/uploads/2023/03/The-State-of-the-Island-2023-1.pdf.

Levin, Michael J. 2010. *The Status of Micronesian Migrants in the Early 21st Century.* Cambridge, MA: Population and Development Studies Center, Department of Public Health, Harvard University.

Lewin, Ellen. 2009. Introduction to *Feminist Anthropology: A Reader.* Edited by Ellen Lewin, 1–38. Malden, MA: Blackwell.

Limtiaco, Steve. 2019a. "GMH Employees, Governor Discuss Ways to Improve Health Care." *Pacific Daily News,* February 11, 2019. https://www.guampdn.com/story/news/2019/02/11/gmh-employees-governor-discuss-ways-improve-health-care/2835234002/.

———. 2019b. "GovGuam to Recalculate the Financial Impact of Regional Migrants." *Pacific Daily News,* April 11, 2019. https://www.guampdn.com/story/news/local/2019/04/11/govguam-regional-migrants-numbers/3444290002/.

Lipsky, Michael. 1984. "Bureaucratic Disentitlement in Social Welfare Programs." *Social Service Review* 58 (1): 3–27. https://doi.org/10.1086/644161.

Lock, Margaret, and Vinh-Kim Nguyen. 2010. "Colonial Disease and Biological Commensurability." In *An Anthropology of Biomedicine,* 79–102. Malden, MA: Wiley-Blackwell.

Lock, Margaret, and Nancy Scheper-Hughes. 1996. "A Critical-Interpretive Approach in Medical Anthropology: Rituals and Routines of Discipline and Dissent." In *Handbook of Medical Anthropology: Contemporary Theory and Method,* edited by Carolyn F. Sargent and Thomas M. Johnson, 31–70. Westport, CT: Greenwood Press.

López, Leslie. 2005. "De Facto Disentitlement in an Information Economy: Enrollment Issues in Medicaid Managed Care." *Medical Anthropology Quarterly* 19 (1): 26–46. https://doi.org/10.1525/maq.2005.19.1.026.

Lum, Thomas. 2023. *Compacts of Free Association.* Congressional Research Service Updated March 17. (Washington, DC). https://crsreports.congress.gov/product/pdf/IF/IF12194.

Lutz, Catherine. 1984. *Micronesia as Strategic Colony: The Impact of U.S. Policy on Micronesian Health and Culture.* Cultural Survival 12. Cambridge, MA: Cultural Survival.

———. 1986. "The Compact of Free Association, Micronesian Non-independence and U.S. Policy." *Bulletin of Concerned Asian Scholars* 18 (2): 21–27.

———. 2006. "Empire Is in the Details." *American Ethnologist* 33 (4): 593–611.

Mack, Ashley Noel, and Tiara R Na'Puti. 2019. "'Our Bodies Are Not Terra Nullius': Building a Decolonial Feminist Resistance to Gendered Violence." *Women's Studies in Communication* 42 (3): 347–370.

Magnussen, Lois, Jan Shoultz, Karol Richardson, Mary Frances Oneha, Jacquelyn C. Campbell, Doris Segal Matsunaga, Selynda Mori Selifis, Merina Sapolu, Mariama Samifua, and Helena Manzano. 2011. "Responding to the Needs of Culturally Diverse Women Who Experience Intimate Partner Violence." *Hawaii Medical Journal* 70 (1): 9.

Mahony, Frank J. 1969. "A Trukese Theory of Medicine." PhD diss., Stanford University.

Maisonneuve, Gisele. 2006. "The Women's Movement in Papua New Guinea as a Vehicle to Enhance Women's Participation in Development." *Contemporary PNG Studies* 4: 10–30. https://search.informit.org/doi/epdf/10.3316/informit.085173867636108.

Malinowski, Bronislaw. 1929. *Sexual Life of Savages in North Western Melanesia.* London: Routledge and Kegan Paul.

Manderson, Lenore. 1996. *Sickness and the State: Health and Illness in Colonial Malaya, 1870–1940.* Cambridge: Cambridge University Press.

———. 1998. "Shaping Reproduction: Maternity in Early Twentieth Century Malaya." In *Maternities and Modernities: Colonial and Postcolonial Experiences in Asia and the Pacific,* edited by Kalpana Ram and Margaret Jolly, 26–49. Cambridge: Cambridge University Press.

———. 2018. "Humans on Show: Performance, Race and Representation." *Critical African Studies* 10 (3): 257–271.

Manderson, Lenore, and Margaret Jolly. 1997. "Introduction: Sites of Desire/Economies of Pleasure: Sexualities in Asia and the Pacific." In *Sites of Desire/Economies of Pleasure: Sexualities in Asia and the Pacific,* 1–26. Chicago: University of Chicago Press.

Marcus, George E. 1995. "Ethnography in/of the World System: The Emergence of Multi-Sited Ethnography." *Annual Review of Anthropology* 24:95–117. https://doi.org/10.1146/annurev.an.24.100195.000523.

Marshall, Leslie B., and Mac Marshall. 1979. "Breasts, Bottles and Babies: Historical Changes in Infant Feeding Practices in a Micronesian Village." *Ecology of Food and Nutrition* 8 (4): 241–249. https://doi.org/10.1080/03670244.1979.9990573.

———. 1980. "Infant Feeding and Infant Illness in a Micronesian Village." *Social Science & Medicine* 14 (1): 33–38. https://doi.org/10.1016/0160-7987(80)90038–1.

———. 1982. "Education of Women and Family Size in Two Micronesian Communities." *Micronesia* 18 (1): 1–21.

Marshall, Mac. 1976. "Solidarity or Sterility? Adoption and Fosterage on Namoluk Atoll." In *Transactions in Kinship: Adoption and Fosterage in Oceania,* edited by Ivan Brady, 28–50. ASAO Monograph Series. Honolulu: University of Hawai'i.

———. 1979. *Weekend Warriors: Alcohol in a Micronesian Culture.* Mountain View, CA: McGraw-Hill Humanities, Social Sciences & World Languages.

———. 2004. *Namoluk Beyond the Reef.* Edited by Edward R. Fischer. Westview Case Studies in Anthropology. Boulder, CO: Westview Press.

Marshall, Mac, and Leslie B. Marshall. 1990. *Silent Voices Speak: Women and Prohibition in Truk.* Belmont, CA: Wadsworth.

Martina, Michael, and David Brunnstrom. 2023. "U.S. aims for over $7 billion in aid for 20-year Pacific islands compacts." *Reuters,* March 23, 2023. https://www.reuters.com/breakingviews/us-aims-over-7-billion-aid-20-year-pacific-islands-compacts-2023-03-23/.

Mason, Leonard. 1983. "The Anthropological Presence in Micronesia." Presented at the 32nd Annual Meeting of the Society for Applied Anthropology, Tucson, AZ, April.

McElroy, Anne, and Patricia K. Townsend. 2009. "Chapter Six: Culture, Ecology, Reproduction." In *Medical Anthropology in Ecological Perspective.* 217–266. New York: Routledge.

McMillan, Karen, Christine Linhart, Hilary Gorman, Myjolynne Kim, Catherine O'Connor, Michelle O'Connor, and Avelina Rokoduru. 2020. *Adolescent Unplanned Pregnancy in the Pacific: Chuuk.* Sydney: UNSW.

McPherson, Naomi, ed. 2016. *Missing the Mark? Women and the Millennium Development Goals in Africa and Oceania.* Toronto: Demeter Press.

Mead, Margaret. 1923. *Coming of Age in Samoa.* New York: Morrow.

Miculka, Cameron. 2014. "Cruz Asks Bordallo for Help on Immigrant Removal." *Pacific Daily News*, March 21, 2014.

Mintz, Sidney W. 1998. "The Localization of Anthropological Practice: From Area Studies to Transnationalism." *Critique of Anthropology* 18 (2): 117–133. https://doi.org/10.1177/0308275X9801800201.

Mitchell-Eaton, Emily. 2016. "New Destinations of Empire: Imperial Migration from the Marshall Islands to Northwest Arkansas." PhD diss., Syracuse University.

Molesworth, Kate, Florence Sécula, Rachel A Eager, Zuhro Murodova, Shakhlo Yarbaeva, and Barbara Matthys. 2017. "Impact of Group Formation on Women's Empowerment and Economic Resilience in Rural Tajikistan." *Journal of Rural and Community Development* 12 (1). https://journals.brandonu.ca/jrcd/article/view/1336.

Moral, Beatriz. 1996. "Conceptualization of Women, the Body and Sexuality in Chuuk (Micronesia)." PhD diss., University of Basque Country, Spain.

———. 1998a. "Changes in Women's Status in Micronesia: An Anthropological Approach." In *Indigenous Women: The Right to a Voice*, edited by Diana Vinding, 65–74. Copenhagen, Denmark: International Work Group for Indigenous Affairs.

———. 1998b. "The Chuukese Women's Status: Traditional and Modern Elements." In *Common Worlds and Single Lives: Constituting Knowledge in Pacific Societies*, edited by Verena Keck, 273–284. Oxford: Berg.

———. 2002. "Erotic Legends and Narratives in Chuuk, Micronesia." *Micronesian Journal of the Humanities and Social Sciences* 1 (1–2): 26–38.

Mountz, Alison. 2011. "The Enforcement Archipelago: Detention, Haunting, and Asylum on Islands." *Political Geography* 30 (3): 118–128. https://doi.org/10.1016/j.polgeo.2011.01.005.

Mountz, Alison, and Jenna Loyd. 2014. "Transnational Productions of Remoteness: Building Onshore and Offshore Carceral Regimes Across Borders." *Geographica Helvetica* 69 (5): 389. https://doi.org/10.5194/gh-69-389-2014.

Mukhopadhyay, Maitrayee. 2014. "Mainstreaming Gender or Reconstituting the Mainstream? Gender Knowledge in Development." *Journal of International Development* 26 (3): 356–367. https://doi.org/10.1002/jid.2946.

Munro, Jenny, Els Tieneke Rieke Katmo, and Meki Wetipo. 2022. "Hospital Births and Frontier Obstetrics in Urban West Papua." *Asia Pacific Journal of Anthropology* 23 (4–5): 388–406. https://doi.org/10.1080/14442213.2022.2115121.

Munro, Jenny, and Alexandra Widmer. 2022. "Reproducing Life in Conditions of Abandonment in Oceania." *Asia Pacific Journal of Anthropology* 23 (4–5): 301–310. https://doi.org/10.1080/14442213.2022.2115543.

Na'puti, Tiara R. 2019. "Archipelagic Rhetoric: Remapping the Marianas and Challenging Militarization from 'A Stirring Place.'" *Communication and Critical/Cultural Studies* 16 (1): 4–25. https://doi.org/10.1080/14791420.2019.1572905.

Na'puti, Tiara R., and Michael Lujan Bevacqua. 2015. "Militarization and Resistance from Guåhan: Protecting and Defending Pågat." *American Quarterly* 67 (3): 837–858. https://www.jstor.org/stable/43823236.

Neechuumeres: Chuukese Women of Guam. 2021. Facebook. Created August 19, 2021. https://www.facebook.com/neechuumeresinguam/.

Notwell, Jessica Alexandra. 2014. "Y Intergenerational Leadership? YWCA Solomon Islands' Feminist Rights-Based Approach to Young Women, Power and Equality." Master's thesis, York University.

Oliver, Douglas, ed. 1951. *Planning Micronesia's Future: A Summary of the United States Commercial Company's Economic Survey of Micronesia, 1946*. Cambridge, MA: Harvard University Press.

Ong, Aihwa. 2006. *Neoliberalism as Exception: Mutations in Citizenship and Sovereignty.* Durham, NC: Duke University Press.

Ong, Aihwa, Virginia R. Dominguez, Jonathan Friedman, Nina Glick Schiller, Verena Stolcke, and Hu Ying. 1996. "Cultural Citizenship as Subject-Making: Immigrants Negotiate Racial and Cultural Boundaries in the United States [and Comments and Reply]." *Current Anthropology* 37 (5): 737–762.

O'Rourke, Dennis. 1980. *Yap: How Did You Know We'd Like TV.* Video. Canberra, Australia: Ronin Films.

Ortner, Sherry B. 1972. "Is Female to Male as Nature Is to Culture?" *Feminist Studies* 1 (2): 5–31. https://doi.org/10.2307/3177638.

Palafox, Neal A., and Allen L. Hixon. 2011. "Health Consequences of Disparity: The US Affiliated Pacific Islands." *Australasian Psychiatry* 19 (1_suppl.): S84–S89. https://doi.org/10.3109/10398562.2011.583072.

Panuelo, David. 2022. "Letter to Pacific Island Leaders May 20, 2022." https://s3.documentcloud.org/documents/22039750/letter-from-h-e-david-w-panuelo-to-pacific-island-leaders-may-20-2022-signed.pdf.

Pels, Peter. 1997. "The Anthropology of Colonialism: Culture, History, and the Emergence of Western Governmentality." *Annual Review of Anthropology* 26 (1): 163. https://doi.org/10.1146/annurev.anthro.26.1.163.

Pels, Peter, and Oscar Salemink. 1994. "Colonial Ethnographies." *History and Anthropology* 8 (1): 352.

Perez, Michael P. 2002. "Pacific Identities beyond US Racial Formations: The Case of Chamorro Ambivalence and Flux." *Social Identities* 8 (3): 457–479. https://doi.org/10.1080/1350463022000030001.

Perry, Nick. 2023. "Micronesia's president accuses China of 'political warfare.'" *AP News,* March 13, 2023. https://apnews.com/article/micronesia-china-political-warfare-taiwan-55ea0ebc5e6580f14e7331acd878e907.

Peter, Joakim. 2000. "Chuukese Travellers and the Idea of Horizon." *Asia Pacific Viewpoint* 41 (3): 253–267. https://doi.org/10.1111/1467-8373.00121.

Petersen, Glenn. 1998. "Strategic Location and Sovereignty: Modern Micronesia in the Historical Context of American Expansionism." *Space and Polity* 2 (2): 179–205. https://doi.org/10.1080/13562579808721779.

———. 2004. "Lessons Learned: The Micronesian Quest for Independence in the Context of American Imperial History." *Micronesian Journal of the Humanities and Social Sciences* 3 (1–2).

———. 2009. *Traditional Micronesian Socieites: Adaptation, Integration, and Political Organization.* Honolulu: University of Hawai'i Press.

———. 2015. "American Anthropology's 'Thailand Controversy': An Object Lesson in Professional Responsibility." *SOJOURN: Journal of Social Issues in Southeast Asia* 30 (2): 528–549.

Pobutsky, Ann M., Lee Buenconsejo-Lum, Catherine Chow, Neal Palafox, and Gregory G. Maskarinec. 2005. "Micronesian Migrants in Hawai'i: Health Issues and Culturally Appropriate, Community-Based Solutions." *California Journal of Health Promotion* 3 (4): 59–72. https://doi.org/10.32398/cjhp.v3i4.1782.

Pobutsky, Ann M., Dmitry Krupitsky, and Seiji Yamada. 2009. "Micronesian Migrant Health Issues in Hawai'i: Part 2: An Assessment of Health, Language and Key Social Determinants of Health." *California Journal of Health Promotion* 7 (2): 32–55. https://doi.org/10.32398/cjhp.v7i2.2012.

Poyer, Lin, Suzanne Falgout, and Laurence Marshall Carucci. 2001. *The Typhoon of War: Micronesian Experiences of the Pacific War.* Honolulu: University of Hawai'i Press.

Price, David H. 2016. *Cold War Anthropology: The CIA, the Pentagon, and the Growth of Dual Use Anthropology.* Durham, NC: Duke University Press.

Puas, Gonzaga. 2021. *The Federated States of Micronesia's Engagement with the Outside World: Control, Self-Preservation and Continuity.* Canberra: Australia National University Press.

Quesada, James, Laurie Kain Hart, and Philippe Bourgois. 2011. "Structural Vulnerability and Health: Latino Migrant Laborers in the United States." *Medical Anthropology* 30 (4): 339–362. https://doi.org/10.1080/01459740.2011.576725.

Quimby, Frank. 2011. "The Hierro Commerce: Culture Contact, Appropriation and Colonial Entanglement in the Marianas, 1521–1668." *Journal of Pacific History* 46 (1): 1–26.

Raidoo, Shandhini, Bliss Kaneshiro, and Paris Stowers. 2021. "Guam: The US Territory Where America's Day Begins but Abortion Access Is Still in the Dark." *Contraception* 104 (1): 33–35. https://doi.org/https://doi.org/10.1016/j.contraception.2021.03.030.

Rainbird, Paul. 2003. "Taking the Tapu: Defining Micronesia by Absence." *Journal of Pacific History* 38 (2): 237–250. https://doi.org/10.1080/0022334032000120558.

Ram, Kalpana. 1998. "Maternity and the Story of Enlightenment in the Colonies: Tamil Coastal Women, South India." In *Maternities and Modernities: Colonial and Postcolonial Experiences in Asia and the Pacific*, 114–143. Cambridge: Cambridge University Press.

Rapp, Rayna. 2001. "Gender, Body, Biomedicine: How Some Feminist Concerns Dragged Reproduction to the Center of Social Theory." *Medical Anthropology Quarterly* 15 (4): 466–477. https://doi.org/10.1525/maq.2001.15.4.466.

Rauchholz, Manuel. 2008. "Demythologizing Adoption: From the Practice to the Effects of Adoption in Chuuk, Micronesia." *Pacific Studies* 31 (3/4): 156–181.

———. 2009. "Towards an Understanding of Adoption, Person and Emotion: The Ideal Norm and the Reality of Life amongst the Chuukese of Micronesia." PhD diss., University of Heidelberg.

———. 2012. "Discourses on Chuukese Customary Adoption, Migration, and the Laws of State(s)." *Pacific Studies* 35 (1): 119–143.

———. 2016. "Masculine Sexuality, Violence and Sexual Exploitation in Micronesia." *Asia Pacific Journal of Anthropology* 17 (3–4): 342–358. https://doi.org/10.1080/14442213.2016.1196724.

Reed, Adam. 1997. "Contested Images and Common Strategies: Early Colonial Sexual Politics in the Massim." In *Sites of Desire/Economies of Pleasure: Sexualities in Asia and the Pacific*, edited by Lenore Manderson and Margaret Jolly, 48–71. Chicago: University of Chicago Press.

Rehuher, D., E. S. Hishinuma, D. A. Goebert, and N. A. Palafox. 2021. "A Historical and Contemporary Review of the Contextualization and Social Determinants of Health of Micronesian Migrants in the United States." *Hawai'i Journal of Health & Social Welfare* 80 (9 suppl. 1): 88–101. https://www.ncbi.nlm.nih.gov/pmc/articles/PMC8504325/pdf/hjhsw8009_S1_0088.pdf.

Reubi, David. 2020. "Epidemiological Imaginaries of the Social: Epidemiologists and Pathologies of Modernization in Postcolonial Africa." *Medical Anthropology Quarterly* 34 (3): 438–455.

Richardson, Eugene T. 2020. *Epidemic Illusions: On the Coloniality of Global Public Health.* Cambridge, MA: MIT Press.

Rogers, Robert F. 1995. *Destiny's Landfall: A History of Guam.* Honolulu: University of Hawai'i Press.

Rosa, Jonathan, and Yarimar Bonilla. 2017. "Deprovincializing Trump, Decolonizing Diversity, and Unsettling Anthropology." *American Ethnologist* 44 (2): 201–208.

Rosaldo, Michelle Zimbalist, and Louise Lamphere, eds. 1974. *Woman, Culture, and Society.* Stanford, CA: Stanford University Press.

Rosaldo, Renato. 1989. *Culture & Truth: The Remaking of Social Analysis.* Boston: Beacon Press.

Roter, Debra L., Moira Stewart, Samuel M. Putnam, Mack Lipkin, William Stiles, and Thomas S. Inui. 1997. "Communication Patterns of Primary Care Physicians." *Journal of the American Medical Association* 277 (4): 350–356. https://doi.org/10.1001/jama.1997.03540280088045.

Rubinstein, Donald H. 1992. "Culture in Court: Notes and Reflections on Abortion in Guam." *Journal de la Société des Océanistes* 94 (1): 35–44. https://doi.org/10.3406/jso.1992.2605.

———. 1995. "Love and Suffering: Adolescent Socialization and Suicide in Micronesia." *Contemporary Pacific* 7 (1): 21–53.

———. 1999. "Staking Ground: Medical Anthropology, Health and Medical Services in Micronesia." In *American Anthropology in Micronesia: An Assessment,* edited by Robert C. Kiste and Mac Marshall, 327–359. Honolulu: University of Hawai'i Press.

Rubinstein, Donald H., and Michael J. Levin. 1992. "Micronesian Migrants to Guam: Social and Economic Characteristics." *Asian and Pacific Migration Journal* 1 (2): 350–385. https://doi.org/10.1177/011719689200100208.

Russell, Toya V., Ann N. Do, Eleanor Setik, Patrick S. Sullivan, Victoria D. Rayle, Carol A. Fridlund, Vu M. Quan, Andrew C. Voetsch, and Patricia L. Fleming. 2007. "Sexual Risk Behaviors for HIV/AIDS in Chuuk State, Micronesia: The Case for HIV Prevention in Vulnerable Remote Populations." *PLoS ONE* 2 (12): e1283. https://doi.org/10.1371/journal.pone.0001283.

Sablan, Jerick. 2014. "Bill Would Prioritize Citizens: FAS Migrants Could Wait Longer for Public Housing." *Pacific Daily News,* June 30, 2014.

Salinas, Johanna. 2020. "Rapid Engagement Team Formed to Fight Covid-19; Gil Baza, Zero Down Subdivisions Identified as Hotspots." *Pacific Island Times,* October 15, 2020. https://www.pacificislandtimes.com/post/2020/10/16/rapid-engagement-team-formed-to-fight-covid-19-gil-baza-zero-down-subdivisions-identified.

Scheper-Hughes, Nancy. 1994. "Embodied Knowledge: Thinking with the Body in Critical Medical Anthropology." In *Assessing Cultural Anthropology,* edited by Rob Borofsky, 229–242. New York: McGraw-Hill.

Scheper-Hughes, Nancy, and Margaret M. Lock. 1987. "The Mindful Body: A Prolegomenon to Future Work in Medical Anthropology." *Medical Anthropology Quarterly* 1 (1): 6–41. https://doi.org/10.1525/maq.1987.1.1.02a00020.

Scheyvens, Regina. 2003. "Church Women's Groups and the Empowerment of Women in Solomon Islands." *Oceania* 74 (1–2): 24–43.

Schuller, Mark. 2009. "Gluing Globalization: NGOs as Intermediaries in Haiti." *PoLAR: Political and Legal Anthropology Review* 32 (1): 84–104. https://doi.org/10.1111/j.1555-2934.2009.01025.x.

Sentell, Tetine, Ann Chang, Hyeong Jun Ahn, and Jill Miyamura. 2016. "Maternal Language and Adverse Birth Outcomes in a Statewide Analysis." *Women & Health* 56 (3): 257–280. https://doi.org/10.1080/03630242.2015.1088114.

Shaw, Susan J. 2010. "The Logic of Identity and Resemblance in Culturally Appropriate Health Care." *Health: An Interdisciplinary Journal for the Social Study of Health, Illness and Medicine* 14 (5): 523–544. https://doi.org/10.1177/1363459309360973.

Shek, Dina M., Rebecca Delafield, James Perez Viernes, Joseph Pangelinan, Innocenta Sound-Kikku, Jendrikdrik Paul, Tulpe Tosie Day, and Shanty Sigrah Asher. 2021. "Micronesians Building Healthier Communities during the COVID-19 Pandemic." *Hawai'i Journal of Health & Social Welfare* 80 (10 suppl. 2): 30. https://www.ncbi.nlm.nih.gov/pmc/articles/PMC8538110/.

Shoultz, Jan, Lois Magnussen, Kay Hansen, Selynda Mori Selifis, and Margaret Ifenuk. 2007. "Intimate Partner Violence: Perceptions of Chuukese Women." *Hawaii Medical Journal* 66 (10): 268–271.

Silliman, Jael. 1999. "Expanding Civil Society: Shrinking Political Spaces—the Case of Women's Nongovernmental Organizations." *Social Politics: International Studies in Gender, State & Society* 6 (1): 23–53. https://doi.org/10.1093/sp/6.1.23.

Smith, Sarah A. 2016. "Migrant Encounters in the Clinic: Bureaucratic, Biomedical, and Community Influences on Patient Interactions with Front-Line Workers." *Social Science & Medicine* 150: 49–56. https://doi.org/10.1016/j.socscimed.2015.12.022.

———. 2018. "Chuukese Patients, Dual Role Interpreters, and Confidentiality: Exploring Clinic Interpretation Services for Reproductive Health Patients." *Hawaii Journal of Medicine & Public Health* 77 (4): 83. https://www.ncbi.nlm.nih.gov/pmc/articles/PMC5883252/.

———. 2019a. "Embracing the Obstetric Imaginary: Chuukese Women, Migration, and Stratified Reproduction." *Medical Anthropology* 38 (4): 342–355. https://doi.org/10.1080/01459740.2019.1587422.

———. 2019b. "Gender, Relationships and Sexual Violence in the Lives of Women from Chuuk, Micronesia." *Journal of Aggression, Maltreatment & Trauma* 28 (2): 146–165. https://doi.org/10.1080/10926771.2018.1494236.

Smith, Sarah A., and Heide Castañeda. 2021. "Nonimmigrant Others: Belonging, Precarity and Imperial Citizenship for Chuukese Migrants in Guam." *PoLAR: Political and Legal Anthropology Review* 44 (1): 138–155. https://doi.org/10.1111/plar.12421.

Smith, Sarah A., and Falyn Katzman. 2020. "The Collective Power of Women's Organisations in Chuuk, FSM." *Global Public Health* 15 (8): 1144–1156. https://doi.org/10.1080/17441692.2020.1751231.

Solovey, Mark. 2001. "Project Camelot and the 1960s Epistemological Revolution: Rethinking the Politics-Patronage-Social Science Nexus." *Social Studies of Science* 31 (2): 171–206.

Spitzer, Denise L. 2004. "In Visible Bodies: Minority Women, Nurses, Time, and the New Economy of Care." *Medical Anthropology Quarterly* 18 (4): 490–508. https://doi.org/10.1525/maq.2004.18.4.490.

Stipe, Claude E., Ethel Boissevain, Ronald J. Burwell, Vinigi Grottanelli, Jean Guiart, Hermann Hochegger, Rodolfo Larios Núñez, Lucy Mair, Martin Mluanda, and William H. Newell. 1980. "Anthropologists versus Missionaries: The Influence of Presuppositions [and Comments and Reply]." *Current Anthropology* 21 (2): 165–179.

Stole, Jasmine. 2016. "Governor Plans More Removals." *Pacific Daily News*, July 13, 2016. https://www.guampdn.com/story/news/2016/07/13/governor-commutes-migrants-sentence-removes-him-guam-executive-order/87052324/.

Stoler, Ann Laura. 1995. *Race and the Education of Desire: Foucault's History of Sexuality and the Colonial Order of Things*. Durham, NC: Duke University Press.

———. 2016. *Duress: Imperial Durabilities in Our Times*. Durham, NC: Duke University Press.

Swartz, Marc J. 1958. "Sexuality and Aggression on Romonum, Truk." *American Anthropologist* 60 (3): 467–486. https://www.jstor.org/stable/666336.

Taitano, Gina E. 2023. "Chamorro vs. Chamoru." Guampedia. Last modified on January 19, 2023. http://www.guampedia.com/chamorro-vs-chamoru.

Taitano, Joe. 2022a. "ACLU Supports Local Abortion Access." *Pacific Daily News*, July 31, 2022. https://www.guampdn.com/news/aclu-supports-local-abortion-access/article_332229d8-0f0f-11ed-9d78-37253a213793.html.

———. 2022b. "GMH Requests $30.5M Budget to Keep Up with Pay Raises, Rising Costs." *Pacific Daily News*, May 19, 2022. https://www.guampdn.com/news/gmh-requests-30-5m-budget-to-to-keep-up-with-pay-raises-rising-costs/article_13b83256-d7ea-11ec-a5d7-f34d2f7e27dd.html.

———. 2022c. "Leon Guerrero Vetoes Heartbeat Act, Lets Burn Pit Ban and Other Measures Become Law." *Pacific Daily News*, December 28, 2022. https://www.guampdn.com/news

/leon-guerrero-vetoes-heartbeat-act-lets-burn-pit-ban-and-other-measures-become-law /article_be977718-868b-11ed-9bdd-d360ebf8ea9b.html.

———. 2022d. "Public Health to Move Back to Single Office Space." *Pacific Daily News*, May 22, 2022. https://www.guampdn.com/news/public-health-to-move-back-to-single-office-space/article_39694066-dbfb-11ec-b784-ef5b3cbfb88d.html.

Taylor, Janelle S. 2003a. "Confronting 'Culture' in Medicine's 'Culture of No Culture.'" *Academic Medicine* 78 (6): 555–559. https://doi.org/https://journals.lww.com/academicmedicine/Fulltext/2003/06000/The_Hidden_Curriculum_in_Multicultural_Medical.3.aspx.

———. 2003b. "The Story Catches You and You Fall Down: Tragedy, Ethnography, and Cultural Competence." *Medical Anthropology Quarterly* 17 (2): 159–181. https://doi.org/10.1525/maq.2003.17.2.159.

Teaiwa, Teresia K. 1999. "Reading Paul Gauguin's Noa with Epeli' Hau'ofa's Kisses in the Nederends: Militourism, Feminism, and the 'Polynesian' Body." In *Inside Out: Literature, Cultural Politics, and Identity in the New Pacific*, edited by Vilsoni Hereniko and Rob Wilson, 249–63. Lanham, MD: Rowman and Littlefield.

Tomas, Jojo Santo. 2016. "Calvo: Feds to Deport Convicts from Philippines, FSM." *Pacific Daily News*, September 4, 2016. https://www.guampdn.com/story/news/2016/09/04/calvo-feds-deport-convicts-philippines-fsm/89859896/.

Torres, M. Gabriela, and Kersti Yllö. 2020. *Sexual Violence in Intimacy: Implications for Research and Policy in Global Health*. London: Routledge.

Trask, Haunani-Kay. 1991. "Natives and Anthropologists: The Colonial Struggle." *Contemporary Pacific* 3 (1): 159–167. https://www.jstor.org/stable/23701492.

Trouillot, Michel-Rolph. 1990. "The Odd and the Ordinary: Haiti, the Caribbean, and the World." *Cimarrón: New Perspectives on the Caribbean* 2 (3): 3–12.

———. 1991. "Anthropology and the Savage Slot: The Poetics and Politics of Otherness." In *Recapturing Anthropology: Working in the Present*, 17–45. Santa Fe: School of American Research Press.

———. 2003. "Adieu, Culture: A New Duty Arises." In *Global Transformations: Anthropology and the Modern World*, 97–116. New York: Palgrave Macmillan.

Tsing, Anna. 2008. "The Global Situation." In *Anthropology of Globalization*, edited by Jonathan Xavier Inda and Renato Rosaldo, 66–98. Malden, MA: Blackwell.

UNICEF. 2016. "The State of the World's Children." June 2016. https://www.unicef.org/reports/state-worlds-children-2016.

———. 2017. *Situation Analysis of Children in the Federated States of Micronesia*. United Nations Children's Fund (Suva). https://www.unicef.org/pacificislands/media/1101/file/Situation-Analysis-of-Children-Micronesia.pdf.

Unnithan-Kumar, Maya, and Sunil K. Khanna. 2014. *The Cultural Politics of Reproduction: Migration, Health and Family Making*. New York: Berghahn Books.

U.S. Army Corps of Engineers. 2020. *Facilities Condition Assessment: Guam Memorial Hospital, Tamuning, Guam*. April 8, 2020. https://www.doi.gov/sites/doi.gov/files/uploads/oia-guam-memorial-hospital-facility-assessment.pdf.

U.S. Census Bureau. 2022. "2020 Island Areas Censuses: Guam." Demographic Profile Dashboard. March 27, 2023. https://bsp.guam.gov/census-of-guam/

USCIS (U.S. Citizenship and Immigration Services). 2018. "Fact Sheet: Status of Citizens of the Freely Associated States of the Federated States of Micronesia and the Republic of the Marshall Islands." July 23, 2018. Washington, DC.

Valenti, Jessica. 2010. *The Purity Myth: How America's Obsession with Virginity Is Hurting Young Women*. Berkeley, CA: Seal Press.

Vance, Carole S. 1991. "Anthropology Rediscovers Sexuality: A Theoretical Comment." *Social Science & Medicine* 33 (8): 875–884. https://doi.org/10.1016/0277-9536(91)90259-F.

Vine, David. 2015. *Base Nation: How US Military Bases Abroad Harm America and the World.* New York: Metropolitan Books.

Ward, Martha C. 1989. *Nest in the Wind: Adventures in Anthropology on a Tropical Island.* Long Grove, IL: Waveland Press.

Weiner, Annette B. 1980. "Reproduction: A Replacement for Reciprocity." *American Ethnologist* 7 (1): 71–85. https://doi.org/10.1525/ae.1980.7.1.02a00050.

———. 1995. "Reassessing Reproduction in Social Theory." In *Conceiving the New World Order: The Global Politics of Reproduction*, edited by Faye D. Ginsburg and Rayna Rapp, 407–424. Berkeley: University of California Press.

Wendland, Claire L. 2016. "Estimating Death: A Close Reading of Maternal Mortality Metrics in Malawi." In *Metrics: What Counts in Global Health*, edited by Vincanne Adams, 57–81. Durham, NC: Duke University Press.

Willen, Sarah S. 2013. "Confronting a 'Big Huge Gaping Wound': Emotion and Anxiety in a Cultural Sensitivity Course for Psychiatry Residents." *Culture, Medicine, and Psychiatry* 37 (2): 253–279. https://doi.org/10.1007/s11013-013-9310-6.

Willen, Sarah S., and Elizabeth Carpenter-Song. 2013. "Cultural Competence in Action: 'Lifting the Hood' on Four Case Studies in Medical Education." *Culture, Medicine, and Psychiatry* 37 (2): 241–252. https://doi.org/10.1007/s11013-013-9319-x.

Wolf, Eric, and Joseph G Jorgensen. 1970. "Anthropology on the Warpath in Thailand." *New York Review of Books* 15 (9): 26–35.

Wong, Vanessa S., and Crissy T. Kawamoto. 2010. "Understanding Cervical Cancer Prevention and Screening in Chuukese Women in Hawai'i." *Hawaii Medical Journal* 69 (6 suppl. 3): 13–16. https://www.ncbi.nlm.nih.gov/pmc/articles/PMC3123140/.

Wood, Kathryn M., and Kristine Qureshi. 2017. "Facilitators and Barriers for Successful Breastfeeding among Migrant Chuukese Mothers on Guam." *SAGE Open Nursing* 3:1–9. https://doi.org/10.1177/2377960816688909.

Workman, Randall, and Donald Rubinstein. 2019. "Suicide in Micronesia: Guam's Historical Trends and Patterns." Guampedia. https://www.guampedia.com/contemporary-guam-suicide-in-micronesia/.

Xu, Tom K., Tyrone F. Borders, and Arif Ahmed. 2004. "Ethnic Differences in Parents' Perception of Participatory Decision-Making Style of Their Children's Physicians." *Medical Care* 424:328–335. https://www.jstor.org/stable/4640746.

Yamada, Seiji. 2011. "Discrimination in Hawai'i and the Health of Micronesians." *Hawai'i Journal of Public Health* 3 (1): 55–57.

Yamada, Seiji, and Ann Pobutsky. 2009. "Micronesian Migrant Health Issues in Hawai'i: Part 1: Background, Home Island Data, and Clinical Evidence." *California Journal of Health Promotion* 7 (2): 16–31. https://doi.org/10.32398/cjhp.v7i2.2012.

Yamin, Alicia Ely, and Vanessa M. Boulanger. 2013. "Embedding Sexual and Reproductive Health and Rights in a Transformational Development Framework: Lessons Learned from the MDG Targets and Indicators." *Reproductive Health Matters* 21 (42): 74–85. https://doi.org/10.1016/S0968-8080(13)42727-1.

Young, Marti, and Renee Storm Klingle. 1996. "Silent Partners in Medical Care: A Cross-Cultural Study of Patient Participation." *Health Communication* 8 (1): 29–53. https://doi.org/10.1207/s15327027hc0801_2.

INDEX

ABOUT THE AUTHOR

SARAH A. SMITH is chair and associate professor of public health and co-director of the Health Disparities Research Institute at State University of New York (SUNY) Old Westbury. She earned a PhD in applied anthropology and a master of public health from the University of South Florida. She has published research on migration, identity, and exclusion; sexual violence and human trafficking; stratified reproduction; women's organizations; and clinical environments. She has also worked on interdisciplinary teams focusing on life-span approaches to women's health; human papillomavirus identification, treatment, and vaccination knowledge among healthcare providers; cancer prevention in Micronesia; and adolescents seeking online sexual health information. Smith is a feminist medical anthropologist; her work situates public health and health care in the context of U.S. imperialism, benign neglect, gender inequality, and transnational migration.

Available titles in the Medical Anthropology:
Health, Inequality, and Social Justice series

Carina Heckert, ***Fault Lines of Care: Gender, HIV, and Global Health in Bolivia***

Joel Christian Reed, ***Landscapes of Activism: Civil Society and HIV and AIDS Care in Northern Mozambique***

Alison Heller, ***Fistula Politics: Birthing Injuries and the Quest for Continence in Niger***

Jessica Hardin, ***Faith and the Pursuit of Health: Cardiometabolic Disorders in Samoa***

Beatriz M. Reyes-Foster, ***Psychiatric Encounters: Madness and Modernity in Yucatan, Mexico***

Sonja van Wichelen, ***Legitimating Life: Adoption in the Age of Globalization and Biotechnology***

Andrea Whittaker, ***International Surrogacy as Disruptive Industry in Southeast Asia***

Lesley Jo Weaver, ***Sugar and Tension: Diabetes and Gender in Modern India***

Ellen Block and Will McGrath, ***Infected Kin: Orphan Care and AIDS in Lesotho***

Nolan Kline, ***Pathogenic Policing: Immigration Enforcement and Health in the U.S. South***

Ciara Kierans, ***Chronic Failures: Kidneys, Regimes of Care, and the Mexican State***

Stéphanie Larchanché, ***Cultural Anxieties: Managing Migrant Suffering in France***

Dvera I. Saxton, ***The Devil's Fruit: Farmworkers, Health, and Environmental Justice***

Siri Suh, ***Dying to Count: Post-Abortion Care and Global Reproductive Health Politics in Senegal***

Vania Smith-Oka, ***Becoming Gods: Medical Training in Mexican Hospitals***

Daria Trentini, ***At Ansha's: Life in the Spirit Mosque of a Healer in Mozambique***

Mette N. Svendsen, ***Near Human: Border Zones of Species, Life, and Belonging***

Cristina A. Pop, ***The Cancer Within: Reproduction, Cultural Transformation, and Health Care in Romania***

Elizabeth J. Pfeiffer, ***Viral Frictions: Global Health and the Persistence of HIV Stigma in Kenya***

Anna Versfeld, ***Making Uncertainty: Tuberculosis, Substance Use, and Pathways to Health in South Africa***

Tanja Ahlin, ***Calling Family: Digital Technologies and the Making of Transnational Care Collectives***

Sarah A. Smith, ***Forgotten Bodies: Imperialism, Chuukese Migration, and Stratified Reproduction in Guam***

Printed and bound by CPI Group (UK) Ltd, Croydon, CR0 4YY

09/06/2025

14685725-0001